Cat Care, Naturally

Cat Care, Naturally

Celeste Yarnall's Complete Guide to
Holistic Health Care for Cats

Charles E. Tuttle Co., Inc.
Boston ❖ Rutland, Vermont ❖ Tokyo

First published in 1995 by Charles E. Tuttle Company, Inc.
of Rutland, Vermont and Tokyo, Japan, with editorial offices at
153 Milk Street, Boston, Massachusetts, 02109.

1 3 5 7 9 10 8 6 4 2   00 99 98 97 96 95

The chart of a cat's age vs human's age on page 20 is ©1995 Race Foster, D.V.M. and Martin R. Smith, D.V.M. and is reproduced by their permission.
    "Taurine Content of Selected Food" on page 55 is reprinted by permission from *Nutri-
ent Requirements of Cats,* revised edition, © 1986 by the National Academy of Sciences.
Courtesy of the National Academy Press, Washington, D.C.
    Text by Dael on pages 227–229 is from *The Crystal Book* by Dael, © 1983 Dael Walker,
and is reprinted by kind permission of the author
    "Ideal Schedule of 66 of the Most Common Remedies," on pp. 175-76 is ©1990 Raul
Ibarra, M.D. It is reprinted by kind permission of the author and of the *Townsend Letter for
Doctors,* 911 Tyler Street, Port Townsend, WA 98368-6541.
    Text by John H. Fudens, D.V.M., on pages 123-126 is reproduced by permission.
    Illustrations on pages 225 and 226 by Imelda Casper.

Library of Congress Cataloging-in-Publication Data

Yarnall, Celeste,
    Cat care, naturally : Celeste Yarnall's complete guide to holistic health care for
cats / by Celeste Yarnall ; illustrations by Imelda Casper.
        p. cm.
Includes bibliographical references and index.
ISBN --8048-3025-8
1. Cats. 2. Cats—Health. 3. Cats—Diseases—Alternative treatment. 4. Holistic
veterinary medicine. I. Title.
SF447.Y37 1995
636.8'0893—dc20   94-39373
                                                          CIP
Book design by Jill Winitzer
Cover design by Kathryn Sky-Peck
Printed in the United States of America

Note

Material for this book has come to me over years of study. Every effort has been
made to credit sources, but if any omissions were made, I will be happy to make
the correction once it is made known to me.

Contents

Foreword

WHEN I finished reading *Cat Care, Naturally*, only one word came to mind: Wow! Celeste Yarnall has challenged a Mount Everest of information and has conquered it. She has done what most of us in the field of holistic medicine have contemplated, but few have dared to do—taken a multitude of complicated healing systems and boiled them down to their essences. Her writing is easy to understand and beautifully accented with poignant personal experiences. *Cat Care, Naturally* is certain to become a standard in the libraries of natural animal enthusiasts. It is without a doubt the most up-to-date compilation of what is happening in the growing world of natural animal care. Anyone who loves cats must follow it.

When I first graduated veterinary school nearly a decade ago, those practicing holistic alternatives such as herbology and homeopathy were considered quacks by nearly everyone in the field of animal health. I used to feel the same way. However, life has a way of leading us on fascinating journeys. As a result of my own chronic health problems, I began investigating nonconventional health approaches. On my path I found that veterinary schools do not teach the maintenance of well-being, or even true healing. Instead, they teach the restoration of the appearance of health. With most chronic and acute health disturbances, drugs and surgery merely make things look better. But all healing comes from within the body, so the true key is to help the body heal itself. Anything else is an insult to the very essence of the individual and generally leads to more serious problems.

As we move into the twenty-first century, many physicians are recognizing the value in healing alternatives. A tremendous number of mainstream practitioners are opening up to other approaches. The reason is simple: chronic degenerative diseases are appearing in epidemic proportions in the human and animal populations. Conventional medicine has no answers to the growing list of health questions we face. Increasingly, people are taking health care into their own hands and finding answers in holistic methods. *Cat Care, Naturally* will help animal owners do just that.

Many mainstream doctors are ignorant of this information, but most will pay attention when they see enough positive results. The real problem is that most of my colleagues are afraid. In order to accept the principles of holistic medicine, they must be willing to throw away many of their beliefs about how the world works. What could be more frightening?

Health care practitioners need to understand that humans and animals are more than bags of chemicals and physical components. We are a vital energetic force with an inborn intelligence that knows how to react to various stresses and insults. What we call "diseases" are simply the body's attempts to heal itself. We should not suppress diseases, but honor them, use them as guides to discovering energetic disturbances and their appropriate remedies. Once the vital forces are balanced, the physical symptoms heal. Yarnall has written about many different energy healing systems. Initially, some readers may have difficulty with these concepts, but that's okay— most of us had trouble at the beginning. Take it from one who has been there, persistence pays!

My favorite section—and the one I feel is most important—is the one on vaccinations. Yarnall's description of vaccine-induced damage should be required reading in veterinary schools. If we could only get mainstream veterinary medicine to understand and accept that section and the chapter on natural nutrition, the remainder of the material in this book would hardly ever be needed. Doctors need to face the fact that most damage to animals is caused by vaccinations and commercial foods. Unfortunately, both are the products of multibillion-dollar industries. Since the shift from conventional to holistic medicine usually means a large financial loss, many practitioners are not willing to change. Despite these obstacles, those truly interested in healing are discovering the fulfillment it brings.

We are on the edge of a health care revolution, and our survival depends on it. Celeste Yarnall has stepped forward to be a general in this battle. If we are to be victorious, each and every soldier needs to pull his or her own weight. Ultimately, animal owners are in control of their companions' health care options. We must speak up if we want alternatives, and must vigorously seek out and support those who offer them. And we must report the benefits to those who are skeptical. If each of us who reads *Cat Care, Naturally* were to stop vaccinating our animals and change to natural feeding, the impact would be far-reaching. By spending money on holistic alternatives rather than conventional foods and treatments, we can send a thundering message to the veterinary community, and eventually they will respond. After all, it was our desire for "magic bullets" and quick "cures" that got us into our current situation. Only we can get ourselves out.

I once heard a learned rabbi say, "Every thought affects the cosmos." *Cat Care, Naturally* makes my universe a better place. Thank you, Celeste Yarnall, and may God bless you.

—Russell Swift, D.V.M.

A Letter from
Dr. Chambreau

EVERY ONE OF US wants our adored cats to be truly healthy. We are sad, even sick at heart, when they are ill, unhappy, or misbehaving. When I was a strictly conventional veterinarian, I took care of cats the way veterinary college had taught me. Most seemed to improve under my treatment, but some never did, and others kept returning with the same or more severe problems. The owners liked me a lot, but I felt uncomfortable in the role of expert—somehow, the owners had information about their animals that I did not know how to use to keep them healthy. I began to question the entire philosophy of my veterinary medical training, and my assumptions that vaccination, commercial diets, and the alleviation of symptoms were the best means of keeping animals healthy.

This wonderful book can help you have healthy, happy, long-lived cats. As you read it, you will learn what true health is and how to attain it for your cats—and yourself too. Once I learned the power of homeopathic medicine, a whole new world of health opened up for me, as it will for you. Cats (and all animals, humans included) can be remarkably healthy. They may be treated for a period of time (weeks to months) and then never need further treatment in their lives! Some cats become healthy when their owners merely change their diet to fresh, raw foods. Others are so profoundly ill from vaccinations that, even when on good diets, they need deeper and more comprehensive treatment.

True feline health, as Celeste Yarnall discovered and will teach you in *Cat Care, Naturally*, is far beyond what we have been tolerating for decades. Cats need not vomit hairballs, be picky eaters, have runny eyes (or even discharge in the corners), have oily ears, and so forth. They should be playful, creative, interactive, eat well, glow with vitality, live long, and not need ongoing treatment for anything. Vibrant health—what a wonderful goal to be working toward!

Celeste has covered many aspects of what we need to do to have healthy cats. Her book teaches the underlying philosophical tenets critical for you to understand when working toward health. Sometimes an animal may seem to be getting more ill on the path to healing, so you need to develop the skills to evaluate how your cat is really doing. Perhaps, for instance, some symptoms are worse, but the cat has brighter eyes and a healthier behavior—this would indicate movement toward health.

Cat Care, Naturally also describes a variety of treatments and preventive approaches to choose from—acupuncture, homeopathy, herbs, nutrition, bodywork, and much more. You may select a holistic veterinarian to work with you in curing your cat, or start on your own by changing the diet and supplements, for this may be all your cat needs to become healthy. This book contains so many references that you may need to quit work (or sleep) for a few months to absorb all the new information, including where to contact holistic veterinarians and how to enroll conventional ones in supporting your new choices. Celeste has filled these pages, as well, with touching examples from the lives of her own and others' cats.

If you are already treating your animals holistically, this is still the book for you. It is well written, has been checked by several holistic veterinarians for accuracy, and goes much deeper into the philosophies underlying health than any other book available. The bibliography and resources sections alone make this an incredible reference.

Most importantly, I hope everyone will read the section on vaccinations, as, in my opinion, this practice is bringing our animals to an intolerable level of ill health. If you even begin to question current medical practices, reading this book will have been worthwhile. We all need to reevaluate what we are told by "experts" in all fields, especially medicine. Remember, "conventional" medicine has only been around for a hundred years or so, while "alternative" medicine has been practiced successfully for thousands of years. However, there are some wonderful benefits to be had from conventional medicine, and I do not recommend turning your back blindly on new developments.

Our cats depend on us to choose the healthiest lifestyles for them. They are here to help us heal the planet, and by studying this book and making use of the resources Celeste leads you to, you will be moving down the right path. I strongly recommend that you develop a cohesive health philosophy and employ whatever techniques support that philosophy. Then you and your cats can experience vibrant, creative, long-lasting health.

Thank you, Celeste Yarnall, not only for starting yourself on the path, but for taking the time to share it with others.

—Christina Chambreau, D.V.M.

Acknowledgments

FOR THEIR invaluable contributions to this project I would like to thank:

My devoted friend Imelda Casper for her assistance in the preparation of this book.

Ann Sanson and Mary Mosshammer for their encouragement of me as a new breeder, as well as my cat breeder friends Laurie Schiff and Ralph Shelton, Diane Wells and Michael Troutman, Barbara Honey, Marianne and Tom Caracash, Kathy Merrick, Onita Cox, Ron and Carol Mackey, Michael and Debbie Claeys, Shannon Ramsey, and Lynn Black.

My mentor, Pat McKay, the author of *Reigning Cats and Dogs*—who taught me that uncompromising is the only way to be when it comes to the health of our companion animals—for her friendship and constant support of this effort.

Christina Chambreau, D.V.M., for her detailed review of my manuscript, and for giving so much of her time and providing so much valuable information. Her endorsement and letter introducing this project is greatly appreciated.

Russell Swift, D.V.M, of Pet Friends, for sharing his expertise and for generously providing a foreword to this book.

Melinda Leeson, of Nature's Own Environmental Services, Inc.; and Charles Loops, D.V.M., for their reviews of the manuscript and their useful input.

Richard Pitcairn, D.V.M.; Anitra Frazier; and Norma Eckroate for laying the foundation for this book with their own excellent ones.

Luke Granfield, *Tiger Tribe*; Sis Sewall, *Healthy Pets—Naturally*; and Charlene Smith, *Natural Pet*, for their continuing contribution to the cause of holistic health care for cats.

Jesse Davis for his time, effort, and knowledge of antioxidants and how to use them.

The late John Craige, V.M.D. and Joy Birdsall Craige, O.M., for information regarding therapeutic sound and dowsing.

John Fudens, D.V.M.; Nancy Scanlan, D.V.M.; and Steven Hoot, D.C., for their insights.

Wayne Perry, of Sound Touch Therapy Center, for his contribution through healing with sound.

Virginia Young, of Best Friends, for always being there for me and supporting my efforts to provide my cats with her wonderful supplements.

Carol Wells, of Teamwork Marketing; and L.F.I. for materials relating to colloidal silver and gold.

Systemic Formulas, Inc.; Lydia Hibby, Animal Communication; and John Lowry, Energy Balancing, for assistance in their areas of expertise.

Yolanda LaCombe for her considerable knowledge of flower essences.

Jim McMullan for giving me the confidence to present this material to the world.

My publisher, Peter Ackroyd, president of Charles E. Tuttle Company.

Kathryn Sky-Peck, of the Charles E. Tuttle Company, for her staying power and for providing me with out-of-print research materials regarding astromedicine.

Robin Jacobson, my insightful editor and human dictionary, for her patience during the long hours we spent together revising and polishing the manuscript.

My mother, Helene Yarnall, for teaching me to shoot for the stars.

My daughter, Camilla Forte, for her endless encouragement throughout this project and, indeed, my life.

The companion cats of my family, friends, and colleagues—among them my mother's Ariel, Teddy, Tiffany, and Cassie; Cami's Aladdin and Charlie; and Imelda's Clawed Monet, Tiger Lily, Max, Merlin, and Mica—for the love and inspiration they offer every day.

And, lastly, my special "celestial cats"—Chloe, Celina, Romeo, Colette, Renoir, Judy, Jasmine, Dolly, Isis, and all the precious kittens I've had the privilege to raise.

I am eternally grateful for their enormous contribution to this work, and deeply blessed to have shared my life with them.

This book is dedicated to my mother, Helene, my daughter, Camilla, and to Romeo, the king of my cats.

Introduction

I CAN'T remember a time in my life when I wasn't fascinated by all living things. Butterflies were a special passion and so were birds. My mother and I finger-tamed parakeets, nurturing them from egg to maturity. My father built an outdoor aviary with double chicken wire to protect them from marauding neighborhood cats. I also had a baby chick, which grew up to be a rooster and rode on the handlebars of my tricycle. The lizards flourished in a special box outside the house.

The first tragedy I can recall in my life was the untimely death of that rooster, whose name was Petie, at the "hands" of a neighborhood cat. Next the lizards disappeared, and I suspected the cat got them as well.

One day, while I was mourning the loss of my beloved friends, a big orange tabby cat visited me. I fell in love with this old tomcat at first sight, though I thought he might be the culprit. We had a little talk and I forgave him, learning, at a very early age, that this was just his nature. It was hard to believe people could just let their beautiful animals roam. I begged to keep him, but our neighbors, though they had many cats, refused to give him up.

Eventually, I did get a cat. My sixth-grade teacher found a litter in her backyard incinerator, an antique that had long ago been laid to rest, but made a safe home for the tiny gray kittens. I managed to obtain one by begging and pleading, and I named her Dusty, as she was covered with ashes when my teacher found her.

I dressed Dusty in doll clothes and pushed her about in a baby carriage. She endured these tortures because she loved me unconditionally and was the center of my universe. My mother and I fed Dusty raw liver, which she ate by spearing each chunk with her claw, rinsing it in her drinking water, and raising it to her mouth. It seemed natural for her to eat fresh, raw, whole food.

Dusty was an indoor-outdoor cat because we didn't know any better then, and in the 1950s there were fewer outdoor hazards. But even though I always worried when she went on her nightly escapades, her ultimate fate was even scarier to me. My father had her put to sleep while I was attending my grandmother's funeral in Chicago, but he wouldn't tell me why. Her loss was almost unbearable for me. To this day I don't know what happened.

Still grieving, I turned to birds again—my backyard blue jays. They were wild and free, and I respected that. The one I named Fluffy would swoop down from TV antennas and big trees, and take a peanut from my hand. A neighbor who worked as a photographer for the *Los Angeles Times* took my picture performing this feat. That tiny photo in the paper was the start of my modeling career, and I went on to act in movies, on TV, and in commercials, which I still do today.

I didn't have an animal again until I was in my twenties and separated from my first husband. I decided I wanted a dog, but not just any dog. I had watched every episode of "Lassie" as a child, and, somewhere between the rooster and the first cat, a collie had ventured up to my fence. I, of course, took him in and wanted to keep him, but he had run away from his tormentors (the neighbor's children) and, naturally, he had to go back home.

I simply had to have a collie. I adopted a puppy, named her Lonnie, and eventually bred her with Lassie (actually a "he"!). I met Rud and Betty Weatherwax (then Lassie's owners) one day by driving to their home and introducing myself and Lonnie to them. They loved her and asked me to bring her back when she came into season.

Lonnie had two puppies by Lassie. But shortly thereafter she developed bone cancer and had to be put to sleep. For weeks afterward, I could still feel her presence. I wondered why she had to die so young. Could it have had anything to do with the commercial food she'd been raised on?

It was years before I had another animal companion. I'd loved Lonnie so deeply that while I was pregnant I said to my mother, "I don't think I can possibly ever love the baby like I do this dog!" But, of course, my daughter, Cami, is the dearest thing in the world to me. I'll never forget how afraid she was of Lonnie's puppies until I put one on her little lap and placed her hand on top of it. Thus began her own love of animals.

When I got married a second time, my new husband surprised me on my birthday with a collie puppy. We named him Laddie and bought him a girlfriend named Bonnie. When my husband and I separated, he got custody of the dogs.

I decided I wouldn't have any more pets. Losing them was too heartbreaking. But then, a beautiful black cat visited my backyard. Instinctively, I ran outside and picked up this sweet creature, which wore no collar or tag. Cami and I searched the neighborhood for lost cat signs, even posting some of our own. We bought food, litter, and toys, gave the cat a bath—and fell in love with it. But after three days, signs went up in the neighborhood. The cat lived right next door, and the neighbor's housekeeper had accidentally let him out. Off he went, leaving me catless again.

One day, when I couldn't stand it anymore, I adopted Chloe from my local pet store, asking the salespeople as many questions as I could. At their suggestion I bought a small book on cat care and took her to the veterinarian. Chloe had a serious reaction to her shots and had to go on antibiotics, which she didn't tolerate very well. I filed that information away, vowing to look into a more holistic approach.

Along the way I adopted several more feline friends—Celina, a lilac lynx point, colorpoint shorthair (Siamese); Romeo, a platinum point Tonkinese; Colette, a blue mink Tonkinese; and Renoir, a white oriental shorthair—learning that working with reputable breeders was the best way to acquire a cat.

Though most of the breeders seemed to be aligned with my veterinarians regarding vaccinations, medications, and commercial food, I kept feeling as if something were wrong. On this regime my mother's Balinese came down with pancreatitis. The doctor bills were enormous, and the cat was put on prescription food, which was also very expensive. A biochemist might have been able to identify all the chemicals in that food, but I surely couldn't.

I became determined to figure out a way to keep cats well through preventive medicine—good natural nutrition, herbs, and supplements—just as I did for myself. So I bought every book on the subject that seemed interesting—books on different breeds, tips on grooming, showing cats, breeding cats, when to call the veterinarian, how to cope with the loss of a cat, and several natural cat books. I was dazzled by the magnificent pictures and intrigued by promises of the ultimate cat book, but found many inconsistencies, contradictions, and inaccuracies. Alternative schools of thought were conspicuous by their absence.

After a tremendous amount of reading, I consulted with many traditional veterinarians, but found their knowledge to be quite limited. They routinely prescribed worming medications, antibiotics, and steroids, and they recommended vaccinations and commercially prepared foods. They seemed to know very little about nutrition or alternative therapies. I sought out veterinary clinics for cats only—at least there were no dogs in the waiting room to upset my cats.

At long last I found what I was looking for: a group of holistic veterinarians and practitioners trained in homeopathic medicine, as well as in nutrition and alternative methods—fresh food diets, herbs and supplements from natural sources, and hands-on healing such as chiropractic and acupuncture. I never stopped asking questions, taking notes, and reading everything I could get my hands on. After much trial and error, I put together a program that works for me and my beloved cat companions. And my cats blossomed.

It was then that I knew I had a serious contribution to make. I couldn't bear to see any more cats brought into this world nutritionally bankrupted and abused by the overuse of steroids, vaccinations, and antibiotics. I decided to start a limited program breeding "holistically raised" kittens. Today I breed Tonkinese and oriental shorthairs under the cattery name "Celestecats." They're reared on fresh, natural whole foods and lots of love.

In *Cat Care, Naturally*, you'll find everything that I feel has real merit regarding the "new age," or holistic, feline sciences, along with anecdotes about my own experiences. With the help of my book and its resources section, you can take back responsibility for the health care of your companion animals.

I'm not attempting to prescribe treatment, to interfere with whatever therapeutic course you and your personal veterinarian have chosen, or to suggest that traditional veterinary medicine is not valuable. Of course, it's valuable. It has saved countless lives. Even holistic veterinarians sometimes use allopathic drugs when drastic methods are needed, such as in life-threatening situations or when natural approaches are taking longer than their animal companions may have the strength to endure. I only wish to share what I've learned and what has worked for me—safe, nontoxic methods of healing and maintenance of well-being.

Many people turn to alternative therapies when traditional medicine fails them or has gone as far as it can. But rather than waiting for this to occur, you can start your cats on the road to health now—regardless of their age. We all need to know that alternatives exist, how to find them, when to use them, what questions to ask, and when to say, "Let me check that out!" Remember, your veterinarian works for you. And he or she is not God. To me, the ideal veterinarian is one who practices the holistic approach. Instead of declaring war on entire microbial species, he or she looks to boosting the animal's immune system, developing its resistance to disease. The idea is one of gentle healing and rebuilding.

I trust you will find *Cat Care, Naturally* to be of help. The opportunity to share my work with you is a great honor.

A Note of Caution

THIS BOOK is not intended, nor should it be regarded, as veterinary medical advice. Prior to administering any therapeutic course, please consult a doctor of veterinary medicine or a holistic veterinarian. It is their function to diagnose your cat's medical problem and suggest a course of therapy.

Because my approach to cat care is considered to be alternative by definition, many of the ideas expressed herein have not been investigated or approved by any regulatory agencies. National, state, and local laws vary regarding the application or use of these therapies. Accordingly, the reader should not substitute them for treatment by a doctor of veterinary medicine, but rather may use them in conjunction with veterinary care. Always discuss alternative approaches with your doctor of veterinary medicine before embarking upon them. An increasing number of veterinarians are utilizing alternative therapies, and you may wish to consult one or more of them regarding the treatments they offer. Ultimately, you must take full responsibility for the health of your feline companion.

The author and the publisher expressly disclaim responsibility for any adverse reactions or effects resulting from the use of information contained in the following pages.

Chapter One

Getting to Know Your Cat

A BRIEF HISTORY OF THE CAT

WHEN introducing people to my health regime for cats, I'm often asked, "Aren't our domestic cats different from their wild ancestors?" So before we begin to cover the various holistic methods of cat care and feeding, let's look at the history of this graceful animal.

As Leonardo da Vinci once said, "The smallest feline is a masterpiece." All cats carry with them extraordinary sensory abilities, including verbal and nonverbal communication skills, a sophisticated sense of balance and agility, formidable hunting skills and territorial codes, and complex sexual behaviors.

The domestic cat remains much the way nature designed its forebears, creatures that lived on fresh raw meat and vegetation. From Miacis (the weasel-like ancestor of all carnivorous animals) and Dinictis (the first catlike animal, which appeared ten million years later) descended both the Viverridae (civets, genets, mongooses) and the Felidae (all modern cats, large and small).

Today there are some 30 to 40 species of cats, ranging in size from the African black-footed cat, at 4½ pounds, to the tiger, which can weigh up to 800 pounds. All modern domesticated breeds belong to one species, *Felis sylvestris*, and all are capable of interbreeding both with one another and with the wild *sylvestrises*.[1] For example, today's domesticated Bengal breed is the result of the hybridization of the Asian leopard cat and domestic tabbies.

As an agricultural society developed in Egypt thousands of years ago, the stores of grain naturally attracted mice, giving wild cats a plentiful supply of fresh food and thus beginning a mutually beneficial relationship between humans and cats. As revered as cats were in ancient Egypt, so were they reviled and persecuted in medieval Europe, but they survived to be prized in modern times as a companion to humans.

THE MODERN CAT

THE CAT has become the most popular pet in America. At the time of this writing, cats outnumber dogs 52 to 53 million in the United States, and that number is climbing. More than a hundred pedigreed breeds have been standardized and registered in Europe and North America; however, today we recognize fifty different breeds listed in one or more registries. Though space will not allow me to detail each breed in this book, many wonderful illustrated books on the subject are available.[2]

For simplicity's sake, let's divide domestic pedigreed cats into two categories, those with thick-set bodies, such as the Persian and the British shorthair, which share their ancestry with Felis sylvestris; and those with slender bodies, such as the Siamese, the

Abyssinian, and the oriental and colorpoint shorthairs, which have retained the lithe forms of the African race of cats once called Felis lybica and now recognized as Felis sylvestris lybica.

The first type, the chunky "cobby" type, tends to have a more laid-back personality. The second type, the svelte oriental, is much more active and curious. Many dispositions and body types fall between these extremes, including the semicobby, the semiforeign, the foreign, and still another category called "long and substantial" (including the birman, Maine coon, ragdoll, Norwegian forest cat, Turkish van, and ocicat).

Paradoxically, the needs of modern domesticated cats are the same as those of their wild cousins. However, since domesticated breeds are rarely required to act as guardians of the grain stores, we now provide for their daily needs and comforts, duplicating the natural feline diet and lifestyle as closely as we can within the safety of our homes.

A HOLISTIC APPROACH TO CAT CARE

WHAT IS holistic health care and how does it relate to your cat? To me, holistic care means treating the whole person or animal as a unique individual, a perfect living thing. In the course of upsetting the delicate ecological balance of our planet, we humans have upset the ecology of animals, both wild and domestic.

The term *holistic* was coined in the 1960s by H. Ray Evers, a medical doctor concerned about chronic diseases for which there was no cure and about the growing use of drugs for various complaints. Dr. Evers felt that many of the "wonder drugs" prescribed by *allopathic* (conventional) physicians suppressed symptoms (which he saw as the body's way of expressing itself) that would only resurface later, sometimes in more severe forms, and certain drugs caused side effects worse than the original disease. While studying the New Testament, he discovered the Greek word *holos* (whole); both Saint John and Saint Paul mention it in reference to the whole person—body, mind, and spirit.[3]

Evers began working from the belief that there was more to illness than just germs and the endless quest to annihilate them. He felt that, on every plane, imbalances and stresses were the roots of disease. The cure was not in drugs but in rebalancing patients' bodies, returning them to peace and harmony with their environment. This philosophy could also be used by patients as a powerful tool for self-healing.

It's vital to understand what true health means. Certainly, the cat would have no obvious diseases. Just as important, she'd be free to express herself creatively, to be humorous, playful, angry, sad, happy, exuberant, clever, and agile. In the last few decades we've tolerated many symptoms in our cats that we believe aren't real problems but which actually reflect ill health. The following chart lists early warnings that your as-yet-undiseased cat should be treated preventatively by a holistic practitioner.

If any of these symptoms are present—or any others that make you ask yourself, "I wonder if this is normal?"—please call a holistic veterinarian now rather than waiting for your cat to get sick enough that you have no doubts. Early, deep energetic treatment may extend and enhance the quality of your animal companion's life.

Holistic practitioners offer a myriad of approaches, most of which are covered in the following chapters. These include nutritional therapy, herbs, homeopathy, flower essences, and aromatherapy; chiropractic, acupuncture, and other hands-on

EARLY SIGNS OF DISEASE IN CATS[4]

Excessive timidity, roughness, or standoffishness

Biting when petted too long or for no reason

Hysteria when restrained

Irritability

Indolence

Perching high all the time

Clumsiness

Tendency to roam more than before

Change in voice

Failure to groom well or at all

Freckles developing as cat ages

Dry or oily, thin, dull coat

Flea infestations

Fragile or thickened and distorted claws

Whiskers falling out

Eye discharge, including "sleep" in corner of eyes

Itchy or discharging ears

Slightly oily ears that need to be wiped out frequently

Frequent recurrence of ear mites

Excessive hunger or finickiness

Excessive or insufficient weight

Eating nonfood items such as rubber bands, plastic, paper

Drinking water more than weekly (unless eating dry food[5])

Bad breath

Loss of teeth

Red gumlines, pale or red gums

Vomiting or gagging on hairballs

Getting diarrhea from certain foods, such as milk

Failure to cover stool or to use litter box for elimination

Constipation or hard, dry stools

Stiffness or inability to jump onto counters

Sexual aberrations

Body temperature above 101.5 °F

modalities; and light, sound, crystal, and magnet therapies; and many other alternatives. I have added astromedicine, the study of the twelve sun signs as guides to understanding the needs and behaviors of my cats. I believe that in treating the whole being we should make use of everything nature has to offer.

Finding the right practitioner is a basic part of providing your cat with the right care. The Resource section provides information on finding holistic veterinarians in your area. You can contact the American Holistic Veterinary Medical Association for referrals and information. AHVMA will give you a list of member veterinarians in your area, but no information about their skill or training in a holistic modality, or even their current interests.

You must ask each practitioner about his or her philosophy, watch how they are with your cat, and evaluate your cat's response to therapy (see the Homeopathy section on cure, palliation, and suppression). Only you can determine who is the right practitioner for you and your precious cat. Don't be afraid to interview several, or to change practitioners if you're not satisfied. Ask as many questions as necessary to be sure you understand what's involved before you agree to any treatment.

THE CAT AND YOU

IF YOU'RE about to adopt a cat, I urge you to read this book in its entirety, and to ask yourself the questions below. If you answer no to any of them, you could well be in for some sleepless nights and many lessons learned the hard way. If you're already living with a cat, perhaps considering these questions now will help you improve the existing situation. In any case, I hope to spare you and your beloved feline companion the heartache of hazards that could claim its life.

Begin by asking yourself:

"Am I truly ready to share my life and my space with a cat?"

"Am I prepared to treat the cat as a member of my family and not as a possession?" You can never "own" a cat. You may be its companion, its friend, a member of its human "family," but you'll never be able to possess or control it.

"Am I prepared to keep the cat indoors, "catproof" my house, and purchase items required for its basic needs and comforts?" The hazards of outdoor life for a cat are too great, and no responsible person will risk it unless the yard or patio has been completely enclosed and designed to incorporate a cat run.

"Am I prepared to deal with indiscriminate scratching while I train the kitten, not to declaw it even if an arm of my favorite chair gets scratched?" Remember, declawing a cat is the equivalent of amputating a person's fingertips!

"Am I prepared to undertake the responsibility of having the cat spayed or neutered, unless I have the permission of my breeder, and have the knowledge and ability to breed the cat conscientiously?" If you wish to only have one litter prior to altering, consider rescuing a female cat and her kittens from the pound instead, and then having the mother and her babies altered. (It's an old wives' tale that it's cruel to spay a female cat prior to her having her first litter. It's crueler to bring unwanted kittens into this world, when countless cats and kittens are put to sleep every day because of overpopulation.)

"Am I prepared to clean a litter box a minimum of two times

a day; to provide fresh purified water at all times; to purchase and administer supplements; and to provide holistic veterinary and dental care?" These tasks can be costly and/or time-consuming.

"Am I prepared to make arrangements with a friend or neighbor, to hire a pet-sitting service, or to board my cat with someone who will continue my holistic regimen whenever I'm away from home for more than twenty-four hours?"

"Am I prepared to take on the responsibility of providing holistic care for the cat's entire life span?" The cat could live as long as twenty years, sometimes even longer, requiring almost as much commitment as caring for a child.

"Am I prepared to be legally responsible for the cat's acts against visitors to my home?" You can be held responsible for a guest's injuries, even if the guest provoked the cat.

There's no lack of evidence as to what sharing your life with a cat can do for you. Simply cuddling with a cat will help you live longer and remain healthier, lowering your blood pressure and dramatically reducing stress. Studies have even shown that close contact with a pet may help hospitalized patients wean themselves off sleeping medications. In any event, a cat's companionship and affection must be earned.

The bottom line is, can you be good for and to a companion cat? If you're lucky enough to share your life with one of these noble and elegant creatures, how can you not provide it with everything it needs in order to live a long and healthy life?

Chapter Two

Interacting with Your Cat

NONVERBAL COMMUNICATION

NONVERBAL communication is a gift that all life-forms share, one you'll need to reawaken in order to better interact with and care for your animal companion. Most cat lovers already possess a good working knowledge of feline body language: the subtleties of ear and tail posturing, the dilation of the pupils, the use of the claws, and so on. Through nonverbal communication, you can actually begin to see through the cat's eye and become its voice. You can learn the basics simply by taking a class.

I studied nonverbal communication with Lydia Hibby, who received her training from Beatrice Lydecker, the author of *Stories the Animals Tell Me*. I highly recommend this book, as well as *Kinship with All Life* by J. Allen Boone, the grandfather of this communication technique. Boone describes his relationship with Strongheart, a German shepherd movie dog, explaining that long before we had language, we were able to communicate among ourselves and with animals.

Those of us fortunate enough to have been raised with pets

"talked" to them—they "talked" back—without words. If you remember your own such early experiences, you've probably chalked them up to an extremely active imagination. Or perhaps you once played with a set of twins who told you they each knew what the other was thinking, or you heard your mother say she had "woman's intuition" or "just knew something was wrong." Have you ever had an image of a friend come to mind and then received a phone call from that very person saying, "I was just thinking about you and wanted to say hello"? These are all examples of nonverbal communication.

Try it now with your cat. Start by listening to your heart instead of your mind. Close your eyes. Remember every detail: the feeling of her weight on your lap, her silky fur, her scratchy little tongue licking your hand, those deep trusting eyes staring up at you. Try to visualize her walking toward you or jumping up on your bed. Often, even the first time you do this, the cat will be on your lap before you know it, so happy that you've communicated with her in her own way.

Always communicate in positive terms—what you want your cat to do rather than what not to do. Cats live fully in the moment, so don't ask them if they want to go to the groomer or to a cat show. They don't know how they'll feel until they get there.

When you say, "Don't scratch the couch," your cat sees an image in your mind's eye of herself scratching the couch. So she thinks it's okay to scratch the couch, but your yelling at her sends a mixed signal. Better to say, in a stern tone, "No! Scratch the scratching post!" If you actually take her to the scratching post and reinforce the positive behavior, it's so much the better.

It's impossible to hide your feelings from cats. They can even take on your stresses, fears, and frustrations. In *Behaving As If the God in All Life Mattered*, Machaelle Small Wright suggests that you avoid arguing in front of your companion animals.[1] It's too stressful for them. It's not fair to treat them as if they're not in the room when we lose control of our emotions. Their sensibilities must be respected.

So try visualizing positive, loving pictures rather than worrying in negative, destructive ones. Do you ever wonder why what you worry about happening often seems to happen? Practice positivity instead, and you'll find it spilling over into every aspect of your life.

Have you ever noticed your cat just sitting and staring at you, squinting or blinking slowly and gently? She's just floating on your thoughts and sending you little "kitty kisses!" In her book *The New Natural Cat*, Anitra Frazier describes how to return these kisses by gently blinking your own eyes as you think, "I love you." Your cat will be delighted you're learning her language.

You can practice your newly awakened heart-to-heart communication skills with a brand-new cat at a cat show or pet store. I like to begin by learning the cat's name, if possible, but if you can't obtain the name, use "baby" or "kitty." Try saying the name in a sweet, soft, "feminine" (high-pitched) voice. In the animal world the female voice is nonthreatening, the lower sounds conjure up fear. So if you're a man, or a woman with a deep voice, raise your pitch and speak gently.

Animal communicator Cindy Wood recommends getting down on the floor, at the cat's eye level.[2] Imagine the cat sitting on the floor of your own bedroom. You may get a picture of what *his* home looks like from his point of view; perhaps you can distinguish the outlines of a bed or a coffee table from underneath, and what the cat sees from that perspective. Your image may look like a black-and-white negative.

If you don't get a picture, it doesn't mean you're not doing it right. The cat may just be telling you he's not allowed in the bedroom. Continue to listen with your heart. Read the feelings you do get, and go on. He may be trying to tell you something about what he likes or dislikes. Or he may be content exactly where he is right now. Keep going.

What do his floors look and feel like? Do the cold, slippery floors make him nervous as he skids on them? Do his nails feel good holding onto the carpeted stairs? Now visualize the cat's feeding area. Does he eat dry or moist foods? Do you taste or feel any textures in your mouth? What about clean, fresh water? What has he smelled recently? He may change the picture you get to reflect his truth.

Are there other animals where he lives? Send him a picture of one of your cats. What does he say to that? What does he like to play with—a ball, feathers, ribbons, or streamers? Give him these images and see what you get back. Ask questions of his human companion to help you assess your images.

When I asked my Renoir what made him so frightened when he first came to live with me, he sent me a black-and-white negative image of him cowering in the back of a carrier, with his sister in front of him, and looking out into an abyss through the mesh door. I remembered picking him up at the baggage claim area at the airport—this beautiful nine-month-old male had been locked in his carrier for over eight hours and had wet himself. This experience had made him feel miserable and untrusting of people. He then showed me a beautiful color picture of himself playing with a feather in my bedroom, so I knew he wanted to change the subject. I promised him he'd never have to fly anywhere again.

As you read the visual images your cat friend sends you, along will come feelings of space and expansion if he has room to play and cozy places to rest in—or feelings of contraction if he's been caged or otherwise too restricted.

Perhaps you may feel he's trying to tell you about an aggressive person. Though you may think that this is a man, it could be a woman or child with a strong personality—cats sense human beings as personalities, not as men and women. Ask the cat how he likes this person. He may wish the person would leave him alone, or may enjoy playing with the person but can't understand why he gets scolded for playing too roughly.

It's important to understand that, to cats, play means pouncing, grabbing hold with their mouths, and kicking with their hind legs. They love to jump on dangling toys and "capture" them as if they were prey. This is their favorite sport—they are, after all, predators. However, never encourage them to pounce on your hands or feet.

Many people like to turn their new kittens over on their backs and briskly rub their tummies. Their little feet begin to kick—a natural defense mechanism. Only extremely well-adjusted, trusting cats—most commonly, neutered males—will tolerate having their bellies touched. I don't recommend this activity unless you know the cat enjoys it. The gentle approach is always best.

As you begin to practice nonverbal communication with consistency, you may wonder if the images you receive are fantasy or fact. Here's a story from my own experience. I brought my Romeo in his carrier to one of Lydia Hibby's seminars, which was held at an equestrian center. I set up his pup tent (a child's play tent) and placed his bed and water inside, providing him with his own little den. Then I had to go to the restroom, which was across the grounds. In the brief time I was gone, one of my classmates noticed that Romeo was virtually climbing the sides of his tent and screaming. When I returned, she and the others explained that I'd forgotten to tell him I'd be right back, so he felt abandoned and anxious. Even though he was in a tent, the walls were thin and translucent, and nearby there were dogs, horses, and men with cameras. I learned a valuable lesson that day, and whenever I forget he reminds me: "Just tell me what's going on, okay? I worry when you leave me."

One way you can analyze the overall well-being of an animal is to do a body scan. Just look at the animal, starting with the head and working down the back to the tip of the tail. How do you feel as compared with how you felt before you began? If you feel anything unusual that passes as quickly as you continue your scan, you know you're on to something. Ask the cat, using his name, how he feels as you move along his body.

Once, when I was at a holistic animal clinic, I met a woman who didn't have any idea what was wrong with her ailing cat. While communicating with this animal, I felt his mouth was hurting him, so I told the woman to have the veterinarian check it. Sure enough, the cat had a severe gum infection.

Lydia Hibby tells a story about consulting with a woman whose pet snake wasn't eating. Lydia communicated with the snake and asked its owner if there could be any reason to suspect that paint was the problem. The woman remembered that she had recently painted a tiny screw in the snake's habitat. As soon as she removed the screw, the snake began eating again. The paint fumes had made the snake lose its appetite.

As you practice, your skills will improve. When you do the body scan, you may feel discomfort in certain parts of your own body. If this happens, simply release the feeling and say to yourself, "This animal's feelings are its own. I release them." In your mind's eye, you could wrap the cat in a healing white light or say a prayer or blessing. Then, simply turn off the pain, much as you would the TV when it transmits images that upset you. In any event, don't be the recipient of this pain.

Nonverbal communication seems to come easiest with other people's animals. It's sometimes difficult to practice with our own because we've become so emotionally involved with them, but gradually you'll develop your own proficiency. I do my best communicating with my own cats through play. In this way I talk to them about their day. Sometimes they compete to communicate with me all at once.

I rarely touch other people's cats—and before I do, I always ask the animals' permission. But petting their aura is more subtle. Using this indirect way of laying on hands (the space around the body is referred to as the etheric double), you can often feel the animal's energy. This is a valuable avenue of communication and diagnosis, and through it you can offer much healing to your pet, especially when you use love as the catalyst.

Nonverbal communication can greatly expand your relationship with animals, but remember that some cats are reserved, just like certain people. They simply don't want to converse. Don't be discouraged. And, as I mentioned, some people never get pictures, only feelings—and that's fine. Trust yourself, and proceed with imagination and confidence. You're on your way to being a nonverbal communications expert!

PLAY

THROUGHOUT the field of holistic medicine, practitioners and clients are attempting to create change, to get things moving in the direction of *ease* (as opposed to *dis-ease*). To most of us the idea of change means the possibility we can improve our lives and those of our companions. In order to enhance the life of your cat, you must understand his needs. We've come up with a nutrition program that provides domesticated cats with a reasonable substitute for hunting their own food, but domestication, however well-meaning, has still deprived cats of their birthright as carnivores—the thrill of the hunt.

Kittens and adult cats that live indoors, where they are safe and secure, need play even more than their outdoor cousins. When cats are inside, they go without the exercise and stimulation they'd get if forced to hunt for their dinner. So we must make time to play with them on a daily basis. Kittens, especially, need to be interactive with us and the other animals in our lives. It actually improves their "IQ's."

If you have more than one cat, you're already ahead of the game. You've been an eyewitness to the shenanigans compatible cat companions get into when left to their own devices. They get their exercise this way, improving their circulation and working up their appetites. At my house the mischief usually starts at an appointed hour, about 5:00 P.M. The cats have napped and they're hungry, so the chase begins. It's mock hunting, a release of pent-up hunting energies. This behavior begins with kittens as young as three to four weeks of age. They hide and wiggle their little bodies, focusing those keen eyes on the mark, and *wham!*, they strike and kick, kick, kick. This is how they explore their world, their territory.

In a recent litter, I could easily see teams being formed and friendships made among the siblings. When I pointed out to one of my kitten buyers how closely a brother and sister had bonded, she adopted both of them. Another young woman brought home her "only child," but within forty-eight hours had acquired another kitten as a pal.

It's terribly important for us not to impose limitations of intelligence on these incredibly clever beings. If you think you can't teach or your cat can't learn some tricks, this limitation is coming from you, not the cat. I have cats that walk on leashes, come when called, fetch and retrieve balls, jump into my arms when asked, and I know it's because I do one very simple thing: project the positive result I hope to attain.

My training sessions are fun. I'm paying attention exclusively to the cats, and they love it. Romeo brings his little ball with the bell for me to throw. He'll repeat this as many as twenty times in a row. If I'm not available, he plays by himself or organizes some team sport akin to soccer. When the ball gets stuck somewhere, he calls me to rescue it. He also practices his dexterity by passing the ball back and forth between his front paws like a real soccer player, often talking to the ball (he may be swearing, but I'm not sure).

Some of my other cats throw their toys into the air and pounce on them, sometimes shredding them. Kitty "aerobic classes" are our favorite. That's when I get down the collection of fishing pole toys. You can make your own by tying any toy or feather to a length of monofilament line (single-strand nylon bead-stringing or fishing line) and attaching it to a stick. Just flick it through the air or drag it across the floor. Cats naturally respond to horizontal movements, as this is the way mice scurry when fleeing from them.

You can also add catnip to the playing field. I usually put some on the scratching post, and it lasts about a week. Some cats don't respond to catnip at all—the taste for it may be genetic. I don't recommend giving catnip to kittens under six to eight months of age. Experiment carefully with your cats and supervise the ensuing activities, as some animals may respond aggressively.

Cardboard boxes and paper bags become great hiding places. Even pieces of tissue paper fascinate cats. You can join the fun by instigating a game of hide-and-seek, making little squeaking noises and pouncing from behind walls, doors, or furniture. It's important for cats to have their own furnishings. I believe a "cat tree" is essential, as cats need to climb vertically in order to develop their full strength. If you don't provide this type of feline jungle gym, your drapes could become the "tree" instead.

Many of my clients tell me their cats are hyperactive just before bedtime. While we, their favorite toys, were away at work all day, the cats slept—and now they've got all this energy to vent. This is another great reason to have more than one cat in your house—they play with each other all day while you're gone, then sleep peacefully through the night.

Consider visiting a cat show if there's one nearby. You'll find vendors selling an incredible array of cat fun and games, even including feline tarot cards for us to tell our companions' future! However, toys can be as simple as little bits of paper rolled up and tossed for a game of fetch. Ping-Pong balls are great fun, too. (My editor, Robin, tells me she's sorry she ever started the paper ball game—now Zoot raids her wastebaskets while she's not around, dumping the contents all over the floor!)

You can also overstimulate a cat and, in doing so, become his prey—get bitten or kicked—so be careful. Use a toy, not your hand, to buffer you. I like hand puppets in the form of stuffed animals. I make them talk and move, and the cats can kick all they want. But remember, their fangs and claws can still penetrate!

A note of caution: Items that could be hazardous to toddlers if swallowed are also best kept away from animals, as they too put everything in their mouths. So keep yarn, string, paper clips, pins, needles, rubber bands, and plastic bags in catproofed (child-proofed) cupboards or tightly covered containers. Safely recycle or dispose of other potentially harmful materials, such as plastic shrinkwrap. I recommend avoiding Christmas tinsel and angel hair completely.

Once cats start chewing on something such as string, they're not able to stop swallowing it, and the foreign matter may become life threatening as it works its way through the intestines. If you're lucky, you'll find it in the litter box; if you're not so lucky, emergency measures may become necessary. Contact your veterinarian immediately if such a thing happens.

Finally, always be gentle and include lots of love in your play sessions. This is the magical ingredient in all holistic therapies. As children, we loved to play. Who's to tell us we can't still be children with our cats—they won't tell anyone!

YOUR CAT'S AGE IN HUMAN YEARS

COMPARING the relative age of cats and humans is both important and fun.[3] We've all heard that a calendar year in a cat's life corresponds in aging to seven human years, but this isn't accurate. For example, a two-year-old cat is fully developed and mature, but a 14-year-old human isn't. And 20-year-old cats are not uncommon, but how many 140-year-old humans do you know? This chart will help you calculate your cat's age in human terms.

AGE OF CAT	AGE OF HUMAN
1 year	15 years
2	24
3	28
4	32
5	36
6	40
7	44
8	48
9	52
10	56
11	60
12	64
13	68
14	72
15	76
16	80
17	84
18	88
19	92
20	96

The Dangers of Conventional Care

VACCINATION

THOUGH vaccination has become a highly controversial subject, those who challenge the concept are sometimes treated as if they were against apple pie and motherhood. I consider conventional vaccines to be extremely dangerous. As you'll see in this chapter, many veterinarians agree that vaccination is one of the most harmful things we do to our animals.

Why do we vaccinate? We're afraid our animals will get certain diseases. If we were offered a single vaccine that would protect our cats against any possible ailment, we would welcome that vaccine without question. Christina Chambreau, D.V.M., poses the following questions regarding the practice of vaccination: "What are we doing to the whole animal, the whole immune system of our cats? Why are cats becoming more unhealthy, living shorter life spans, and having smaller litters? New diseases have appeared even since we started vaccinating so heavily. Cats used to get a panleukopenia (cat distemper, a.k.a. feline infectious enteritis) vaccine when they were kittens, occasionally a rabies vaccine, and nothing else for the rest of their lives. What a difference today."[1]

We need to examine three aspects of vaccination: **1.** Are vaccines safe or do they cause harm? **2.** Are they necessary and effective? **3.** And what are the alternatives to vaccinating against specific diseases? This chapter will include stories of cats harmed by vaccines, reports from immunologists and veterinarians, a historical perspective of vaccination, and a discussion of how I myself deal with this issue.

Most veterinarians recommend cats be vaccinated for panleukopenia, calicivirus, chlamydia, and rhinotracheitis (upper respiratory infections). Many also encourage injections for feline leukemia (FelV), feline infectious peritonitis (FIP), Lyme disease, and even ringworm. These combinations are repeated every year until the cat dies. "Where in the natural order of this world do we get more than one infection at a time?" asks John Fudens, D.V.M.[2]

W. Jean Dodds, D.V.M., well known for her research at Cornell University College of Veterinary Medicine states, "Recently, polyvalent [containing different viruses] vaccines have been shown to induce suppression of absolute lymphocyte responsiveness. Previous studies have shown a reduction in platelet count. Can antigenic overload from single or combination vaccines overwhelm the host's immune system? If so, can immunosuppression result?"[3] What Dr. Dodds is proposing is the possibility that inoculating with all these different viruses at one time may weaken our cats' overall health.

Richard Pitcairn, D.V.M., also received a Ph.D. in immunology and has done extensive research with tissue samples. He reports that in the wild, when overpopulation has occurred, there has been a rabies epidemic or a distemper epidemic, but never both at once. Few people get both diphtheria and measles at the same time, yet we vaccinate for both at the same time. How would you feel if your internist recommended you be vaccinated for all the childhood diseases as well as influenza and hepatitis every year for the rest of your life?

Do vaccines cause harm? Dr. Pitcairn has stated that the majority of problems facing veterinarians today stem from vaccines. (The term used in homeopathy for this condition is *vaccinosis*.) He provides wonderful case histories of seriously ill animals that improved when given a homeopathic remedy known to treat vaccinosis. In fact, says Pitcairn, the animals did not respond to other remedies until given the one that counteracted the damage done by vaccines: "The effect of vaccination, besides the physical effects of stimulating an antibody response is to establish a chronic disease . . . resulting in mental, emotional, and physical changes that can, in some cases, be a permanent condition."[4]

Dr. Pitcairn has also shown that, in each animal, vaccination causes a chronic condition with different multiple symptoms. When faced with these symptoms, we often think our cats have contracted a disease or developed a problem, rather than identifying the ailment as vaccinosis. Pitcairn lists many such symptoms, among them: laziness or inaction; finicky or ravenous appetite; poor grooming; hair ball vomiting or cough; cystitis; nephritis; inflammatory bowel disease; chronic upper respiratory infections; increased sexual desire; aggression; destructiveness; sucking on wool; excessive licking; seizures. He warns, "If I may venture to make a prediction, it is that fifty to one hundred years from now, people will look back at the practice of introducing disease into people and animals for the purpose of preventing these same diseases as foolishness . . . a foolishness similar to that of the practice of blood letting and the use of toxic doses of mercury in the treatment of disease."[5]

If you knew, asks Dr. Pitcairn, when you gave a vaccination, that you might save an animal from an episode of an acute disease, and you also knew that you would be sentencing the animal to a lifetime of chronic disease, would you still vaccinate? C. Edgar Sheaffer, D.V.M., has said that, "Vaccinosis in animals is a true disease state."[6] My own research leads me to believe that some vaccines prevent acute disease by presenting a chronic disease in its place, and that the disease will come back in a form that modern veterinary medicine is incapable of curing.

"In many ways, chronic panleukopenia looks like feline leukemia," states Dr. Pitcairn. Jeff Levy, D.V.M., elaborates, "I believe that feline leukemia evolved because of vaccination for panleukopenia. And then with the vaccination for feline leukemia, the cat just came up with a different disease, FIV (a.k.a. Feline AIDS). You can see this in cats that are vaccinated and later turn up with all the symptoms of feline leukemia but still test negative. The disease is coming from the cat. And each subsequent incarnation that is necessitated by vaccination, by taking away a natural form, is more serious."[7]

Drs. Pitcairn and Chambreau as well as many other veterinarians feel poor nutrition and vaccinations are the primary causes of all chronic and most acute health problems our beloved pets experience today. They also believe that, under conditions of optimal nutrition, the number of animals succumbing to infectious disease would decrease dramatically in three to four generations. This would virtually eliminate the pressure to develop and promote vaccines.

The vaccinosis condition (also referred to as a feline *miasm*) can be inherited as well. For example: You adopt a naturally raised kitten, which has gone straight from mother's milk (her mother was raised on fresh food) to her own fresh food diet of raw organic meat, raw organic vegetables, cooked organic grains, and pure water, with the finest whole food supplements available. She has not been vaccinated and appears to be the picture of health, when she suddenly runs a 106° fever and exhibits symptoms of upper respiratory infection. With an optimal diet; clean, healthy surroundings; and no exposure to an infected cat, this just shouldn't happen. Then why is she sick? She has inherited the energy imbalance from her parents. Each generation, unless treated successfully to restore health, will become more and more ill. Fortunately, there are always exceptions.

Why do our doctors recommend vaccinations so vehemently? Why must we be forced to settle for chronic disease conditions in place of optimum health? Western medical and veterinary schools indoctrinate their students in a single belief system, that of allopathic medicine. Graduates of these institutions truly believe they are helping to keep disease under control. In addition, the very schools that teach drug and vaccine therapies are funded by the petrochemical and pharmaceutical industries, which manipulate the human and animal population in order to maximize profits.

Indeed, many veterinarians have told me they no longer believe in the practice of vaccination, but are afraid to go around the system. Some brave souls have condemned the practice in print, but they are few and far between. The public is still largely unaware of the frightening facts associated with vaccines since they were first developed in the mid-eighteenth century.

As a direct result of vaccination, humans have had to deal with cancer, leukemia, multiple sclerosis, autism, lupus, mental retardation, blindness, asthma, epilepsy, cerebral palsy, encephalitis, paralysis, tuberculosis, sudden infant death syndrome (SIDS), arthritis, meningitis, allergies, hyperactivity, mild to severe chronic ear infections, learning disabilities, and damage to the liver, kidneys, and pancreas. Our cats are affected by many of these, as well as by feline leukemia, feline infectious peritonitis, feline AIDS, renal disease, hyperthyroidism, and innumerable other syndromes.

Are vaccines effective? Let's look at some frightening facts regarding vaccination of human beings. A study recently published in the *American Journal of Public Health* "demonstrates that there is a 7.3 fold increase in cases of Sudden Infant Death Syndrome in the interval between zero to three days after immunization with the DPT vaccine."[8] If you or your child is represented by one of these statistics, you've learned a very painful lesson, to say the least.

What about the smallpox vaccine? Smallpox (along with other infectious diseases, including diphtheria and scarlet fever) declined with sanitation reforms instituted in the latter half of the nineteenth century. Government health records from all over the world showed that, during the most intensive periods of vaccination, the incidence and death rate attributed to smallpox increased, though these statistics were actually on the decline when vaccination began.[9]

Before 1903 smallpox was almost unheard of in the Philippines (less than three percent of the population were affected, and then only with a mild form). Then the United States military went in and began vaccinating, and by 1905 the Philippines had its first major epidemic. The mortality rate became the highest in cities where vaccination was most intensive. Japan adopted compulsory smallpox vaccinations at a time when the Japanese people had only experienced a few cases. By 1982 they had the largest smallpox epidemic in their history, 165,774 cases and 29,979 deaths. Australia banned the smallpox vaccine after two children had died as a result of inoculation, and in the following fifteen years only three cases were reported in that country. The smallpox vaccine was discontinued in the United States after Dr. Henry Kempe reported to Congress in 1966 that fewer people were dying from the disease than from the vaccination.

In 1987 a front-page article in the *London Times* headlined "Smallpox Vaccine Triggered AIDS Virus" reported the spread of AIDS through intensive vaccination promoted by the World Health Organization (WHO) in Africa and Brazil. Though this story reached the Associated Press, United Press International, and Reuters news services in the United States, it was never reported to the American public.[10] In 1978 the hepatitis B vaccine was given to thousands of homosexual men in major cities throughout the United States. According to Dr. William Campbell Douglas, the hepatitis B vaccine "exhibits the exact same epidemiology as AIDS" and "homosexual males between twenty [and] forty years of age who were not monogamous were targeted for vaccinations."[11]

And what about polio? Here is a sampling of evidence from 1958 and 1959:[12]

Tennessee:	119 cases of polio before compulsory shots
	386 cases of polio after compulsory shots
Ohio:	17 cases of polio before compulsory shots
	123 cases of polio after compulsory shots
North Carolina:	78 cases of polio before compulsory shots
	190 cases of polio after compulsory shots

By the time the Salk vaccine was replaced by the Sabin oral vaccine, the epidemic had been on a downswing for many years, even in areas where no vaccination centers had been set up. In June 1985 the *Los Angeles Times* reported that the only cases of polio occurring in the United States at that time were being caused by the Sabin vaccine.[13]

At least the Sabin vaccine entered the body through the alimentary canal instead of going directly into the bloodstream. But both the Salk and the Sabin vaccines were "cultured" in monkeys, and macerated monkey kidneys constituted an ingredient of the vaccine. Consequently, cancerous brain tumors containing genetic material from the SV-40 monkey virus have been discovered in people who were so vaccinated and in children born to mothers who received the polio vaccine during pregnancy.

When people contract measles, their overall immune system is strengthened in response to the mild challenge of this simple disease (death as a consequence of measles is generally seen only in undernourished populations). When doctors started routinely vaccinating children against measles, we started to see babies who contracted measles at a dangerously early age because their vaccinated mothers were not able to pass on immunity to them. And what was the medical community's solution to this dilemma? Vaccinate infants for measles even earlier!

Might the whole business of vaccinations be a hoax perpetrated on the world's people? According to a report presented by the British Association for the Advancement of Sciences in 1971, deaths from diphtheria, whooping cough (pertussis), scarlet fever, and measles had declined from their peak in 1860 by ninety percent by the time DPT shots were in common use around 1940. After French children had been inoculated in 1941, diphtheria rates rose dramatically to 13,795 cases by the end of the year. By 1943, the number of cases had increased to 46,750.[14]

But what about vaccination in animals? Remember that humans are vaccinated only a few times in their lives, whereas animals are so treated once or twice a year for life. Pamphlet #3 of the Florida League for Humane Progress in Saint Petersburg, Florida, quotes the Delson Chemical Company as stating that compulsory inoculation of your dog (and, we can assume, by extension, your cat) is unconstitutional, not to mention unnecessarily troublesome and expensive. Careful observations have forced them to conclude that inoculations for canine diseases can be extremely dangerous, and are at best unreliable. Vaccinated dogs frequently develop paralysis, blindness, and convulsions, or even die.[15]

And J.E.R. McDonough, F.C.R.S., has written: "Immunization with an attenuated virus [modified live vaccine] cannot prevent distemper. The author has treated many dogs which have developed distemper despite two to three injections of the preventative agent. He is of the opinion that fits, chorea hysteria, etc., in dogs have become more frequent since the use of distemper vaccine. Successful prevention will never by achieved by inoculation."[16]

The English homeopath, C.E.I. Day, M.A., Veterinary M.B., M.R.C.V.S., tells us "there is an awakening recognition among veterinarians of the connection between immunization and various illnesses" and conditions, including bloat, stained teeth, ulcers, chronic gastroenteritis, and seizures. After conducting controlled studies of the effects of both vaccinations and homeopathic immunizations for kennel cough in dogs, Day has concluded that this vaccine is not an advantage but a health risk.[17]

Many other articles have been written over the years about the relationships between vaccinations and immune system diseases. (See Resources for information about articles by Day, Dodds, Rude, Oehen, Tizard, Wilford, McDonald, Phillips, Bastide, and Frick.)

Most people with chronically ill animals believe they were sold sick animals, but often we can trace their problems to the time of vaccination (or to their parents having been vaccinated). It's true that vaccinosis does not afflict all vaccinated animals; some are lucky enough to have very strong immune systems. But if you or your animals have ever been affected by it, you'll never forget it. You take a risk every time you allow your animals, your children, or yourself to be vaccinated. Remember, it's your decision, unless the laws in your state complicate your freedom of choice.

Ron D. Schultz D.V.M., Ph.D., of the University of Wisconsin School of Veterinary Medicine feels there has been a tremendous overuse of vaccination, as well as of antibiotics, for many diseases. To those who wish to use a vaccination for indoor cats, he recommends a killed distemper (feline panleukopenia) vaccine; a kitten series (one shot followed by another three to four weeks later) provides them with lifetime immunity.[18] Dr. Schultz also feels the feline leukemia vaccine is not necessary, as the cat's natural immunity, after six months, is usually sufficient; laboratory tests haven't been able to produce a persistent sickness (viremia) in older cats. Of course, from a holistic standpoint, Dr. Chambreau tells me that Dr. Pitcairn and others recommend using no vaccines at all, because the risk of chronic disease is too great.[19]

Dr. Chambreau feels that most homeopathic veterinarians have a clientele consisting predominantly of unvaccinated patients. These animals sometimes get panleukopenia or other feline infectious diseases, but most recover, and many much quicker than their vaccinated counterparts. Some do die. Most are much healthier (not all are completely healthy because of inherited vaccinosis) than frequently vaccinated animals.

Moreover, injectable vaccines do not work all the time. In both human and veterinary medicine, there are many recorded instances of no immunity developing, or of so-called vaccine breaks occurring, whereby the stimulation of antibodies isn't sufficient to protect against the natural disease. Conventional medicine claims those are body faults and problems. Dr. Fudens states, "It is the fault of the vaccines, as conventional vaccination treats all humans and animals the same."[20] Our cats, for example, get the same vaccines, the same number of virus particles in the vaccines, regardless of how much they weigh or how old they are. They all (and we too) get inoculated with the same combinations of viruses, on the same schedule, and then the same boosters whether the animal needs them or not.

But even when injectable vaccines do work to create immunity, the body still pays a very serious price. Tissue damage may be caused by massive amounts of adjuvant (the substance used to stabilize the vaccine) and antigen (the actual virus particles, which allopathic practitioners believe stimulate immunity), which overload the system. When large quantities of antigen, combined with particles of the carrying agent (usually aluminum hydroxide) enter the body, cysts and tumors often form at the site and become cancerous.[21]

W. Jean Dodds, D.V.M. and others have raised many additional questions: How can you declare a vaccine safe with a test group of only fifteen animals? Why is the same dose (1cc) given to any animal weighing between one pound and twenty pounds? Are booster vaccinations needed annually? Is it safe to vaccinate geriatric animals? Drs. Ron Schultz and Tom R. Phillips, writing in *Kirk's Current Veterinary Therapy* (a book even your conventional veterinarian will have on his shelf) say: "A practice that was started many years ago and that lacks scientific validity or verification is annual revaccinations. Almost without exception there is no immunologic requirement for annual revaccination. Immunity to viruses persists for years or for the life of the animal. Successful vaccination to most bacterial pathogens produces an immunologic memory that remains for years allowing an animal to develop a protective anamnestic (secondary) response when exposed to virulent organisms. Only the immune response to toxins requires boosters (e.g., tetanus toxin booster, in humans, is recommended once every seven to ten years), and no toxin vaccines are currently used for dogs or cats. Furthermore, revaccination with most viral vaccines fails to stimulate an anamnestic (secondary) response as a result of interference by existing antibody (similar to maternal antibody interference). The practice of annual vaccination in our opinion should be considered of questionable efficacy unless it is used as a mechanism to provide an annual physical examination or is required by law"[22] (for instance, certain states require annual revaccination for rabies).

Dr. Schultz vaccinates his puppies for distemper and parvo, then tests their titers (a quantitative measure of the concentration of an antibody or antigen in the bloodstream) annually; he has found that the dogs still have titers in old age. He does not revaccinate his dogs, except for rabies. Even the rabies vaccine, though legally required every three years (or annually, in some states), is probably good for a longer period—laboratories have not challenged animals with the rabies virus over a long period of time to see if the vaccine would be good for as long as ten or even twenty years. Because these tests haven't been conducted, veterinarians continue to vaccinate every one to three years for the rest of the animal's life.

Testing titers is certainly a way to see if your cat has any protection against panleukopenia. A blood sample is sent to a lab, which measures the amount of antibodies present against a disease. These antibodies may have been formed either as a result of vaccination or owing to healthy, natural exposure. Many people report that their animals have maintained titers against panleukopenia for as many years as they've been tested.

Dr. Schultz reminds us we don't know what level of antibodies (what titer) is needed for an individual cat's protection. Some cats need just a few antibodies; some need many more. Says Dr. Chambreau, "The best thing to do is to boost your cat's overall health using the techniques described in this book—and not to worry."

The following are but a few personal examples of problem experiences related to vaccinations. A breeder friend of mine told me about how, when one of her buyers took a naturally raised, unvaccinated kitten for a checkup, the veterinarian talked her into going against her breeder's advice and she allowed him to vaccinate the kitten. The kitten died in its carrier on the way home.

My own Romeo had an upper respiratory infection before I adopted him, and needed antibiotics before he could come home with me. Thereafter, he contracted an upper respiratory infection after every vaccination my veterinarian gave him (this was before I knew about the dangers of conventional vaccines). It would take two weeks of antibiotics before the symptoms seemed to disappear. The second to last time Romeo was vaccinated, he ran 105° fever and was almost comatose four hours after receiving the shot. I helped him by giving him fluids, syringe feeding him broth for days. The next year the veterinarian insisted on vaccinating him again, giving him a dose of the antihistamine Benedryl first, thinking he was simply allergic to the adjuvant. Four hours later he was running a fever of 105.5° and staring into space. Once again I rushed him to the emergency hospital, where he was given 10 mg of prednisone and fluids, with instructions from the emergency veterinarian never to vaccinate him again!

Allopathic veterinarians will tell you that Romeo's reaction was rare, but I'm hopeful that eventually they'll recognize, just as holistic veterinarians have, that the possible long-term effects (such as chronic disease) are just as dangerous as Romeo's immediate and acute reaction. Vaccinations, in my opinion, actually gave him the disease against which they were supposed to be protecting him.

My first Tonkinese litter contained four of the healthiest, most beautiful kittens I'd ever seen. The evening of their first kitten series of three-way modified live vaccine, they all ran a 105° temperature. One kitten's eyes crossed from the acute conjunctivitis and high fever. Another's eyes were damaged as a result of the infection, and a third's eyes still run to this day. Coincidence? Genetics? I don't think so. My veterinarian didn't make the connection to the vaccine, and inoculated them three more times, completing the kitten series. The last two vaccinations were four way, including immunization for chlamydia. I thought this was extraordinarily risky because it was my understanding that cats were never supposed to be vaccinated when sick.

The terrible and costly ordeal continued: Consultations with eye specialists mounted into thousands of dollars. Extensive blood work was performed. Steroids and antibiotics were administered. All these procedures only made matters worse. It took me over a year to restore health to these precious kittens through the use of homeopathic remedies.

To make matters even worse, after this episode Chloe developed a cyst at the site of her last vaccination. Celina's hair fell out in a big round patch at her vaccination site, and several other cats suffered from a general malaise. Conventional veterinarians consider a symptom or condition to be a side effect only if it occurs within seventy-two hours of the vaccination. But holistic veterinarians tell me that vaccinosis can occur any time during the life of our cats.

To understand the concept of vaccination, imagine if I handed you a glass of bovine urine to drink and told you it was good for you, and would keep you from getting sick. This is, in effect, what we're doing when we subject our cats to these suspicious substances. The vaccines we so readily inject into our animals' bodies and our own may contain any of the following noxious ingredients: decayed animal or animal embryo proteins, pus, blood, diseased mucus, urine, feces, formaldehyde, acetone, mercury derivatives, aluminum, carbolic acid, glycerine, and even antibiotics (in order to protect the virus particles from bacterial contamination). And to think this is what we've been convinced produces resistance to disease!

The bottom line is that unhealthy animals should not be vaccinated, and healthy ones don't need to be because they can probably resist infection, or may be successfully treated holistically even if they do get infected. This is not, of course, a 100 percent guarantee. But even vaccines don't provide 100 percent protection, and with them, as you've seen, come long-term consequences to overall health.

I hope by now you're at least willing to question the practice of vaccination, especially the whole area of massive, repeated (booster) vaccinations. I encourage you to read Sue Marston's *The Vaccination Connection* and any other publication you can find which presents the other side of the vaccination question. Find out as much as you can—not only for your own sake, but for the sake of our animals, our children, and future generations.

For instance, do you know what vaccines you, your children, or your animals have been injected with? When shopping for a car or a computer, we investigate the manufacturers, their integrity, their warranties, their maintenance and service policies, what it costs to insure the item and what it takes to keep it running. But when it comes to our own bodies and those of our precious animals, do we ask for the credentials of the pharmaceutical company? What's in a medication? What its side effects are? How it was tested? How long it's been in use? What the alternatives are? What the chances are that our animals will get these diseases if we keep them indoors and don't vaccinate? How many times doctors have seen "new and improved" vaccines? And do we consider the fact that viruses and bacteria, despite our best efforts, are programmed for survival?

Isn't it time to take responsibility not for only our own health, but for the health of our companion animals? Every medical system since prehistory has acknowledged the power of a higher being, of spirit, and of the life force. But have the

American Medical Association, the Veterinary Medical Association, the American Dental Association, the National Institute of Health, the Center for Disease Control, the World Health Organization, and the Food and Drug Administration become our new gods? Perhaps all living things were put on this earth with everything they need for survival. Where did we get the idea that we knew better and could tamper with something as precious and complex as the immune system?

Perhaps we can have healthy animals simply by making lifestyle changes (to fresh raw foods, purified water, natural supplements, fresh air, regular exercise, proper hygiene, reduced exposure to stress and pollutants, and keeping them indoors). With this regimen, who'd need vaccines?

If we just continue to accept the practice of vaccination and do not speak out when we see the effects of vaccinosis, a new and safer system (such as the use of immune boosters rather than immune suppressors) will never be developed. I feel we're on the right track when we work holistically to keep both ourselves and our cats healthy in the first place. What a concept—a healthy immune system simply supported to do the job for which nature designed it, to keep us well naturally!

If all this has had as much impact on you as it had on me, you've probably decided to not vaccinate your animal (or to vaccinate him less). But there are still many questions to be answered: Will my veterinarian still examine and treat my cat? Can he be boarded or groomed? Should I isolate him at home? How do I help my already vaccinated cat? If I want to protect him with homeopathic vaccination or nosodes (homeopathic substitutes for conventional vaccines), what should I do? If a rabies vaccine must be administered by law, is there any help I can give my cat?

First, as always, I recommend you become the client of a holistic veterinarian. Interview several to find out their philosophy regarding treatment and vaccinations. Let them know you want to do the absolute best for your cat and ask what they recommend. After this process, if you still wish to vaccinate your cat, the choice is yours. If you do have your cat vaccinated, please make sure she's as healthy as possible at the time, and that she does not receive any other treatment, such as surgery or even a bath, during the same visit.

If you must vaccinate, I recommend (as Dr. Schultz does) only the single (not the three- or four-in-one) killed distemper (feline panleukopenia) vaccine for kittens nine weeks of age, followed by a booster three to four weeks later. Use homeopathic remedies for any side effects that may occur, and remember that a vaccine is supposed to provide lifetime protection. Further boosters, as previously mentioned, are of little or no benefit. I've found most veterinary clinics want automatically to update vaccinations when animals are brought in for their annual visits, so you must tell your veterinarian why you wish to stop this practice, and make sure he puts a note to this effect in your cat's records.

If you must bring a sick cat to a veterinarian you don't know and that veterinarian wants to vaccinate, I urge you to refuse, reminding him of the manufacturer's instructions accompanying the product—that it is to be administered to healthy cats only.

Animal nutritionist and author Pat McKay warns not to vaccinate cats during pregnancy.[23] For that matter, it's not a good idea during any time of stress on the immune system, such as when you have to board your animal at a kennel. Even the simple act of bathing a cat lowers the body temperature and thus creates stress. So if you choose to vaccinate, please follow the advice of the pharmaceutical companies and of your holistic veterinary practitioner regarding administration.

To me, there is no safe time. How do we know whether our cats are incubating a disease or are immunosuppressed? I can only suggest you consult with a practitioner well versed in veterinary homeopathy and then weigh the risks. I hope this information will help you make your own decision, rather than having one forced upon you—out of fear, habit, or ignorance—by your breeder or veterinarian.

If a rabies vaccine is required for cats by law, either in general or for travel, please use only a killed virus vaccine. Most states only require this vaccine every three years, but several insist on annual vaccinations. Many states still don't legally mandate rabies vaccines for cats, so check with your local holistic veterinarian. Drs. Chambreau and Pitcairn highly recommend giving the homeopathic nosode Lyssin 30C two hours after the rabies vaccine has been administered, but only if the animal isn't under deep homeopathic treatment. Again, be sure the cat is as healthy as possible at the time of vaccination. If she isn't well, try obtaining a letter from your holistic veterinarian saying that a health risk would be incurred if the animal were to be vaccinated in its present condition. This letter may allow you time to build up the animal's constitution before risking another vaccination.

What about animals that have already been vaccinated? Some may have not been negatively affected at all. Most will be showing subtle signs of energy imbalance. And many will be obviously ill with any or several of numerous ailments. It's best to contact a holistic practitioner as soon as you observe any problem, and begin treating the observable signs. Of course, at this and any other time, you may enhance your cat's overall health through the suggestions in this book.

And even if you become certain that vaccination made your cat ill, please don't feel guilty. Remember that you did your best, based on the advice of experts, the veterinarians to whom you entrusted the care of your animal.

NOSODES

IF YOU feel your cat needs immunizations and are now fearful of conventional vaccines, you may wish to consider nosodes, homeopathic remedies made from diseased tissues or discharges from an infected but unvaccinated and untreated animal, which are potentized in the same manner as all homeopathic substances. Many people think of nosodes simply as homeopathic vaccines (see chapter 5), but this is not their only function. Nosodes can be administered either therapeutically (in order to treat a disease) or prophylactically (in order to prevent a disease).

Though nosodes do contain a causative organism, their efficacy doesn't depend on the presence of the organism itself. It is the substances formed by the animal's immune response to invasion by bacteria or viruses that make nosodes effective. In homeopathic terms, the substance was taken from an animal suffering from a disease that manifests in a certain symptomatic picture, so we can administer the nosode to an animal whose condition resembles that picture. For instance, the nosode distemperinum may be used to treat distemper. Nosodes made by this method are actually classified as isopathic[24] rather than homeopathic because the substance was taken from an animal suffering from a disease.

Many nosodes have been proved and have an established drug picture, but most veterinary nosodes have only recently been developed, and there have been no *provings*.[25] These nosodes are used solely for the prevention of a given disease or in its treatment. In some cases, the use of nosodes has brought out symptoms of a latent disease, but I don't know of them ever having produced the disease itself.

Please note that, just as with conventional vaccines, nosodes should be administered only to healthy animals when used as a preventive protocol. When they are given to sick cats (even those with only subtle symptoms such as thirst, a red line on the gums, or a dry coat), some may actually exhibit deeper signs of existing illness.

How do we administer nosodes? At the time of this writing, there is controversy on several grounds: Should nosodes be used at all? Should they be administered in combinations, or one at a time with a break in between? Should they be used routinely for prevention, only after exposure to a particular disease, or as a remedy when the animal has actually contracted the disease? For what length of time do they protect? And so on. Dr. Chambreau agrees with those who say that much more work needs to be done to evaluate and standardize the use of nosodes.[26]

You may want to consult various practitioners (such as Drs. Pitcairn, Loops, Lemmon, and Fudens—see Resources). Some practitioners advise that you boost immunity with nutrition and supplements only. Others prefer homeopathic treatment. And some promote the use of nosodes not only as perfectly safe, but as the best alternative to conventional vaccination. Of course, nosodes are not always effective—but neither are conventional vaccines.

The homeopath C.E.I. Day has shown very good evidence that homeopathic vaccines may protect against kennel cough.[27] An outbreak of kennel cough in a kennel of forty dogs showed the use of conventional vaccination to be ineffective. Eighteen of the forty dogs had been previously vaccinated with P13 and Bordetella before the outbreak. Every one of the vaccinated dogs became ill with a cough (100 percent), but only nineteen of the remaining twenty-two unvaccinated dogs developed symptoms (86 percent). The symptoms were severe, and the owners decided to try the kennel cough nosode. Over the next several months, a total of 214 dogs were so treated and observed. After use of the nosode, the incidence of kennel cough decreased in the previously unvaccinated dogs.

Historically, nosodes and homeopathic remedies have been used most successfully in the midst of human epidemics. This is probably the best use of these remedies in animals as well. Dr. Chambreau suggests the following scenario: "You've put your new cat on a fresh food diet consisting of raw meat, raw vegetables, cooked grains [see chapter 4, "Nutrition"] and supplements. Your holistic practitioner has treated her with homeopathy or other holistic therapies in order to eliminate any of the subtle signs of underlying energy imbalance. Then you go to a cat show or bring home a stray you've rescued from an alley, and soon after you hear of an outbreak of panleukopenia at the show or in the alley cat population. You give one 200C dose of the nosode for panleukopenia, as well as herbal or dietary supplements to stimulate the immune system, and wait to see if any symptoms develop. If they do, you treat them homeopathically with the help of your holistic veterinarian.

"Unfortunately, the notion of using nosodes on an ongoing basis is slipping into our modern rationale of 'protecting the body because it can't be healthy enough to protect itself.' But far better than using vaccines or even nosodes supposedly to prevent or control disease is to have your cat be so healthy that you don't feel the need to protect against any specific disease."

Indeed, there's a trend among many holistic veterinarians to use the nosodes in place of vaccines. I feel they're far less risky than conventional vaccines as a preventative protocol. Though most often given orally, they may be injected as well; however, I'm opposed to the all-too-common practice of injecting things into the body. If you decide to use nosodes prophylactically, contact your homeopathic veterinarian for her recommendations as to how and when to administer them.

Even though Dr. Pitcairn seems to have had no problems with using nosodes in combination, he admits that single nosodes are probably a better bet.[28] Drs. Loops, Hamilton, Chambreau, and others recommend a protocol of ascending potencies (30C, 200C, and 1M) of individual nosodes be given, according to the following protocol:

One dose is 3 granules given orally.

For cats of any age (kittens can be started at three weeks of age, even as early as one day old if in a poor environment):

- One dose of 30C twice in one day.
- One week later, one dose of 30C.
- One week later, one dose of 200C.
- One month later, one dose of 200C.
- One month later, one dose of 1M.
- Six months later, one dose of 1M.

This may be continued for life, every six months, if your homeopathic veterinarian feels it's necessary. Your veterinarian will advise you on an individual basis as to what is the best regimen in your particular case.

Start with the feline enteritis (cat distemper, panleukopenia) nosode. Wait until you are at step 3 with this nosode before starting at step 1 with any other nosode you feel is needed for your cat. Nosodes for upper respiratory infection (URI), feline leukemia (FeLV), and feline infectious peritonitis (FIP) are not needed unless your household has a serious problem, and your homeopathic veterinarian concurs.

Warning: I've heard that some holistic veterinarians have recommended oral administration of nosodes, with follow-up doses put in the cat's water bowl. This can be a very dangerous practice. Nosodes are not food supplements but extremely energetic remedies. They should be used, if at all, only under the strictest guidelines, so seek a second opinion if this manner of administration is suggested to you. When used in a haphazard way, nosodes may cause an aggravation (symptoms that actually mimic the remedy, that is, look like the disease you're trying to prevent).

Keep reading the holistic animal care magazines, such as *Tiger Tribe* and *Natural Pet*, to get updated information on nosodes. I've found that all the practitioners in the holistic community care deeply about the welfare of your companion animals. Feel free to share information with them and to network actively. If you experience a problem with nosodes, please report it to Drs. Pitcairn, Chambreau, Loops, and Hamilton, or the America Holistic Veterinary Medical Association (AHVMA) (all telephone numbers and addresses are listed in Resources section).

Remember, the jury is still out on nosodes. Opinion is deeply divided at present. To reiterate my personal feeling about the use of any substance, conventional or not: A healthful lifestyle, with plenty of fresh food and proper hygiene is what keeps our immune systems at their peak. Let's encourage research dollars to be spent on natural ways to build up the immunity of both ourselves and our companion animals.

TOXINS IN YOUR HOME

THERE ARE many reasons to create a nontoxic environment in your home—obviously, health of self, family, and companion animals being at the top of the list. Over time, exposure to toxic chemicals can contribute to the development of cancer, birth defects, genetic changes, allergies, and other disorders and illnesses, to say nothing of a generally weakened immune system.[29]

Another reason to detoxify your home is cost. The use of toxic chemicals in the home indirectly costs billions per year—about one billion in medical bills and five billion in lost work time. Furthermore, many household items on the market are mislabeled or lack adequate warnings.

Owing to their size and physiology, children and animal companions are the most vulnerable to toxicity. They inhale more air per body weight than adults because their respiratory rate is 10 percent higher. Many pollutants are heavier than air and are therefore found in greater concentration lower to the ground, so children and animals receive much higher exposure. Finally, their bodies are not as well equipped as adults' to process toxic chemicals.

Cleaning products are among the most hazardous materials found in the home. The following is a list of a few products you should consider replacing with those made from nontoxic, biodegradable ones. Check your local health food store for safe products:

Air freshener (especially those in aerosol dispensers)
Ammonia
Liquid dish detergent
Dishwasher detergent
Disinfectant
Fabric softener
Furniture polish
Glass cleaner
Insecticides
Scouring powder
All heavy-duty chemicals

Beware that clumping litters containing sodium bentonite clay can be extremely dangerous to kittens and even adult cats. Remember that cats ingest anything that collects on their paws or fur. If they ingest clumping litter, it clumps in their intestines. So look for natural alternatives to this type of product (see Resources section).[30]

Also note that many companion animals' levels of toxic metals have reached dangerous proportions. If you wish to have a heavy metal or mineral analysis (by methods of atomic absorption rather than flame photometry, which is not as exacting) done on a sample of your companion animal's fur, you may contact Analytical Research Labs (see Resources).

Warning: Be sure to read labels on everything that goes into your companion animal's mouth. For instance, the preservative sodium benzoate, which is added to such products as Stat and

Nutrical as well as many brands of aloe vera juice, is known to be poisonous to cats. Look for brands free of this dangerous preservative.

TOXINS AND DEFICIENCIES IN COMMERCIAL FOODS

IN HER book *Natural Healing for Dogs and Cats,* Diane Stein recounts some six years of intensive testing she performed on pet food, bottled water, and some human foods routinely fed to animals both at home and in veterinary clinics.

Her work began when her own cat became ill. She sent off a sample of its hair for analysis to Analytical Research Lab. The deranged mineral levels detected prompted a heavy metal screening test. They found heavy levels of lead and mercury, and also extremely high levels of aluminum (.45 ppm [parts per million]—whereas .05 ppm is the allowable level in humans). They were amazed that the animal was still alive under these conditions.

The cat's food and water were then tested. It turned out that the popular prepared food Stein had been feeding—which was highly touted as both complete and natural—contained several thousand times more aluminum than was allowable for humans! She treated her cat with homeopathically prepared substances and started making her own food, and the cat recovered.

To be sure, aluminum is a very serious cause of chronic degenerative diseases; for example, it has been found in the brains of victims of Alzheimer's disease during autopsy. Stein found high levels of aluminum in Gerber's baby food (veal, chicken, and beef varieties), Starkist tuna, and every dog and cat food marketed during 1985. The dry food contained the highest levels (even higher than food canned in aluminum) because of the methodology used in processing.

Stein's study concluded that twenty-eight of the sick dogs and cats she tested had toxic levels of aluminum. She reported the following symptomology: central nervous system symptoms such as chewing wall boards and doorknobs, trying to catch imaginary objects in the air, and aggressive, violent behavior; suppressed immune system; chronic dermatitis; coryza; nasal discharge; endocrine dysfunctions such as hypothyroidism, hyperactivity of the parathyroid due to lowered calcium levels, adrenal hyperfunction as continued chemical stress influenced the medulla of the adrenals.

She also found that hypothyroidism, diabetes, lack of pancreatic digestion enzymes, lowered hydrochloric acid in the stomach (needed for protein digestion) resulted in signs of poor nutrition such as dry, lusterless hair and coat; dry, flaky skin; increased intestinal fermentation; constipation; dehydration; low-grade fever; and liver, kidney, and heart pathologies. Blood tests showed increased BUN (blood urea nitrogen) and creatinine levels (indicating kidney damage), decreased platelets (needed for blood clotting) in the circulating blood, and elevated cholesterol levels (indicating liver and pancreas damage).[31]

Following her strict detoxification program and supporting this with homeopathic treatment, Stein was able to restore balance and health to the tested animals. For four years she tried to share her findings with the Food and Drug Administration (FDA), but to no avail.

Once you begin challenging what's in commercial pet food, you'll be amazed at what you'll find. One of the things that convinced me to begin preparing the fresh food diet for my cats was the video *Holistic Pet Care*, in which Joanne Stefanatos, D.V.M., tells of a visit to a meat-packing plant, where she saw tumors being cut out of animal carcasses, then placed along with the animals' livers and anything else not salable for human consumption (so-called meat by-products) into a separate container. When she asked what this was all about, plant personnel told her not to worry because this material was only going to be sold to pet food manufacturers! [32]

According to Ann Martin, in *Natural Pet* magazine, "Animal proteins consist of diseased meat, road kills, contaminated material from slaughterhouses, fecal matter, euthanized cats and dogs, poultry feathers, all prepared together as rendered material."[33] Then there are the moldy grains and other rancid foods, such as spoiled processed meats. At one time a particular pet food company used as a source of fiber peanut shells contaminated with fungus that produced a lethal toxin. In 1983, researchers at the University of California, Davis alerted veterinarians to be on the lookout for a potentially serious skin disease traced to consumption of several generic dry dog foods in supermarket chains.

A ground-up array of disease-ridden tissue containing high levels of hormones and pesticides (which may have contributed to the animal's death) wind up in a concoction called meat meal. P. F. McGargle, D.M.V., a veterinarian and federal meat inspector, observes that feeding such waste products to pets increases their chances of getting degenerative diseases and cancer.[34]

Many people use the term *starvation diet* to describe this nutritional nightmare. How can anyone consider this to be a healthy diet for our animals? It doesn't remotely resemble the food they'd eat in the wild!

Why, then, have we been feeding our domestic cats such an inferior diet? For years pet food manufacturers have worked to convince us that only they possess the proper formulas to give our companion animals a balanced diet. That's like telling you you're not qualified to prepare a nutritious meal for your own child (which is exactly what the baby food companies try to do!). The pet food industry is making a profit of some $9 billion a year,[35] and we Americans have been spending twice as much on pet food as we do on cereals and grains for ourselves, and four times as much on pet food as on baby food[36] (you can make your own baby food too, by pureeing organic fruits and vegetables in the blender).

Today, you need to be a chemist just to identify half the ingredients in a can or bag of pet food. Since I'm not, I'd rather prepare food for my animals from scratch. At least I know what's in it! At first this seemed like a lot of work. Now I really enjoy it and feel a tremendous sense of satisfaction in knowing my animals are eating high-quality natural food. I even make up food for my kitten buyers and other natural food clients, and deliver it right to their doors, along with supplements and many of the natural products mentioned throughout this book (see Resources).

Pet food manufacturers cook the meat they include in their products in order to sterilize it and supposedly prevent disease (they also add chemicals to sterilize and preserve the meat), but this is necessary because they're using inferior and spoiled animal remains. However, when animal fat is cooked, it becomes grease, which isn't any better for your animal's arteries than it is for your own! Cats do, however, need the essential fatty acids found in raw meat. Furthermore, cooking destroys many of the valuable enzymes found in raw meat and vegetables. Suffice it to say, the best diet you can feed your cat is the fresh food diet.

For those interested in scientific research to help justify the time needed to prepare the fresh food diet, consider this: In 1932 Francis M. Pottenger, Jr., M.D., began a ten-year experiment in which he fed a diet of two-thirds raw meat, one-third raw milk and cod liver oil to a group of cats.

Generation after generation of cats on this program maintained regular broad faces with prominent malar and orbital arches, adequate nasal cavities, broad dental arches, and regular dentition; inflammation of the gums was seldom seen. The male skull remained different in formation from the female; in fact, throughout their bodies, each sex maintained its distinct anatomical features. Their tissue tone was excellent, and their fur of good quality, with very little shedding. The calcium and phosphorus content of their femurs was consistent, and all internal organs were fully developed and functioned normally.

Over their life span, they were resistant to infections, and to fleas and various other parasites; they showed no signs of allergies. They were gregarious, friendly, and predictable in behavior. They produced healthy litter after litter, with few miscarriages, and the mothers nursed their young without difficulty.

Dr. Pottenger fed another group of cats a diet consisting of two-thirds *cooked* meat, one-third raw milk and cod liver oil. Those cats produced offspring in which each kitten in the litter had a different size skeleton. There were almost as many variations in the faces and dental structures of the second and third generations as there were animals—the effects of a deficient diet were literally written all over these kittens' faces. In addition, their long bones tended to increase in length and decrease in diameter, with the hind legs being longer than the front. The internal structure of their bones became coarser, and they showed evidence of calcium loss.

By the third generation, their bones had become as soft as rubber, and bone infections were common, as were heart problems; nearsightedness and farsightedness; marked irritability; parasites, skin lesions, and allergies; underactive or inflamed thyroids; infections of the respiratory system, kidneys, liver, genital organs, and bladder; arthritis and inflammation of the joints, inflammation of the nervous system, paralysis, and meningitis. By this time the cats were so physiologically bankrupt that none survived beyond their sixth month, thereby terminating the strain.

Some of the cooked-meat-eating females were dangerous to handle, including a trio nicknamed Tiger, Cobra, and Rattlesnake for their proclivity toward biting and scratching. The males, on the other hand, became more docile, often to the point of being unaggressive, and their sex drive was "slack or perverted." This diet seemed to have caused a role reversal, with the females becoming the aggressors and the males becoming passive; there was also evidence of "increasingly abnormal activities between the sexes." Such sexual deviations were never observed among the raw-meat-eating cats.

The average weight of kittens born to cooked-meat-eating mothers was nineteen grams less than the raw-meat-nurtured kittens. Diarrhea and pneumonia took a heavy toll on the cooked-meat group of kittens, and they developed all kinds of allergies. They sneezed, wheezed, scratched, and were irritable. In autopsies the intestinal tract of cooked-meat-eating cats measured seventy-two to eighty inches long (six feet or more), whereas the normal length for an average cat is forty-eight to forty-nine inches (approximately four feet).

Dr. Pottenger summed up his study by saying that the elements in raw food, which activate and support growth and development in the young, appear easily altered and destroyed by heat processing and oxidation. Just one year of a diet considered adequate for human consumption could so reduce the vitality of cats that it could take them as much as three years to recover, if they could recover at all. It took three to four generations on the raw meat diet to reverse these problems genetically.[37]

So you can see how vital this information is to us breeders and to those of you who share your homes with cats. We can't blame genetic deficiencies and chronic diseases simply on luck. We have a responsibility to provide each new generation with what it needs to be better than the last, or we won't have our animal companions around much longer.

At the time of Pottenger's research, the nature and composition of the vital elements in raw food was unknown, but it was known that ordinary cooking denatures proteins, making them less digestible for carnivores. The modern pet food industry would argue that all of the essential amino acids destroyed by cooking are added back in the form of supplements. It is true that if that study were repeated today, all kinds of vitamin and mineral supplements would be added to the cooked diet, and we now have antibiotics, which might save or prolong those nutritionally deprived cats' lives.

The fact remains that cats get benefits from raw meat that they can't get from cooked, bagged, or canned foods. For even if a cooked food diet could provide essential nutrients, it doesn't necessarily follow that they can be absorbed by the body. They may have been rendered unabsorbable by the use of excessive heat in the presence of sugar and fat, exposure of protein to strong alkaline solutions, and oxidation of protein when stored with polyunsaturated fat—means by which the industry routinely processes pet food ingredients.[38] It's a tricky business trying to replicate the structure of a living thing, and the living thing (raw whole food) is what the cat was designed to hunt and eat.

How can we trust the feeding of our beloved companions to an industry driven by profit? Robert Pett of Pett Foodco says one of the reasons commercial and veterinary pet foods are nutritionally bankrupt is economic competition. Keeping the price competitive dictates the use of cheap ingredients, and appeal of these inferior ingredients is enhanced through the use of chemicals (artificial colors and flavors). You save money in the short run, but ultimately the veterinary bills are enormous.[39]

My own research has shown that the majority of commercial pet food companies label their products misleadingly, referring to corn husks and peanut shells as "vegetable fiber," and hydrolyzed chicken feathers as "poultry protein products." The percentages of protein, fat, and carbohydrates listed on the labels provide no useful information on biological values (the actual utilization quality of ingredients). Dr. Plechner makes this challenge: "Can our animals really use this so-called food? Can they even digest it and process it into the necessities of life?"[40]

If our cats keeled over and died after they ate a single can of commercial food, there would be no doubt about its danger, but since it takes years to develop cancer and other degenerative diseases, most allopathic veterinarians just blame these occurrences on fate. They'd certainly never blame their own, expensive veterinary brands. These foods may sustain life, but they don't promote health.

How quickly pet food manufacturers and veterinarians have forgotten about a taurine deficiency causing eye problems (lesions and central retinal degeneration, as well as reduced reproduction in queens, reduced growth of kittens, and dilated cardiomyopathy) in cats all over the country.[41] Labs tested top brands of cat food and found them deficient in this valuable amino acid (though these brands had been labeled and advertised as nutritionally complete). Sufficient taurine is provided naturally in a fresh food diet—primarily in raw meat and poultry—but the pet food manufacturers had destroyed this nutrient by cooking their

TAURINE CONTENT OF
SELECTED FOODS *in mg/kg, wet weight*[a]

Item	Uncooked Mean	Uncooked Range/±SE	Baked[b] Mean	Baked Range	Boiled[c] Mean	Boiled Range
Beef Muscle	362	150-472	133	96-125	60	58-63
Beef Liver	192	144-270	141	68-184	73	36-95
Beef Kidney	225	180-247	138	130-144	76	68-88
Lamb Muscle	473	446-510	257	220-284	126	91-184
Lamb Kidney	239	128-440	154	81-290	51	47-55
Chicken Muscle	337	300-380	229	140-310	82	71-180
Milk, cows, colostrum[d]	38	+-7				
Milk, cows[d]	1.3	+-0.3				
Milk, cats[d]	359	+-0.42				

[a]Potential significance of free taurine in the diet. Adapted from Roe and Weston, 1965.
[b]Homogenate baked 30 min. at 177°C.
[c]Homogenate boiled 15 min. in deionized water. Very high proportions of tissue taurine may be recovered in the cooking fluid.
[d]Taurine concentrations in mg/l. Adapted from Rassin et al, 1986.

meats. So they added taurine back to the depleted food, but tout-ed it as some magical ingredient in their new and improved product, turning the disaster they'd created into just another mar-keting ploy! Was the food now 110 percent complete?

The canning process alone appears to influence the levels of dietary taurine found in the food, so canned cat food must contain a higher level of taurine than dry food. A thousand ppm for dry food and 2500 ppm for canned are currently added to processed cat foods (see chart on previous page to see how taurine is dimin-ished by baking or boiling).[42] This is only one example of how commercial processing denigrates the quality of our animals' food.

You can see from the previous chart how beautifully nature provides taurine in raw meat and mother cat's milk for the feline diet. Taurine is sold in health food stores as a supplement, and must be added to a cooked meat diet for cats. Raw heart meat is extremely high in taurine and feeding raw meat, including heart often, gives cats the right amount of this essen-tial amino acid.

You're probably wondering how pet food companies can use ingredients not fit for human consumption and still claim their products are nutritionally complete. A governmental body called the National Research Council (NRC) has been established for the purpose of defining nutrient levels; these levels are estab-lished on the basis of feeding studies using isolated nutrients. Differing diets are fed to animals, the results are observed and recorded. If a particular diet seems to prevent disease, it's used as the basis to establish minimum levels of nutrients that must be present for a food to be considered complete.[43] Another group, the American Association of Feed Control Officials (AAFCO), performs a feeding trial in which a so-called complete diet is fed to animals for a few weeks in order to determine if it prevents obvious diseases or malnutrition.

State and national regulatory bodies permit foods that have passed these two tests to claim and advertise to be nutritionally complete. Another popular method measures the digestibility of a pet food by measuring the nutrients ingested and those eliminated in the stool. The company tries to prove that its food contains nutrients that are digested and absorbed into the body to a degree believed to be adequate.

Many feeding trials are performed by the manufacturers themselves, so we only see the studies the industry wants us to see. Besides, the duration of their tests is insufficient to prove anything. Just because a cat doesn't get sick or die during a few weeks' time doesn't mean the diet is good for the cat. It's the subtle deficiencies that occur over long periods of time that concern me. And how about the excretion test? Is nutrition now a lesson in subtraction—the difference between what is eaten and what is excreted? Many substances, including outright toxins, may be absorbed by the body. Simple digestibility is not an adequate test for nutritional value.

NRC levels seem ridiculous to me because over forty essential nutrients are known at this time and over fifty more are under investigation. How then can commercial pet food be truly complete? Minimum levels represent the bottom of an average. Would you be satisfied eating no fresh food, but only a processed ration that met NRC levels?

So, once again, we're expected to turn over responsibility for the well-being of our companion animals to someone else, just as we've done with our own medical care and nutritional needs. R. L. Wysong, D.V.M., (a well-respected pet food manufacturer) calls us the "turn-it-over society," which makes promoters of fast food—for both humans and animals—rich. When huge financial concerns are at stake, we can't trust that our individual best interests are being served.

At least Dr. Wysong's company has had the courage to admit that its food, and every other manufacturer's, is incomplete without the addition of fresh raw meat and vegetables, grains, and supplements. The Wysong Institute has put out a pet health alert to the human companions of dogs and cats, warning that veterinary research has shown that thousands of pets have become ill and thousands have suffered needlessly from improper nutrition. In the booklet *Fresh and Raw* (see Resources), Dr. Wysong tells us there's no such thing as a complete and balanced commercial pet food, whether bagged or canned, and that supplementation to such food is absolutely necessary.

The Wysong Company recommends, of course, that you buy their processed food and supplements. However, at least they state that fresh, raw whole foods should be added to their canned and bagged products. Dr. Wysong admits that cooking destroys, alters, or depletes many vital nutrients, and that heat can initiate chemical reactions that turn food into toxins and carcinogens. He states that the ideal protein source in the wild is "prey" animals, and that for domesticated animals, muscle and organ meats are the best substitutes. [44]

The horror stories recounted above are only a few of the compelling reasons to change your cat's diet to fresh, homemade food (see the following chapter, "Nutrition," for further information). I'm grateful to those who've had the courage to do unprecedented research and bring us this vital information.

NEVER MICROWAVE ANYTHING!

STATISTICS now indicate that something very serious happens to food heated in microwave ovens, an appliance many cats' owners use on a daily basis to warm their cats' food. A study conducted last year in Germany indicated that human consumption of microwaved milk and vegetables was associated with a rise in cholesterol and a decline in hemoglobin levels, and low levels of hemoglobin are associated with anemia (which may results in rheumatism, fever, and thyroid insufficiency).[45] The study also concluded that eating microwaved vegetables was associated with a major drop in lymphocyte (a type of white blood cell) counts, showing that the subjects tested were responding to the food as if it were an infectious agent.[46] The subjects' radiation levels of light-emitting bacteria were higher as well, which indicated that microwave energy was being transmitted from food to person. Stanford University Medical Center no longer uses microwaves to warm breast milk, and Minneapolis Hospital tells new mothers not to microwave their babies' milk, as it has been found that microwaved breast milk loses 98 percent of its immunoglobulin A antibodies.[47]

All this indicates that a pathological change occurs in human blood when microwaved food is consumed—to say nothing of the nutritional damage done to food when it is vibrated 2.5 million times per second. But what about cats? In September 1993 a rumor circulated at the AHVMA Conference regarding a study done on microwaved food with cats as subjects. All the cats in this supposed study were said to have died after a short period of eating all microwaved foods. The experiment was allegedly funded by a microwave manufacturer, which, when the results proved disastrous, shut down the study and buried the data.[48]

Fact or fiction—who knows? But what *is* clear, is that the powers that be in the food industry want to turn us all into fast food junkies. Remember, millions of dollars are spent convincing us we can't live without this or that modern convenience, without regard for the consequences to our health. The microwave is high on the list of these lethal "conveniences."

Nutrition

NUTRITION AS PREVENTIVE MEDICINE

THE FIRST departure holistic medicine took from allopathic medicine was in the area of nutrition, which became the foundation of all alternative healing therapies. Twenty-five hundred years ago Hippocrates said, "Thy food shall be thy remedy." In 1965 Henry G. Bieler, M.D., entitled his landmark book *Food Is Your Best Medicine*, and Anitra Frazier, in *The New Natural Cat*, refers to diet as a "magic wand."

For many years nutrition experts have repeated what we must all instinctively know, that "you are what you eat." We humans add bananas and strawberries (raw fruit) to our cereal on a daily basis. We order a salad (raw vegetables) with our dinner. Even if we don't, we know we should. What person wants to eat exclusively out of cans and or bags the rest of her life? So why should it be different for our cats?

In *Reigning Cats and Dogs*, Pat McKay tells us that 90 percent of disease in animals is related to poor nutrition.[1] Why is this so? Cats are carnivores. Supermarket cat food and expensive veterinary brands are not what nature intended them to eat (see Toxins and Deficiencies in Commercial Foods, in chapter 3, "The Dangers of Conventional Care"). Felines in the wild eat mice, birds, reptiles, insects and small amounts of vegetable matter and grains. They don't carry around little Bunsen burners to cook their meals, nor do they nibble all day on bits of kibble.

As the caretakers of our animal companions, we can do some very simple things to insure their long life, optimum health, and resistance to disease.[2] I'm not suggesting that we provide them with field mice and small birds, but that we duplicate in our kitchens, as closely as possible, the cat's natural diet. Basically, we must try to re-create a mouse! Remember, cats that hunt in the wild eat, as Anitra Frazier says, the whole animal, "right down to the whiskers."[3] They even get their grains and vegetables from the innards of their prey.

This is Nature's plan, and a whole cadre of holistic veterinarians agree. Dr. Christina Chambreau feels, "A natural diet consisting of raw meat and vegetables, cooked grains, natural supplements, and pure water is so necessary for overall health that it's difficult to cure a cat if a raw diet is not being fed." This special combination of ingredients is the foundation of what I refer to throughout this book as "the fresh food diet."

There are very few physiological differences between our domesticated cats and their wild relatives—large and small. A diet of raw food makes sense for all cats because they have sharp tearing teeth, short small intestines, and highly acidic systems to protect them from most of the parasites and bacteria found in raw meat. Meat eating is deeply ingrained in the feline nature, causing the bodies and emotions of all cats to be the way they are today, even among domesticated breeds.[4] Deprive your animals of their birthright, and you'll have ill-tempered, sickly companions.

I have spoken with John Briscoe, a senior animal keeper at the Los Angeles Zoo, to get an idea of what he feeds their cats. Every feline, from the black-footed cat (which is smaller than our domestic cats) to the lions and tigers, is fed raw meat every day. This is supplied in five-pound feeding tubes and is supplemented with a bit of soy grits and with vitamins and minerals.[5] As a treat, the smaller cats get a couple of mice a day, and the big cats get raw bones to gnaw on several times a week.[6] The adults are fed only once a day. If these cats are fed canned or dry food, they "burn out" and refuse to eat.

Everyone who has been introduced to the fresh food diet initially protests: "But my cat has been eating an inferior diet all his life. What can I expect if I start feeding him raw meat? What about the effects of microbes such as salmonella on my animal, which hasn't had the opportunity to develop the 'right stuff' in his digestive tract?"

John Briscoe doesn't seem at all concerned about dangers from raw meat, and Rich Freitag of Spectrum Foods (suppliers of raw feline and canine food to the majority of American zoos) says the only animals he would worry about are those that have been fed sterile diets or animals with highly compromised immune systems. Dr. Chambreau even finds that feeding raw meat to very sick animals that are also under holistic treatment helps them recover much faster.

She says it's safer to use naturally raised meat, as the animals from which it came were not filled with steroids or forced to live and breed in deplorable conditions, and were therefore themselves more resistant to parasites. You may ensure the safety of the fresh food diet by taking the necessary precautions to guarantee freshness. Make sure you know about the techniques of proper refrigeration and kitchen hygiene, and use the meat sterilization technique detailed in How to Prevent Contamination and Spoilage, on page 90 for perhaps the first year your cat is on this program (though you may continue to sterilize indefinitely if you wish).

Russell Swift, D.V.M., explains that, though commercial processing of pet food with heat destroys many harmful parasites and bacteria, a healthy cat's digestive system possesses a strong, naturally occurring defense mechanism capable of destroying these organisms on its own.[7] Feeding cats cooked meat products weakens this system, making them more susceptible to parasites and infections from sources such as tapeworms (transmitted via fleas)—those who fear what's in raw meat should be more concerned about what's in those cans and bags!

When we feed fresh food, the cat's intestinal tract remains clean and strong. The digestive secretions are potent, and the environment within the bowel is inhospitable to worms, salmonella, and so forth. In fact, the entire body, including the immune system, remains healthier as a result of improved nutrition, and is thus more resistant to *all* disease.

Raw meat, Dr. Swift continues, contains enzymes that helps cats digest it. Cooking destroys these vital compounds, so the cat's pancreas must secrete more of its own enzymes in order to compensate. Such artificially created stress is a precursor for a great number of chronic and acute health problems. Cooking also reduces the water content and alters the protein structure of meat, making it even more difficult to digest, further damaging the animal's health and vitality. I hope by now you can see that proper nutrition is the best preventative medicine—the key to your cat's health!

Before You Begin

AT THIS point you may be considering the idea of adding fresh foods to your cat's commercial diet—thinking this might help, at least a little. But listen to a cautionary tale: Nancy Scanlan, D.V.M., has come across cats that developed rickets (from insufficient calcium or vitamin D, or an excess of phosphorus) owing to all-meat diets or diets of fresh meat added to canned food.

If you wish to add fresh foods to commercial ones, says Dr. Scanlan, it's vital to prepare the complete diet (meat, vegetables, grains, and supplements—in the proportions shown in the chart on page 70). Many people start by mixing their present commercial food fifty-fifty with the fresh food diet, and then wean their cats to all fresh food. See the section on bribe foods (page 89) for more about helping your cat make the transition.

NUTRITIONAL CHECKLIST

I HAVE put together a checklist, based on one prepared by Dr. Fudens,[8] so you can keep track of the components so important to your cat's health (for more detailed information on each of these items, see the Shopping List and Suggested Weekly Meal Plan on pages 71-73):

Protein: Raw meat should be the cornerstone of your cats' diet. But remember, too much of a good thing—that is, a meat-only diet—overworks the kidneys and liver (see Proper Proportions chart on page 69). For cats over five months of age, milk products should be given in moderation, if at all. See below for information about other protein sources.

Carbohydrates: Whole grains should be your cat's primary source of energy, not refined sugar, corn syrup, malt, white flour, or other refined grain products, all of which are found abundantly in commercial pet foods.

Fats: Cooked fat, as previously mentioned, clogs arteries. But the fat in raw meat as well as cold-pressed oils supplies highly beneficial essential fatty acids. Such fat also keeps furballs under control.

Fiber: In the wild, cats get fiber from plants, feathers, hair, beaks, and so on. Their stool thus has ample volume, preventing them from developing anal gland problems, as the gland is squeezed every time they have a bowel movement. Fiber supplements such as bran are okay to use occasionally as a colon cleanse. However, routine inclusion of whole grains in the diet is preferable. Most pet food companies use cheap and indigestible sources of fiber such as cellulose (wood pulp, beet pulp, or peanut hulls) and even feathers and beaks. Yes, it's true that these may be a part of the wild cat's natural diet, but who wants to find it disguised as meat?

Vitamins: Most vitamins are destroyed in cooking, so pet food manufacturers add back synthetic substitutes. Chemical farming has left our soil depleted, most vegetables and fruits are picked when not yet ripe and often reach our markets overripe or rotten, not to mention the dose of carbon monoxide they get being transported by truck. So we must supplement our own and our pets' food, as it simply doesn't contain all the nutrients we need.

Minerals: Minerals act as coenzymes; without them, vitamins don't work. Minerals from chelated plant minerals and colloidal minerals are the most useful. There are some seventy-odd essential trace minerals of major importance. You won't find many of them in canned or bagged cat food.

Enzymes: We know enzymes are not a part of the bags or canned fare, because heat and processing kill them. Cats manufacture enzymes naturally from the basic raw materials in the fresh food diet, and the simple addition of enzymes to sick or geriatric animals' food often causes significant improvement. I always add Dr. Swift's Florazyme food enzymes to each of my cats' meals.

Air: Air, of course, is an essential nutrient because without oxygen, we cannot survive. However, in major cities, owing to pollution, we have 40 percent less oxygen to breathe than our grandparents had. Molds, dust, pollens, ammonia, and chemicals contaminate our air, though the use of air filters, ozone, and ionizers does help. It's unfortunate that we must confine our pets indoors for their safety, but screened sunny windows or porches and cat enclosures provide some outdoor air. You may also leash train your cat for a little "walk on the wild side."

Electromagnetism: A nutrient is defined, in part, as any substantial particle, and electromagnetic currents are considered particles by modern physics. The earth has a natural resonance of which we're deprived when we spend our time indoors with microwave ovens and television radiation, which dose us with harmful human-induced electromagnetic particles. When we touch the earth barefoot or in leather-soled shoes and take our animals out on a leash, we get the benefit of the earth's natural resonance.

Light: The need for full-spectrum light for health and reproduction was documented by John Ott, of Walt Disney stop-
motion photography fame. Scientists tell us that the pineal gland
needs a minimum of fifteen minutes of sunlight daily. So don't
hide your cat behind window shades. Try to create some cozy
spot where she can bask each day. Also, most hardware stores
carry full-spectrum light bulbs, which I place strategically all
over my house for an extra boost.

Water: Distilled, purified, or spring water, as well as water
subjected to reverse osmosis, is the only way to go in a world
where our water has become so chemically polluted.

Love: Without love, babies and animals die, so prepare the
fresh food diet with love. Your cat might be finicky at first, but
wait and see what happens when they finally dig in! How much
love can you put into opening a can or bag?

While assembling this checklist, I've been taking a few
moments out throughout the day to help a four-week-old kitten
eat her fresh food. I started with a morsel on the end of a baby
spoon, so she could get the taste, and then she dove into a
mound in the palm of my hand. What a blessing it is to share my
life with happy, healthy, organically raised kittens—loved by their
mother and human companions from the moment of concep-
tion; given mother's milk followed by fresh raw foods and pure
water; and raised without drugs.

As for the rest of our cats, which have adopted us in different
ways, all we can do is the best we can from now on. With a little
extra time and lots of love and patience, we can provide them
with our personal best. They deserve it, don't they? Make today
your day to begin anew!

THE FRESH FOOD DIET

PAT MCKAY originally formulated the fresh food diet I prepare for my cats in her book, *Reigning Cats and Dogs.* I have modified it slightly after testing it on my own cats. If you're not prepared to provide your cats with fresh prey, I feel Pat's diet comes as close as possible to what they would catch themselves if they were in the wild. What's more, it's fun once you get the hang of it, and you'll be delighted with the results!

Now, let's look at the basic components of the fresh food diet: fresh raw meat or poultry, naturally raised whenever possible; organically grown fresh vegetables; cooked organic grains; and natural supplements. The ratio of raw meat to vegetables and cooked grains[9] is extremely important:

Proper Proportions of Food Groups in the Fresh Food Diet

	Kittens and Pregnant/Lactating Females	Adults
Proteins	70%	60%
Vegetables	15%	20%
Grains	15%	20%

Proteins may be reduced to accommodate special conditions. Contact your holistic practitioner for advice.

All the meats I use and recommend pass inspection for human consumption. I prepare the very same vegetables and grains for myself and my cats. The supplements I give them, albeit in different proportions, are human-quality supplements. And I use only purified, spring, or distilled water for mixing the ingredients together (see Pure Water, page 92). Why feed your cat something you wouldn't eat yourself? Please try to obtain organic ingredients, especially if your animal is ill. I know this isn't always easy, but do the best you can.

My Basic Fresh Food Recipe for Adult Cats

Please Note: Whenever you prepare and serve fresh food, make sure to follow all storage and hygiene precautions outlined in How to Avoid Contamination and Spoilage, pages 90-92. No matter how good your raw ingredients are, if you don't handle them properly, you can make your cats ill!

The recipe below is for normal adult cats, based on a ratio of 60 percent meat to 40 percent vegetables and grains. You will need to adjust the proportions for kittens, pregnant or nursing queens as noted in the Proper Proportions chart on page 69. Protein may also need to be reduced for other special conditions; contact your holistic practitioner or animal nutritionist for advice.

Supplementation in this recipe is also based on adult needs (see My Special Supplements on page 102 and the Resources section for further information on the vitamins, minerals, and enzymes included; see Pure Water for types of water safe to use).

You may make up large quantities and freeze serving portions. I use a measuring cup for the vegetable and grain content in this recipe.

16 oz. (1 lb.)	raw meat or poultry (a mixture of ground and bite-size chunks, pretreated in 8 oz. of purified water and 4 drops of standardized grapefruit extract.)
6 oz.	raw vegetables and fresh herbs (food-processed)
6 oz.	cooked whole or flaked grains
8 fl. oz. (1 cup) (or as needed)	purified water, or homemade/health-food brand chicken broth
1-2 tbsp.	bonemeal (with red marrow)
1 tbsp.	MinerAll Plus or $1/2$ tbsp. MinerAll Plus with $1/4$ tsp. Super Blue -Green Algae
1 tsp.	Bio-C

Optional ingredients (per lb. of meat unless noted):

Begin with 1 tbsp. and work up to 4 fl. oz.	aloe vera juice (without sodium benzoate) Do not use during first trimester of pregnancy.
1/2 tsp.- 4 tbsp.	expeller-pressed vegetable oil (soy, safflower, peanut, wheat germ oil: equal parts of each three times a week)
1 dash Kyolic garlic	
1/4-1/2 tsp. (per cup of food, as directed on label)	Florazyme food enzymes (added at serving time)

Blend all ingredients until you get the consistency of a thick chili. Add additional water or broth if needed. Read on for further details on how to shop for, make up, store, and feed this recipe.

Sample Weekly Meal Plan

THE FOLLOWING meal plan is meant only as a suggestion—to give you an idea of what you can do with the fresh food diet. Within each food group, rotate foods often (see the Shopping List on page 73 for suggested variations)—don't forget: variety is the spice of life! And be sure to add the appropriate supplements in the proper proportions to the proteins, vegetables, and grains listed in this plan!

You may feed the same combinations of vegetables and grains several days in a row as long as you include a wide variety. Feed only one protein source at a time.

WEEKLY MENU

Day	Raw Protein	Raw Vegetables	Cooked Grains
Monday:	ground chuck (beef), beef kidney chunks	carrots, celery	oatmeal
Tuesday:	ground chicken backs, necks (pulverized)	zucchini, yellow squash	multigrain cereal
Wednesday:	ground chicken, chicken liver chunks	broccoli, cauliflower	brown rice or millet
Thursday:	cottage cheese, tofu, or coddled eggs	carrots, zucchini, yellow squash	amaranth or barley flakes
Friday:	ground lamb, lamb heart/kidney chunks	brussels sprouts, pumpkin	leftover whole-grain pasta or mashed potatoes, or baked potatoes with butter
Saturday:	ground beef, beef heart chunks	green beans, carrots, cauliflower	couscous
Sunday:	ground turkey, turkey gizzard/heart chunks	bok choy or Chinese cabbage	kasha or teff

Suggested Shopping List

Organic Raw Meats and Other Organic Proteins: Ground chuck (beef—you can grind meat yourself with the meat grinder attachment of your food processor), lamb (ground), chicken (ground and in chunks), turkey (ground and in chunks). Whole or sliced organ meats, such as beef hearts, kidneys, and livers; lamb kidneys; chicken livers; turkey gizzards, livers, and hearts. Ground chicken backs and necks. Tofu, fertile eggs, raw cottage cheese, nonfat or low-fat plain yogurt (from cow or goat's milk).

Organic Raw Vegetables:[10] Carrots, pumpkin, zucchini, yellow squash, broccoli, green beans, celery, brussels sprouts, peas, sprouts, sweet potato, dandelion greens, wheatgrass, parsley, sage, rosemary, thyme, and other fresh herbs. Frozen vegetables may be substituted if fresh are not available (preferably organic).

Organic Raw and Processed Grains: Brown rice, barley flakes, millet, quinoa, teff, couscous, spelt, amaranth, rolled oats. Multigrain cereals, whole grain pasta.

Other organic foods: Sunflower seeds and/or almonds ground in a food processor. Some cats even enjoy a bit of fruit, especially apple or melon.

Bribe Foods: Baby food (lamb, beef, chicken, or creamed corn).

Water-packed canned chicken, salmon, or mackerel; canned sardines. Canned chicken or beef broth. Raw butter, raw cream.

Water and Supplements: Distilled or purified spring water. Bonemeal, MinerAll Plus, Bio-C, and Florazyme food enzymes. I also include Super Blue-Green Algae. (See Resources section for information on where and how to order.)

Raw Meat Treatments: Nutribiotics or Imhotep brand of standardized grapefruit extract (available at health food stores or through distributors).

Equipment: Food processor or blender (meat grinder is optional).

Some Guidelines for Serving Fresh Foods

PAT MCKAY recommends you use only one protein food per meal. After all, the carnivore in the wild, if lucky, makes one kill a day. You may mix muscle and organ meats, but mix beef only with beef organ meats, turkey with turkey organ meats, and so on. I recommend alternating beef, lamb, chicken, and turkey—but never feed pork. The fat globules in pork are so large, they can clog your cat's blood vessels, which are fifteen times smaller than a human's.[11] You don't need to buy expensive, lean cuts of meat or poultry, as the essential fatty acids in uncooked fat are actually beneficial to cats.

Organ meats, including kidney, liver, and heart, may be fed twice weekly. Because the liver is the body's "detox central," Dr. Chambreau cautions against feeding it more than once a week unless it's organic. Drs. Swift and Chambreau feel that the heart meat is one of the best protein foods. My cats love a little organ meat in their meals. Don't forget, each mouse has kidneys, a liver, and a heart!

Dr. Wysong recommends feeding one part organ meat to five parts muscle meat, cut into chunks your pet can chew. I agree with these proportions, but use a combination of ground meat and chunks, since ground meat mixes better with the vegetables and grains. When I use only chunks, my cats eat the meat and leave the rest. However, chewing is important on a regular basis to help clean teeth and keep them free of tartar buildup. Remember, all meats must include bonemeal, one to two tablespoons per pound of meat.

Pat McKay avoids fish, although it's an excellent protein food, because our waters have become so polluted that finding a safe source of fresh fish is difficult. However, she has recently found an organic tilapia, which I serve—raw, of course—mixed with the usual proportions of vegetables, grains, and supplements. I call it my kitty sushi!

Please don't feed canned tuna! Cats become tuna junkies and sometimes refuse to eat anything else. More importantly, tuna cat food, according to a Cornell University study, has unusually high levels of the toxic metal methylmercury.[12] The tuna used in canned cat food comes from the red meat of the fish, which contains more of these toxins than the white meat tuna sold for human consumption. However, a high level of mercury is still present in the white meat, so please don't feed this either. Try canned mackerel if you must use fish as a bribe food to help your cat get started on the fresh food diet. Sardines in tomato sauce are also wonderful—cats love the strong smell.

Try raw cottage cheese as an alternate source of protein. Nonfat or low-fat organic plain yogurt (from cow's or goat's milk) is a treat for some cats and is excellent for kittens during the weaning period. If you need another good bribe food, raw butter is also fine or even a shot of raw cream once in a while. Pat McKay feels cats over five months old should not have dairy products, as they may cause diarrhea or other digestive upsets, but Dr. Chambreau doesn't have a problem including some raw dairy foods in most cats' diets.

You may also feed a raw fertile or organic egg yolk, or a whole coddled or soft-boiled two-minute egg. Be careful with raw egg white. Many practitioners prefer you cook the white; others feel there is no problem with serving it raw. I'd prefer you make an egg white omelette for yourself, and serve only the raw yolks to your cat. Use them as kittens' first food at weaning time, mixed with brown rice baby cereal, food-processed raw carrot, and a little raw goat's milk, yogurt, or kitten formula. I use Kitty Lac or Goat A Lac (see Resource section).

Some folks have tried tofu. It's hard for me to imagine my cats preying on soy food, but I'm sure I'll try it on them one of these days. However, Dr. Chambreau cautions that cats aren't vegetarians—they must have raw meat regularly. So feed tofu, dairy products, and eggs no more than once a week to normal adult cats.

Vegetables may be used in any combination (try using color as a guide, as you would for yourself), as may grains. Pat McKay reminds us the nightshade vegetables (which include white pota- toes, tomatoes, peppers, and eggplant) should be included only occasionally and need to be cooked (sweet potatoes are okay raw). You should never feed nightshades to animals with symp- toms of arthritis, inflammation, parasites, respiratory problems, or other conditions marked by symptoms such as swelling or mucus.

You may substitute frozen (preferably organic) vegetables if you can't get fresh, but never use canned vegetables, as they are very high in salt and/or sugar and have lost their nutritional value through overcooking. Then, of course, there's the lead imparted from the can. Our cats can do without any more of that!

Wysong recommends raw, organically grown rolled oats or barley flakes; I use a six-grain rolled/flakes mix. Wysong further recommends vegetables, fruits, and nuts grated or finely diced (any varieties you'd eat yourself). Nuts should be fresh, raw, and unsalted. Grasses are also recommended for aiding digestion and cleansing the system. I grow little pots of wheatgrass and keep them available at all times for my cats to nibble.

The whole grains I recommend beginning with are the same ones we eat. Barley, rye, corn, buckwheat, oats, millet, and yellow corn grits are great choices, and Pat McKay recommends amaranth, bulgur, couscous, triticale, quinoa, teff, and spelt as well. But go easy on the corn, as it's a bit hard to digest. My grain mix includes sunflower seeds, and I grind raw almonds occasionally and include them from time to time. Again, variety is the keynote.

I don't like to use bran by itself. I prefer the whole grain—which contains adequate fiber—or bran in conjunction with whole grains (whole oats with added oat bran). Pat McKay also warns that bran, by itself, can be irritating to the colon. Try adding a pinch or two to the food for a week—but only if you feel your cat really needs it—and then go back to using the whole grain by itself. Let the cat's stool be your guide.

Some nutritionists suggest that we be cautious of wheat, too, as it's a common allergen in cats as well as humans. If you rotate foods as often as possible rather than getting into a rut, you shouldn't have problems with food allergies. However, if you're presently dealing with allergies, choose foods you think your cat can tolerate, in combinations of one from each food group at a time. Try starting with barley flakes, ground lamb, carrots, and zucchini, and proceed cautiously from there. I find that food allergies just seem to disappear on this diet, so I've already added wheat back into my cats' diet.

I was worried initially because I had been told that Tonkinese cats are notoriously allergic to wheat. But, then again, Tonk breeders—and breeders in general—have only just begun to switch to this diet. So who knows? The cats may have simply been reacting to the poor quality of the wheat used in commercial pet food. As breeders become enlightened as to the benefits of the fresh food diet served in rotation, fewer and fewer allergies will be experienced. If you're worried about food allergies, you may also work with your holistic veterinarian or animal nutritionist to heal this limitation.

Broth is wonderful for binding together the ingredients of the fresh food diet. It's also a good bribe food for the unconverted, and is great for fasting days (see Fasting, page 86).

Once in a while it's okay to feed table scraps such as roast chicken and rare beef and lamb. But forget about chocolate, which contains theobromine, a known poison to both cats and dogs. They can become addicted to chocolate, so if you've been feeding it regularly, they may actually suffer withdrawal symptoms. Never leave open boxes of chocolate around your house, as your cat or dog might actually die after eating large amounts. Fortunately, cats are usually fastidious eaters and won't have anything to do with chocolate, but be careful anyway. Junk foods (especially deep fried) are taboo. Cats will usually beg for a potato chip but please don't give in. A whole-grain cracker or rice cake from the health food store is a great treat instead.

These are all good reasons for you to improve your own diet as well. You and your cat can eat many of the same things.

Shopping will become easier because you won't need to walk down the pet food aisle (except to buy toys).

Preparation Tips—Keeping Things Simple

I RECOMMEND preparing a large quantity of the fresh food recipe ahead of time and freezing it. You may actually save money this way, especially if you can find a wholesale supplier of naturally raised meats and poultry (if you can't find a reliable local source, check the Resources section for mail-order ideas). My supplier packs for me coarsely ground muscle meats and cubed organ meats. I stock up with as many one-pound packages of various ground and sliced meats as my freezer will hold.

If I run out of meat from my supplier, I go to a local health food store that carries naturally raised meats. I ask the butcher to freshly grind organic chuck with 22 percent fat, and to wrap my order in one-pound packages; I do the same with chicken, turkey, and lamb. As mentioned, I also feed organ meats (remember the ratio: one part organ meat to five parts muscle meat, or feed muscle meat five days a week and organ meats two days a week), and I also use ground chicken backs and necks.

I buy eggs laid by free range hens that haven't been given steroids. Don't keep eggs for longer than two weeks and keep them covered in their original package in the fridge. You can test for freshness by submerging a raw egg in its shell in a bowl of water. If the egg sinks to the bottom, it's fresh; if it floats, throw it away!

At the health food market,[13] I buy a medley of raw vegetables and rotate the combinations often. We all know organic vegetables are best, but if you can't get them, you may soak nonorganic ones for fifteen minutes in a gallon of purified water with a few drops of standardized grapefruit extract, or in a gallon of water with two tablespoons apple cider vinegar. This will help remove residues from pesticides and chemical fertilizers. Frozen organic vegetables, which your health food store may carry, are another alternative if raw can't be found; these are okay to use even though most are blanched prior to freezing. They may be partially defrosted and then run through the food processor just as you would with raw.

I puree my vegetables as finely as I can in my food processor, since cats have a short digestive tract and no grinding teeth, and whole vegetables pass through undigested. I place the pureed vegetables in plastic bags or containers, and freeze or refrigerate them. You may also freeze your cooked grains in containers or freezer bags, or mix the vegetables and grains together and freeze them. Just be sure to label packages with contents, and their weight in ounces, so you can mix the fresh food diet in accurate proportions from food defrosted later on.

I also prepare and freeze homemade chicken broth.[14] Though I prefer homemade, for convenience I keep my shelves stocked with beef, vegetable, and chicken broth in lead-free cans, which many health food stores carry. Pat McKay's favorite broth recipe consists of one tablespoon of raw ground beef and three to four ounces of pure water pureed in a blender (you may also make raw chicken broth with one tablespoon ground chicken, six ounces of water, and four drops standardized grapefruit extract). Administered with a feeding syringe, this broth is ideal for a sick cat, but you'll need to strain it through a sieve to avoid clogging the syringe.

You may take the chill off the fresh food by placing it briefly in a pan on the stove. Or warm the food by adding a little heated purified water, herbal tea (such as slippery elm, raspberry, or fenu-greek brewed very weak for flavor or medicinal use), or chicken broth. Don't cook the food, just make it tepid to the touch.[15]And never use the microwave, as it not only destroys nutrients but may cause other problems as well (see the Never Microwave Anything section in chapter 3). I serve my fresh food right out of the refrig-erator. If it's too cold for the cats they wait a little while before diving in!

I cook my grains in purified water on the stovetop or slow cook them in a Crock-Pot. Many grains are prepared using a ratio of one-third grains to two-thirds water, but read the pack-age instructions (or cookbook recipes) for each grain, as more or less water may be required for certain grains. You may also bring the grain and liquid mixture to a boil and then turn off the burner; let the mixture soak overnight in the refrigerator.

The 6 Grain Rolled Flakes mix I presently use requires only that I boil $2^1/2$ cups of purified water, remove it from the heat and mix in 1 cup of grains. You should cool it before adding it to food. You may also substitute chicken or vegetable broth for the water. Pat McKay suggests adding a few drops of Russell Swift's AniMinerals mineral supplement formulation to water if it is dis-tilled, purified, or treated by reverse osmosis (in the amounts rec-ommended on the bottle—see Supplements and Resources).

Putting a bay leaf in your uncooked grains can keep insects from hatching (but bay leaves are toxic to cats, so don't let your animals eat them). Pat McKay recommends storing uncooked grains in the refrigerator and cooking them within three months.

If your animal nutritionist or holistic veterinarian suggests that you add fiber, try one tablespoon of Miller's Unprocessed Bran per pound of meat. Sometimes a little bran helps pregnant queens, but you'll find the fresh food recipe produces a more compact stool, with less odor, than commercial food. Just be sure to add enough water or broth to make the food the consistency of a thick chili. The rule of thumb is six to eight ounces of liquid per pound of meat.

I never use onions as they are too difficult for animals to digest, but include Kyolic aged garlic, available at health food stores (or see Resources). It smells wonderful, as does a pinch of fresh herbs. However, Melinda Leeson, of Nature's Own Environmental Services, swears by fresh garlic to help boost the immune system. She places fresh garlic inside a capsule that's been lightly dipped in the fresh food mixture, then pops it into her cat's mouth at mealtime. You might also try Anitra Frazier's recipe for "Delicious Garlic Condiment."[16]

Best Friends offers an essential fatty acid recipe formulated by Pat McKay, which consists of equal parts of cold pressed soy, safflower, peanut, and wheat germ oils. I add this two to three times per week to the basic fresh food recipe to prevent hairballs and promote a lustrous coat. I use one tablespoon per pound of meat. This recipe is not complete without the inclusion of bonemeal, MinerAll Plus, Bio-C and food enzymes, so for further information on other items to add see My Special Supplements on page 102.

Feeding Schedules and Quantities

FOR YEARS veterinarians have been telling us to stick with one food, to open a can morning and night, and to leave the dry food out for the cat to nibble on all day (rather like raising a child on Spam and Coco Puffs!). And how would you feel about eating this boring diet left out all day to spoil? Would you ever dream of even tasting it? Of course not. It's not fit for human consumption. No wonder cats get a bad rap about being finicky! With their food left out all day to go rancid, some cats may never show interest in their regular meals.

Remember, cats are carnivores, not grazing animals—and they need time between meals to fast so their system can become acidic. Smelling food and nibbling all day keeps cats' systems alkaline, which is a condition that lowers their immunity. Feline Urological Syndrome (FUS) is directly related to this nibbling. Studies show that dry food fed free-choice causes the urine to be more alkaline for longer periods of time, creating an environment conducive to the formation of urinary crystals and calculi.[17]

Adult cats that have been freely fed (dry food left out throughout the day) should be cut back to one to two meals a day. If you notice your cat has a better appetite at one meal or the other, you can even feed only once a day; just discontinue the meal of less interest.[18] Fasting is also something to consider (see section on Fasting, page 86). Cats that are ill or very old may not fare well with any change in meal scheduling, so consult an animal nutritionist or holistic practitioner for special problems.

Kittens usually start to eat fresh food at between four and five weeks of age. Once weaned, they need to eat six to eight times daily until they are between eight and twelve weeks of age, when they may be cut back to four meals a day. From twenty-four weeks to one year, feed them twice daily, and after one year, once or twice daily, depending on health, breed, and so on. Let their appetite and constitution be your guide. I feed my adult cats twice daily, but the pregnant, lactating queens eat more often, usually three to four times a day.

If you have an especially finicky cat, start by mixing small portions of fresh food into your present cat food. You can begin with as little as one teaspoon of fresh food and work up from there, or offer just the fresh food itself. Most cats love it and dive in; others are addicted to their fast food diets and take longer to convert. Be creative with bribe foods (see page 89). This was extremely helpful to me with a few of my cats.

How much should you feed your cat at each meal? It's simple: If she's left any food in her dish, she's probably had her fill. If the platter is licked clean, she didn't get enough, so give her a little more. Her appetite may vary slightly from time to time, but if she refuses to eat, this could be a sign of illness, not just finickiness. She may simply require a day to fast and heal.

Leave food down no longer than forty-five minutes per meal. This is a good rule on two counts: you'll guard against spoilage, and you'll get your cat used to being fed at specific times rather than free-feeding on kibble all day long.

Getting Started—Some Hints to Help You Make the Transition

YOU'VE READ the chapter. You're a believer, but you're not rushing out to the health food store. Why not? Perhaps, though you'd like to improve your cat's diet, you're feeling a little overwhelmed.

Okay, let's compromise a little—and ease into the fresh food diet. Know that you won't see substantial improvements in your cat's health until you make the switch completely. But you can start right now to improve his present diet, the goal being to get to fifty-fifty for starters. If you can get that far, the rest will be easy. Holistic veterinarians and nutrition experts offer the following collection of tips to get you started.

Wean your cat off his current food immediately if the label states it contains one or more of the following: meat or poultry by-products; meat, poultry, or fish meal; artificial coloring or flavoring; BHA, BHT, ethoxiquin, MSG, propylgallate, propylene glycol, sodium nitrate, or sodium nitrite. Switch to canned health food lines of pet food such as Wysong, Precise, or Pet Guard. Read the labels. You can begin the transition to a natural diet by adding the fresh food ingredients to the higher quality canned food.

Please do not feed dry food. Store it in an airtight container and save it in case of a power failure or major emergency. If you insist on feeding it, then at least moisten it with purified water or broth. Many cats are so addicted to their dry food that weaning them off it may be your toughest job. But as your cat's guardian, you must be compassionately determined. She'll soon learn you mean business. Try adding fresh, raw food to the dry food to begin your conversion, or crushing the dry food and sprinkling it on top of the fresh.

Feed healthy adult cats only once or twice a day. Pick up food bowls after forty-five minutes and wipe up spills, so they can't smell the food when it's not mealtime. Remember, you want your cat's system to concentrate on cleansing and rebuilding between meals, not on digesting all day.

Switch everybody in your household, including you, to purified water. You'll love the taste of spring water or filtered water from which harmful chemicals and heavy metals have been removed.

But distilled water has no taste and is devoid even of valuable minerals, so you may add Russell Swift's AniMinerals to your cat's distilled water for a mineral boost.

Leave out little pots of kitty greens, wheatgrass, or cat-friendly fresh herbs such as catnip for her to nibble on.

Add high-quality supplements, starting with small amounts. Use a natural food enzyme with the canned food you are currently feeding because canned food is virtually devoid of enzymes. I add food enzymes to my fresh food at serving time, just to be sure my cats absorb and assimilate all the healthy ingredients.

Make love and play a daily routine, just as with the fresh food diet. Most of all, don't obsess. No one is perfect. Everyone I know occasionally slips up. If your recipe isn't exactly right, you'll make up for it at the next meal.

Cats pick up on our negative attitudes, so program yourself for success at this new regimen. You can do it! Your cats will love you even more for providing them with the foods nature intended them to eat.

FASTING, VOLUNTARY
AND INVOLUNTARY
and More Tips to Get Cats to Eat Fresh Food

AN AGE-OLD practice, fasting is one of the most overlooked and yet valuable modes of healing. It relieves the body of the task of digesting foods and allows the system to rid itself of wastes and toxins while encouraging gentle healing. Many holistic practitioners encourage *therapeutic fasting* the first day or two of an illness, especially if there is a fever (and/or, I would add, diarrhea). This is a type of *involuntary fasting*. Cats in the wild fast when they're ill, instinctively allowing their bodies to cleanse and detoxify.

Many experts, including Pitcairn and Frazier, recommend routine involuntary fasting once a week for internal cleansing. Fasting from breakfast to the following breakfast can be of help in converting cats to one meal per day and in controlling weight.

I only fast my cats when I have time to give them special care—extra love, and lots of broth and water. If you choose to fast your cat, the fasting day is a wonderful time for grooming and cuddling. Do not fast your cat when you are not home. She needs the extra attention when deprived of her food!

Healthy wild cats gorge on their fresh prey, then sleep and bask in the sun. They may not catch another meal for a day or two. Their bodies are designed for fasting between meals, allowing their systems to become acidic. When they smell food, their system turns alkaline, and a constant alkalinity leaves the immune system vulnerable. So allow your cat to get really hungry between meals, and exercise them to work up a good appetite.

As you switch your cat over to the fresh food diet, you'll probably observe what Pat McKay refers to as *voluntary fasting*. You put the food down. Your cat circles it, sniffs it, shakes a paw at it, and tries to bury it (this doesn't usually mean the cat doesn't like the food, but is a ritual version of burying it for later, when he's really hungry). You've added a bribe food or two, and still no results. No "clean plate club." Your cat simply doesn't recognize the smell of this new food, and smell is what attracts cats to their food.

Since I usually feed most everyone together, I initially got a mixed bag of reactions. It took four months to convert all my cats to the diet. I did, however, resort to feline aerobics before dinner to help them work up an appetite (see Play in chapter 2,

"Interacting with Your Cat"). Often, the love and affection your cats show at feeding time is not only food hunger but hunger for love and attention.

Holistic physician and author Deepak Chopra, M.D., tells about a study done with two groups of laboratory animals. One group was provided daily with an optimum diet by a technician who merely put their food down but never touched them. The other group was fed the equivalent of a fast food diet, but loved and stroked at feeding time. The animals that got the good food but no love died, and those that got the bad food and the cuddles lived.

We can continue to accept the voluntary fast for up to four meals (forty-eight hours).[19] At each scheduled mealtime, put down the dish (including bribe foods if you feel you need to), and pick it up and clean the area forty-five minutes later—whether your cat has eaten or not. Show her you love her, but also that you really mean business. If she doesn't eat, let her fast. No more junk food! Provide kitty greens for them to nibble on and cleanse their systems, keep a bowl of fresh purified water with a few drops of AniMinerals down at all times.

Broth (see recipes above) is wonderful during fasts. Serve it three to five times per day, but leave it down each time for only forty-five minutes. You can include a pinch of vitamin C with bioflavonoid complex and food enzymes.

Since dry food eaters are used to nibbling, they may not at first think you mean business when you pick up the dish. They think that, if they sit by the cupboard where you keep the old bag of kibbles (they know you kept it), maybe you'll break down. If you make it through four meals of this siege, you deserve a pat on the back. Most cats will dive into their fresh food by meal four. You can help by popping a little raw "meat-ball" into their mouths so they get the taste of it.

With very stubborn cases, it's time to drag out your bag of tricks (bribe foods) but please, if your cat is addicted to tuna, dry food, or some other no-no, don't use it! Try something from Anitra Frazier's list, which includes lamb baby food spread on top of the fresh food like a frosting, or an inch of sardine in tomato sauce or raw chicken liver. I like using raw chunks of organic beef or lamb liver, or half a can of the cat's favorite commercial canned food. If repeated tries at homemade food still fail, Dr. Chambreau feels your cat may have an underlying energy imbalance and be in need of some holistic treatment (such as acupuncture or homeopathy) to develop a good appetite.

If your cat is over seven years old, pregnant, nursing, or seriously ill, most holistic veterinarians will recommend that you don't allow an extended fast. Get him eating as best you can. These cats will need extra bribes and "T.L.C." If your cat normally gobbles up his fresh food diet and suddenly refuses to eat and shows any other unusual symptoms, this may be an involuntary fast. Consult your holistic veterinarian as soon as possible.

If your cat refuses to eat and your holistic veterinarian wants you to force-feed, Dr. Chambreau recommends Dr. Pitcairn's recipe for long-term force-feeding:[20]

Blend 2/3 cup raw chicken,
1/4 cup half-and-half,
1/4 tsp. cod liver oil,
10mg vitamin B-complex, and
1/4 tsp. bonemeal, with water or chicken broth.

Feed one cup per eight-pound cat per day (adjust for the weight of your cat).

To force-feed, place your cat comfortably on your lap wrapped in a towel and use a feeding syringe. Repeat every six hours, or as directed by your holistic practitioner. Pat McKay's broth recipe is extremely useful for short-term force-feeding: simply puree ground beef and water, strain, and feed by syringe.

For more on fasting, I recommend Anitra Frazier's *The New Natural Cat* as well as *Dr. Pitcairn's Complete Guide to Natural Health for Dogs and Cats*, and *Reigning Cats and Dogs* by Pat McKay. All three authors advocate fasting under controlled circumstances.

HOW TO PREVENT CONTAMINATION AND SPOILAGE

TO MAKE sure you're giving your cats only the freshest food, you'll need to follow some basic rules of storage and hygiene. Keep your fresh food mixture no more than three days in the refrigerator, or freeze portions and thaw them in the refrigerator the night before feeding. Date the frozen packages and never use them more than six months after freezing. Keep meat out of the refrigerator just long enough to prepare the recipe or serve it. Finally, always smell the meat before you feed it; when in doubt, throw it away!

Ninety percent of spoiled meat problems happen right in our own kitchens. Besides improper storage, spoilage may occur when cutting boards and other preparation surfaces aren't cleaned properly. Clean countertops and floors where your cats eat with diluted hydrogen peroxide, a citricidal cleanser, or a dilute bleach mixture, and then rinse thoroughly with hot water.

To further guard against problems, Pat McKay feels that raw

food should be left out for your cats to eat no longer than fifteen to twenty minutes. Forty-five minutes is my time limit. Use your own best judgment. Again, this will help not only to prevent spoilage but also to ensure that your cat's digestive system gets the fast between meals that it needs (see Feeding Schedules and Quantities).

Standardized grapefruit extract controls salmonella bacteria and acts as a natural preservative. Both Pat McKay and I recommend treating raw poultry (both muscle and organ meat) as follows:[21]

6 to 8 oz. purified water mixed with
4 drops standardized grapefruit extract (liquid concentrate)[22]
and added to 1 lb. poultry

Pour the solution over *ground* poultry and mix thoroughly until the liquid is completely absorbed. The antibacterial action on ground meat is immediate; however, if treating chunks or whole pieces of poultry, you must marinate them for an hour in a covered glass bowl in the refrigerator.

Caution: Keep standardized grapefruit extract away from eyes and sensitive areas. If accidental contact occurs, flush with water for ten minutes. Irritation is temporary, but may last up to forty-eight hours.

If you wish, you may treat any other kind of meat, or even raw egg yolk, in this manner, especially if you're worried about your cat's immune system. This method is also safe to use on meat and poultry you cook for yourself.

In addition, refrigerate all oils immediately after opening as oxidation begins upon contact with air. My editor, Robin Jacobson, suggests keeping oil from becoming rancid by adding water to the oil container as you use the oil up. This displaces the air, and since the oil floats on the water, it can be poured out without pouring out any water.

Never store opened cans of food in the refrigerator, as contamination with lead can be severe.[23] Canned pet food can contain as much as 0.9–7.0 ppm of lead, a daily intake that's considered potentially toxic for children. So store canned food in glass containers. Also, serve food and water in glass or porcelain serving bowls, not plastic. Food interacts with plastic, encouraging feline acne. And never microwave anything (for further precautions regarding food preparation, see chapter 3, "The Dangers of Conventional Care").

PURE WATER

KEEP a bowl of fresh distilled, spring, or purified water available at all time. I have always used distilled or purified water for both myself and my cats. Dr. Henry G. Bieler, author of *Food Is Your Best Medicine*, says that, just as you'd never put tap or mineral water in a steam iron, your kidneys appreciate the same courtesy. I personally use distilled water for that reason. When mixing distilled water with my cats' food, I add Dr. Russell Swift's mineral supplement, AniMinerals. There is another school of thought that suggests that distilled water actually leaches out minerals from our systems. Follow your holistic practitioner's advice. As long as you use bottled water, I'm content with whichever philosophy you choose.

The natural habitat of many wild cats is the plains or savannahs. Cats in the wild drink water only occasionally, getting most of the water their bodies need directly from the flesh of their fresh prey. When you switch to the fresh food diet, you'll notice your cat will naturally consume less water. A healthy cat on this diet may drink once a week or less, even never, according to Dr. Chambreau. When the weather is dry, you'll find your cat drinking more water than usual, even on the fresh food diet.

But cats that eat dry food really tank up, as the kibbles contain only about 2 percent moisture. This is extremely taxing to their kidneys. For cats that insist on eating dry food, try mixing it with purified water or broth, then gradually adding fresh raw food and deleting the dry. At least they'll be getting some fluids this way, and you'll be preparing the way for full conversion to fresh food.

You're providing a most efficient way for your cat to assimilate pure water when you add it to her food. However, cats can die very quickly from dehydration, so it's essential to keep a dish filled with fresh, pure water twenty-four hours a day. Still, most dehydration is caused by not eating rather than not drinking. I strategically place little bowls of fresh purified water around my home.

One day, at my local pharmacy, I happened upon a product called Willard Water (Catalyst-Altered Water, or CAW, developed by the late Dr. John Willard, a professor of chemistry). I bought a four-ounce bottle and a small pamphlet about it.[24] I was told by the pharmacy staff that this water cleanses the intestinal tract and is perfectly safe to drink, bathe in, and mix with food for children, adults, plants, and animals.

Willard Water is described in the literature as "wetter," more reactive, and more efficient. After my first sip, the notion of the water being wetter seemed a great description. It really quenched my thirst. I liked the taste, and it gave me a feeling of being centered, as opposed to stressful or sleepy.

CAW is water that has been altered by a silicone colloidal particle called the *micelle*, one of the most powerful reducing agents (antioxidant) for organic substances. Like the living cell, the micelle, under the proper stimuli, will reverse its polarity and act as an oxidizing agent. The CAW micelle has a negative charge on the surface, which helps remove most of the toxins, harmful bacteria, pollutants, and carcinogens from air, water, and foods, which have a positive charge. The micelle takes electrons from the water and atmosphere, and therefore has an infinite source of electrons to replenish those lost through its action as a reducing agent. The micelle acts like a catalyst, which is why Dr. Willard named this substance catalyst-altered water.

Dr. Willard believed there to be two causes of illness, both concerned with water, air, and food: either that something is needed by the body which is not there, or that something which is not needed by the body is there. In both instances, the use of CAW has an effect.

Rather than a nutrient, CAW (like all water) is the vehicle by which nutrients are carried to the cells and by which waste is carried away from the cells. Because it is a more biologically active form of water, it is said to do a better job of transportation. The micelle is a high-energy particle with a powerful negative magnetic field. It can speed up a chemical reaction without changing the natural result, a phenomenon that allows plants to grow faster and wounds to heal more rapidly.

Willard Water is available in two forms, the clear CAW and the dark CAWXXX. Reputable labs have tested both kinds of Willard Water and classified them as nontoxic, noncorrosive, noncarcinogenic, and incapable of causing harmful side effects. You can safely drink CAWXXX and use it the same way as clear

CAW—just remember to follow the package directions (they differ for each kind) for diluting both these products for drinking and other general domestic uses.

The clear form contains a larger percentage of the catalyst and so is more reactive. The dark CAWXXX contains not only the catalyst but lignite organics. *Lignite* is the fossilized remains of plants, trees, and microorganisms that lived long before humans made their debut on earth. The internal chemistry of these plants enabled them to survive under hostile conditions. Lignite is 60 to 65 percent carbon, and contains hydrogen, nitrogen, and oxygen as well as trace minerals, all invaluable for life processes. There is also evidence of antibacterial, antifungal, and antiviral agents in addition to unidentified growth stimulants for plants and animals. When lignite is treated with Willard Water, the valuable nutrients are made available as conditioners and normalizers, and all undesirable components are eliminated.

You can mix dilute CAWXXX with your cat's food in place of normal purified water. It helps quiet nervous and excitable animals, so I even use it to shampoo my cats, adding one part shampoo to nine parts CAW. A rinse with CAW helps reduce itching, and I've also used it to bathe stuffy noses or irritated eyes, and on wounds, both punctures and abrasions, along with the appropriate homeopathic remedies.

VITAMINS AND MINERALS—
A Guide to Nutritional Supplements

THE FOLLOWING information is just that, for informational purposes only. Basic supplements are definitely needed when feeding a fresh food diet (see Fresh Food Recipe, page 70), but do not attempt other than basic supplementation without first consulting with a qualified feline nutritionist or a holistic veterinarian well versed in nutrition. From time to time, your practitioner may choose to augment your cat's diet with additional supplementation. Find a reliable source for your supplements, as you must be able to count on the integrity of the manufacturers (see Resources).

The key thing to remember is that, in administering supplements, you're trying to achieve balance in your cat's nutrition. Minerals and vitamins work hand in hand, and both are necessary to maintain a healthy body. Our animals' bodies know best what vitamins and minerals they need at any given time. As their guardians, all we can do is try to make sure all the bases are covered. What the body doesn't need at the moment will be stored or eliminated, depending on the type of supplement.

The safest way to provide minerals is through food and other natural substances such as bonemeal, herbs, antioxidants, and montmorillonite clay. Soluble minerals act as:

- Ionized conductors of the electrical current necessary for all bodily functions.
- Catalysts and activators of other nutrients.
- Building blocks of enzymes, hormones, and other natural chemicals used by the body to perform specific functions.
- Equalizers and balancers of body fluids, fluid pressures, and pH. (In the absence of certain trace minerals, certain heavy minerals, such as lead, are more likely to accumulate and cause poisoning.)
- Aids to digestion and assimilation.

No single supplement is a cure-all. Pat McKay recommends not giving any specific vitamin or mineral on an ongoing basis.[25] Just because a friend tells you to try vitamin E for a cat that scratches, doesn't mean you want to give it every day for the rest of your cat's life. The animal may not have a vitamin E deficiency at all, and vitamin E administered without the appropriate amounts of A and D won't do much good and may even be detrimental to your cat's health. So please don't give megadoses of one vitamin or mineral just because it seems to benefit a particular condition.

The chart that follows includes vitamins and minerals found to be necessary through research. Exact requirements of supplements are variable, so utilizing the nutrients in live foods and whole food supplements is a more beneficial option.

VITAMIN AND MINERAL GUIDE CHART[26]

SUPPLEMENT	RECOMMENDED DOSAGE	HEALTH BENEFITS
Vitamin A	10,000 IU weekly	Prevents cataracts, weakness in hind legs; aids tissue development; promotes healthy skin and fur
Vitamin C	250-3,000 mg daily, or to bowel tolerance	Promotes healing of wounds; used to treat arthritis, and chronic/degenerative diseases from stress due to high fever, cigarette smoke, pollution; prevents kidney stones
Bioflavonoid	500 mg for each 1,000 mg vitamin C	Supports vitamin C and is essential to its absorption
Vitamin D	Daily sunlight	Prevents rickets and hypocalcemia; essential for normal growth of bones and teeth; helps behavioral problems and endocrine imbalances
Vitamin E	30-400 IU once a week	Maintains balance between oils/fats and amino acids; great antioxidant; slows again; improves skin, muscles, and nerves; important for healing, especially burns
Vitamin B-complex	Water-soluble and sheds easily so must be continually replenished; exact amount required not known	Helps hyperactivity; improves appetite; used as flea repellent; helps nervous animals; essential for mental and emotional health

INTERACTIONS	BEST FOOD SOURCE
Caution: Excess as harmful as deficiency; confirm exact dosage with holistic practitioner before using. Absorption blocked by use of mineral oil, sugar, or cortisone, or through liver disorders.	Eggs, cod liver oil, raw butter, yogurt, raw meat. Cats do not absorb vitamin A from vegetables
Depleted by cigarette smoke, baking soda, high fever	Leafy vegetables, cruciferous vegetables (such as broccoli), lentils, sprouts, most fruits
	Grapes, raisins, rose hips, white inner skin of citrus fruits
Depleted by excessive or insufficient calcium and phosphorus. Deficiency caused by insufficient sunlight	Cod liver oil, raw butter, cheese, eggs, organ meats
Absorption hindered by mineral oil, chlorine, iron, synthetic hormones	Wheat germ oil, leafy greens and other raw vegetables, seeds, whole grains, raw meat
Depleted by cold weather, stress, antibiotics; megadoses of vitamin C and folic acid decrease B_{12} levels and destroy many B-complex vitamins	Raw liver, wheat germ, unprocessed brown rice, organ meats, cottage cheese, sardines

SUPPLEMENT	RECOMMENDED DOSAGE	HEALTH BENEFITS
Vitamin F	Exact amount required not known	Helps prevent heart problems; essential for skin and coat conditions; essential to thyroid and adrenals; aids in flea problems and dermatitis
Biotin	Exact amount required not known	Promotes thyroid and adrenal health and hair growth, cures feces eating problem; vital for food metabolism. Early sign of deficiency is scaly dermatitis
Folic Acid —Vitamin B_9	Exact amount required not known	Prevents birth defects, weight loss, anemia, eye discharge. Signs of deficiency are anemia and leukopenia
Pyridoxine —Vitamin B_6	Exact amount required not known	Essential for metabolism of protein, healthy nervous system, red blood cell production, strong immune system
Vitamin K	0.02 ug per kcal. Supplementation needed rarely, only when antivitamin K components in diet	Regulates formation of several factors involved in blood clotting; prevents hemorrhaging. Large intakes produce anemia; however, does not appear toxic
Calcium and Phosphorus	500 mg per 100 g meat	Deficiencies lead to nervousness, lameness, muscle spasms, heart palpitations, seizures, bone fractures
Magnesium	Normally obtained in regular diet—deficiency unlikely	Important for nervous system and enzyme function. Signs of deficiency include heart arrhythmia and depression

INTERACTIONS	BEST FOOD SOURCE
Absorption blocked by cooking of fats and oils	Cold-pressed vegetable and fish oils (cod liver oil); oleic, linoleic, linolenic, and arachidonic acids; raw meats and vegetables
Antibiotics decrease production	Bulgur wheat, lentils, tofu, legumes, brown rice
Depleted by cortisone, cigarette smoke, antibiotics	Cod liver oil, tofu, wheat germ, sprouts, fruit
Depleted by pesticides, sugar, laxatives, synthetic hormones	Herbs, raw liver and other organ meats, whole grain cereals
Depleted by drug treatment, especially anticoagulants	Obtained through bacterial synthesis in intestine
Vitamin D required to activate calcium. Deficiencies may be brought on by high-meat diets	Bonemeal most natural source of calcium and phosphorous; mix with raw meat (see Fresh Food Recipe)
Depleted by noise stress. Excess associated with increased incidence of feline urinary syndrome. Vitamin C needed to best utilize calcium/magnesium	Tofu, broccoli, dairy products, sardines

SUPPLEMENT	RECOMMENDED DOSAGE	HEALTH BENEFITS
Zinc	With normal dietary intake of iron and copper, concentrations of up to 8 times minimum requirement will not produce adverse effects Minimum requirement unknown.	Enhances skin and coat condition. Signs of deficiency include poor growth, emaciation, testicular atrophy
Potassium and Sodium	Need for supplementation very rare	Use in cases of exhaustion
Chromium	Exact amount required not known	May help diabetes, as it regulates blood sugar
Iron	Approx. 5 mg daily—exact amount required not known	Fights lead poisoning from commercial foods; builds immunity and energy. Iron oxide far less dangerous form than ferrous sulfate

MY SPECIAL SUPPLEMENTS

I INCLUDE the following supplements, which were formulated by Pat McKay, daily. (See the Resources section for information on how to obtain them.)

Bio-C. One teaspoon of Bio-C formula provides 1000 mg vitamin C with rosehips, 500 mg of bioflavonoid complex including rutin, and hesperidin. I give vitamin C and other water-soluble nutrients in frequent small doses, as they pass through the system in three to four hours. For this reason, putting Bio-C in the food is an ideal way to administer it. Use one teaspoon per pound of raw meat for adult cats.

The primary function of vitamin C is to maintain collagen, a protein necessary for the proper formation of connective tissue, ligaments, tendons, muscles, skin, and bones. Other functions

INTERACTIONS	BEST FOOD SOURCE
Vegetable protein-based diets may dramatically increase requirement; phytic acid (in cereals) decreases availability	Beef liver, chicken, oats, Swiss cheese, some nuts and seeds
Potassium depleted by cooking	Apple cider vinegar (1 tsp. per pint of drinking water)
Depleted by white flour and white sugar	Calves' liver, vegetables, fruit
Too much dairy, eggs, yogurt block absorption	Citrus fruits, tomatoes, broccoli, cantaloupe, beef liver, poultry, beans

include the formation of adrenaline (needed for stressful situations); protection of other vitamins from oxidation; formation of red blood cells; stimulation of the production of interferon; stimulation of the immune system, enabling the body to resist disease, including cancer; inactivation of viruses and bacteria.

Found abundantly in the inner white pulp of citrus, bioflavonoids (vitamin P) are very important to the support of vitamin C. Rutin is part of the bioflavonoid complex, and it strengthens capillary walls. Hesperidin is a crystalline glycoside.

Bonemeal. Bonemeal should be mixed with the fresh raw meat because the meat stimulates acid production in the digestive system and aids in calcium absorption. Mix one to two tablespoons into each pound of meat.

I use Best Friends bonemeal formula with red marrow for two reasons: it contains less than 5 ppm of lead, and it includes, in balanced proportions, all the nutrients necessary for the proper assimilation of calcium. In fact, this product is the only supplemental form of calcium that Pat McKay feels is complete and, therefore, safe for both dogs and cats.

MinerAll Plus. Excellent for flea control and skin allergies, this powder is a unique blend of montmorillonite clay, alfalfa, kelp, dandelion root, and garlic. Collectively, the ingredients in MinerAll provide vitamins A, B-complex, C, D, E, G, K, P, and U, as well as seventy-two trace minerals. McKay recommends one tablespoon per pound of meat.[27]

Montmorillonite clay is a natural source of many trace minerals.[28] Alfalfa contains calcium, choline, magnesium, potassium, phosphorus, silicon, and sodium. Dandelion root contains taraxacin, inulin, gluten, gum, and potash. These substances are useful for remedying chronic disorders of the kidneys, and liver, gallstones, anemia, and diabetes. Kelp contains iodine, iron, potassium, calcium, sodium, choline, sulfur, and silicon. Garlic contains protein, carbohydrates, calcium, iron, potassium, phosphorus, traces of sodium, and vitamins B_1, B_2, B_3, and C, as well as thirty-three sulfur compounds. It is also one of the best vegetable sources of selenium. Both selenium and vitamin E are antioxidants, which act to retard oxidation.

Aloe Vera Juice. Another ingredient in the fresh food diet designed by Pat McKay is food-grade aloe vera juice. It helps combat allergies, arthritis, colitis, constipation, diarrhea, dental problems, hairballs, indigestion, liver, and kidney disease, as well as viral and yeast infections. Pat McKay recommends not using aloe during the first month of pregnancy, as the body naturally undergoes a detoxification during this time, and augmenting that condition can be overwhelming to the cat's system.

Pat McKay warns us to read the label carefully before purchasing aloe vera juice. Be sure it doesn't contain the preservatives sodium benzoate or benzoic acid, which extend the shelf life of the product but are poisonous to cats! Keep unpreserved aloe vera (such as Pure Comforts brand—see Resources) in the refrigerator once it's opened. Freeze-dried aloe vera is also an option.

Vitamin E. I also add a 400 IU capsule of high-quality vitamin E (I like alpha tocopherol) once weekly, as recommended by Anitra Frazier. Sometimes I use a few drops of liquid vitamin E oil, which I keep refrigerated at all times.

I use the following supplements less frequently:

Fatty Acids. Fatty acids, available in raw meat and uncooked oils, are essential to the cat's diet. I use only high-quality, cold-pressed nitrogen-sealed oils, and never cook them, as cooked fat clogs arteries. Under normal circumstances I include oils two to three times weekly in my cats' food to keep hairballs under control and promote luxurious coats.

Pat McKay offers the following formula for making your own fatty acid mixture.[29]

> 3/4 cup Hain's All Blend (a cold-pressed vegetable oil
> available in health food stores)[30]
> 1/4 cup cold-pressed, unrefined wheat germ oil

Mix and refrigerate immediately, as oils begin to oxidize the minute they are opened, and may become rancid quickly. You may add one to two tablespoons to the fresh food to help with dry, flaky skin and coat problems. Or just give your cat a little bit with an eye dropper or syringe; 1cc is about right for hairballs if your cat is troubled by them. Raw, unsalted butter keeps hairballs under control as well.

Melinda Leeson offers an alternative formula:[31]

3/4 cup flaxseed oil
1/4 cup cod liver oil
1/4 dropper vitamin E oil (to retard spoilage)

She recommends two teaspoons daily for cats between five and fifteen pounds or as directed by your nutritionist .

Herbs. From time to time, I use fresh herbs, but just a pinch for aroma and flavor. Sage, thyme, and marjoram smell wonderful and are nice additions, among other savory herbs. I also use a pinch of Sunrider Simply Herbs in my cats' food and my kittens' formula now and then,[32] and I grow little pots of wheatgrass and other herbs and grasses, including catnip, for my cats to nibble on. Don't be concerned if they regurgitate—it's a natural cleansing process that rids them of hairballs.

Acidophilus. This substance is most commonly produced by fermenting milk with lactobacilli (bacteria beneficial to digestion). I keep vegetarian acidophilus (either liquid or capsule form) in my refrigerator. If a cat or kitten has been on an antibiotic,[33] I recommend giving acidophilus during the course of the drug treatment and for several weeks to a month afterward. The lactobacilli replaces many of the friendly bacteria in the intestinal tract which have been wiped out by the antibiotic. Such therapy utilizing friendly bacteria is called *probiotic*. I also often use enzymes containing friendly bacteria (see Food Enzymes, page 110).

Bee Products. Pat McKay also recommends using bee products (bee pollen, bee propolis, royal jelly) from time to time,[34] as do many nutrition experts. Bee propolis is the natural antibiotic the bees use to keep their hives free of bacteria. Combination products are available, but please be stingy with bee substances, as they've been known to cause allergic reactions in sensitive individuals. I don't use them on a daily basis, but have had good results reported. Try one-quarter teaspoon of bee pollen per pound of meat in your fresh food mixture and see how your cats tolerate it. It's a good idea to clear its use with your animal nutritionist first, as royal jelly, for example, can cause allergic reactions.

Biogenetics Supplements. This company produces an impressive line of supplements (see Resources). Their Feline Vitality,™ an antioxidant nutritional supplement for cats, contains a trademarked ingredient called Bioguard Sprouts, which fights free radicals. The use of antioxidants seems to improve the overall well-being and immune response of cats. Bioguard includes vitamins C and E, beta carotene, selenium, and beef liver, which provides B_{12} and other B-complex vitamins; it's blended with beef broth, which makes it palatable to cats. You can crush the tablets with a mortar and pestle and put the powder into the fresh food. However, most of my cats love the tablets as a treat.

Biogenetics also makes Feline Balance which, as the name implies, helps promote alertness, well-being, and composure in stressful situations such as boarding, training, showing, estrus, and illness. Their Bioguard Plus, which comes in both tablets and granules is for people and animals. I use the granules in my own cereal and mix it in the cats' food several times a week.

What about yeast? Perhaps you've noticed that I don't include yeast in the fresh food recipe or as a supplement for my cats. One of the reasons for this omission is that it tends to cause or aggravate allergies. Alfred Plechner, D.V.M., lists yeast, yeast-containing foods, and brewer's yeast (given to animals for supposed flea protection) in his allergic "hit list."[35] Apparently, the DNA and RNA in yeast don't break down completely in the intestines, and when absorbed through the intestinal wall may cause adverse autoimmune responses and weaken organs such as the liver and kidneys. If you're feeding yeast and observe your cat itching and scratching excessively, with the appearance of patches of red skin, please discontinue use.

According to Pat McKay allergies may cause hair loss, itchy rashes, watery eyes, stuffy nose, nausea, diarrhea, flatulence, asthma, bronchitis, coughing, sore throat, arthritis, fatigue, eczema, and depression.[36] She further states that cytoxic tests done several years ago on animals with skin allergies showed that nine out of ten were allergic to yeast. It stands to reason that carnivores would have such an intolerance because their digestive systems, which were designed to digest raw prey, don't have the length (and, therefore, the time), the enzymes, or the proper acid/alkaline balance to break down and assimilate yeast, so they can't benefit from its nutrients.

McKay feels that yeast is a popular filler in food supplements because it's inexpensive! That's why it's in everything from supplements to flea care. She recommends aged and concentrated garlic for repelling fleas, and feels that all the vitamins, amino acids, and minerals in yeast can be obtained from fresh, natural sources. When feeding fresh raw meat, vegetables, and cooked grains along with bonemeal, alfalfa, dandelion, kelp, garlic, and montmorillonite clay supplemented by vitamin C and bioflavonoids (see bonemeal, MinerAll Plus and Bio-C, pages 102-104), your cat is dining at The Ritz.

Melinda Leeson has had results quite the opposite of Pat McKay's. In Leeson's experience, only one in a hundred or more animals exhibits an allergy to brewer's yeast, so she feels it's a shame to blacklist this supplement. However, in case of an allergic reaction, she suggests substitution.

Many other people in the holistic community recommend yeast, including Richard Pitcairn, D.V.M., who suggests a mixture called Healthy Powder; Anitra Frazier, who includes it in her Vita-Mineral mix; and the Wysong Company, which puts it in the supplement Feline Biotic. If you read labels, you'll find yeast in many other pet supplements.

Frazier suggests that, if a cat becomes gassy or bloated (the most common symptoms caused by the use of yeast), you may 1. stop feeding yeast completely; 2. eliminate all toxic, synthetic, and chemical substances from your cat's regimen; 3. give a charcoal capsule morning and evening for two days to absorb putrefaction; 4. add $1/2$ to $1/4$ teaspoon liquid chlorophyll each meal; 5. add acidophilus; 6. add digestive enzymes.[37]

Michael Lemmon, D.V.M., advises that, if yeast obviously causes allergies or other problems such as skin or digestive disorders, that you simply refrain from using it. Otherwise, he feels that yeast, in one or more of its forms, is good for pets, supplying high-quality proteins, B-complex vitamins, and trace minerals.[38]

Yeast comes in various other forms besides brewer's, such as torula yeast, lactic acid yeast (available from Standard Process Laboratories—see Resources), and kefir, which is a milk product made from kefir grains cultured from milk-fermenting yeasts and bacteria. Kefir can be found in cheese and beverage form. Kombucha tea (see page 112) also contains a form of nutritional yeast. Zell oxygen yeast, says Dr. Lemmon, may be used to help the body better utilize oxygen. Finally, Bio Strath yeast (and its animal counterpart, Animal Strath yeast) combines yeast with sixteen herbs.

As always, consult your holistic practitioner, or conduct your own feeding trial and see what happens. From the results of my own experiments, I chose not to include yeast in my fresh food recipe.

Food Enzymes (digestive enzymes). I personally feel that enzymes are an important addition to the diet, especially if you suspect your cat is not digesting her food thoroughly (check her stool for color and consistency; if abnormal, contact your holistic veterinarian or feline nutritionist). Also, freezing and refrigeration, even of the fresh food diet, may cost us some enzyme loss. Since enzymes are destroyed by cooking, commercial pet foods are missing these vital substances (yet another reason to switch to the fresh food diet).

Russell Swift, D.V.M., reports that the routine use of food enzymes is beneficial to cats suffering from asthma, allergies, diarrhea, constipation, gastritis, colitis, obesity, poor weight gain, arthritis, liver and bladder problems, excessive shedding, and oily or dry coats, to name but a few ailments.[39]

Enzymes aren't exotic substances. They're mandatory for proper digestion and absorption of nutrients. If enzymes aren't present in adequate amounts in food, the body tries to make up the difference, increasing the risk of acute and chronic disease. By improving digestion and bowel function, the use of enzymes relieves a large variety of physical symptoms.

I have had excellent results with Dr. Swift's enzyme formulations, both Florazyme LP, which contains liver and pancreas enzymes, and Florazyme EFA, an herbal formula. Florazyme contains enzymes that are highly active at body temperature and

throughout a wide pH range, as well as lactobacillus acidophilus, and lactobacillus bifidus. The Florazyme enzymes
begin to aid in digestion as soon as they are released in the act
of chewing.

I've found that approximately $1/4$ to $1/2$ tsp. of Florazyme LP
per cup of food at each meal is about right for my cats. You'll
need to experiment, but follow Dr. Swift's instructions or those
of your holistic practitioner.

Digestive enzyme products I previously used in my cats'
fresh food contained pancreatic enzymes, papain, and aspergillis
cultures. According to Dr. Swift, pancreas extracts, or pancreatin
(marketed under the trade name Viokase™), aren't the most
effective enzymatic substances because they function only in an
alkaline environment. They do improve digestion in the intestinal tract, but since they're not designed to work in an acidic
environment such as the stomach, they don't start the digestive
process early enough to spare the pancreas overwork. Raw glandular pancreas extracts do help the cat's pancreatic function,
however.

Aspergillus fungal cultures are active throughout a wide pH
range. Plant enzymes such as papain don't need higher than
body temperatures to perform effectively.

Another product to consider is Bio-Culture 2000, a probiotic supplement containing lactobacillus salivarias (a modified
microorganism). You can open a capsule and sprinkle it on the
cat's food along with Florazyme. Many people use it themselves
before traveling abroad, as it doubles the population of viable
organisms every twenty minutes, thus protecting the digestive
tract from infection by exotic organisms. If your cat is an international traveler, he may appreciate it too.

Dr. Chambreau notes that Nu Cat, a supplement from Vetri-science Labs contains enough digestive enzymes for many cats. However, I haven't personally used this product. I understand it contains yeast, which my cat population doesn't tolerate.

Kombucha Tea. Pat McKay has been having wonderful results with kombucha tea, which she brews herself from a starter of regular black tea (such as Lipton's) and white sugar, along with a fungus she cultivates in her kitchen. The fungus, which looks like a thick, soggy pancake, is sometimes called the "Manchurian mushroom," according to Laurel Farms, which ships it to customers all over the country (see Resources). McKay's animals seem to be blooming on this beverage, which she adds to their food.

The kombucha phenomenon has its origins in the Far East some two thousand years ago. Kombucha arrived in the United States via Germany, where entrepreneur Gunther Frank runs a thriving business selling the tea.[40] Russian studies claim to have found that the mold used in the fermentation process produces glucosonic acid, which purportedly detoxifies the liver.

I have heard amazing stories about this beverage, and I feel good about my own results with it. However, when introducing anything new into your own health regime or your cat's, be conservative. Start with small amounts. And check with your holistic practitioner to see if she feels kombucha will benefit you and your cats.

Super Blue-Green Algae. Dr. Chambreau introduced me to Cell Tech's Super Blue-Green Algae for animals.[41] When her own fresh-food-eating cat was off her food a bit and suffering from a kind of lethargy, she offered this algae and the cat bounced right back.

Super Blue-Green Algae is a special strain that grows in the pristine, mineral-rich waters of upper Klamath Lake, high in the Cascade Mountains of Oregon. The lake is fed by streams in over four thousand square miles of volcanically formed mountains; some believe crater lake waters contribute via underground springs.

This algae is acclaimed for its wealth of vitamins, minerals, enzymes, amino acids, and chlorophyll, all in raw organic form. A noncellulose cell membrane makes its nutrients highly assimilable.[42]

The recommended dosage is $1/3$ tsp. per pound of food, or $1/16$ to $1/8$ tsp. per meal. However, as with all new substances, introduce it cautiously, beginning with just a pinch and increasing the dosage over a three-week period to learn your cat's tolerance. Also, when you use Super Blue-Green Algae, either omit your other vitamin/mineral supplementation or use half the normal dosage of MinerAll Plus (see page 104) along with a pinch of the algae. My tribe dove right in to their food when I sprinkled these brilliantly colored granules on top. I presently combine $1/2$ tbsp. of MinerAll Plus and $1/4$ tsp. of Super Blue-Green Algae.

Pycnogenol. Perhaps the most exciting food supplement I've come across is Pycnogenol, a special blend of a type of bioflavonoid called proanthocyanidins. This superantioxidant has many benefits.[43] It seems to enhance the effect of the other antioxidants (such as vitamins A, C, E, and zinc) I use it in my nutritional program. Proanthocyanidins potentiate vitamin C, and some biochemists see evidence that Pycnogenol helps vitamin C enter cells. I certainly feel much better as a result of its inclusion in my own health program, and see increased vigor and immune response in the cats.

Maritime pine bark Pycnogenol seems to give the best results, but grape seed extract (another bioflavinoid) is beneficial too. I myself take several tablets a day, and I crush tablets and mix Pycnogenol into the cat food when I feel they need an extra antioxidant boost.

Colloidal Silver. Colloidal silver is a powerful natural prophylactic and antibiotic. The term *colloid* is defined as a substance consisting of ultrafine particles suspended in a medium of a different matter. All living things exist in the colloidal state, so the body can more readily use medications already in colloidal form. However, most medications are in crystalline form, which the body must convert to colloidal.

A catalyst that disables the particular enzyme that all one-celled bacteria and fungi as well as many viruses use to metabolize oxygen, colloidal silver has been used for thousands of years, apparently with no harmful effects on the body. The Environmental Protection Agency's Poison Control Center reports no toxicity listing for colloidal silver. Research has shown that traces of silver in the body act almost like a second immune system, and that silver is often not present in people with diseased systems. Owing to the high absorption of silver in the small intestine, the friendly bacteria in the large intestine appear not to be destroyed by its action.

Silver has been valued throughout history for its preservative and therapeutic properties. The Romans kept their milk fresh in silver vessels. On their journeys west, American pioneers preserved their milk and water by dropping a silver dollar in the containers. Hospitals used to place a drop of a silver solution in newborn babies' eyes to prevent blindness from harmful bacteria.

Silver was at one time a trace mineral in the soil, so we used to obtain this metal naturally in our vegetables. But owing to the use of chemical fertilizers, this is no longer true. These fertilizers kill most of the living organisms that under normal circumstance would break down the soil, providing minerals to plants in an assimilable form.

Don't confuse colloidal silver with the homeopathic remedy *Argentum nitricum* (see Homeopathy, page 142). They are completely different substances.

An early form of colloidal silver was in common usage until 1938, when it became too costly to produce (it was $100 an ounce in 1930). However, through modern advances we can once again experience its incredible curative power. Silverloid™ (a product marketed under various brand names, including Ultra Colloidal Silver from Threshold's Source Naturals) is a pure mineral supplement composed of minute particles of silver electromagnetically charged and suspended in pure demineralized water.[44]

When using colloidal silver prophylactically, people have reported getting fewer colds and flus. It has been tested successfully against more than 650 diseases and disorders,[45] has been employed to fight canine parvovirus and in other veterinary applications, as well as a leaf spray against bacterial, fungal, and viral attacks on plants. It seems to be effective against antibiotic-resistant strains of bacteria and fungi, which means it may be used against many types of disease-causing organisms simultaneously. Most pharmaceutical antibiotics target specific strains of bacteria. Colloidal silver seems to provide broader coverage.

Used both internally and externally, colloidal silver is reported safe enough to be dropped straight into the eyes (for conjunctivitis) and nose (for sinusitis), or dabbed topically onto the skin for treatment of such conditions as skin cancer, eczema, itchy areas, ringworm, and bites. You may even purify water using colloidal silver: add 1 oz. per gal. water, shake well, wait six minutes, shake again, wait six minutes more, and then drink. I have added colloidal silver prophylactically and therapeutically in my personal regimen as well as my cats'. It doesn't seem to have interfered with any other therapy, either human or feline.

The cats have tolerated colloidal silver extremely well, as it has very little taste and doesn't sting. I just reduce the human dosage in proportion to the cat's weight. I've given it orally to my newborn kittens (one drop each morning) and dropped it in their eyes (one drop in each eye) to prevent infections, as the newborns sometimes scratch each others' newly opened eyes while nursing.

I recommend administering colloidal silver on an empty stomach. If you wish to put it in your cat's drinking water, use distilled water only. I start out with only a few drops in order to determine my cat's reaction. For an acute condition, try seven drops for an adult cat three times daily for the first three days, then once daily for the next seven days. You may then discontinue or cut the dosage in half as a daily maintenance. But, as always, follow the advice of your holistic practitioner. Colloidal silver is also available in a salve form for easier topical application.

Colloidal Gold. Long used for medicinal purposes, colloidal gold has remarkable effects on the human body in both health and sickness. I have no information at this time as to how gold, in this form, may be beneficial to cats. This section has been included for information purposes only, as many people interested in silver also want to know about gold. Don't administer colloidal gold to your cat without consulting first with your holistic practitioner.

The use of gold in medicine is believed to have begun in Alexandria, Egypt, where, a skilled group known as *alchemists* developed an elixir of liquid gold, which they professed had the ability to restore youth and perfect health. Paracelsus, who was one of the greatest known alchemists, founded the school of *iatrochemistry*, the chemistry of medicines, which was the forerunner of modern pharmacology. He developed medicines from metallic elements, including gold. Later, alchemy became more widespread and gold was often used for its healing properties.

About 1857, English chemist Michael Faraday first prepared colloidal gold in a pure state. In the late nineteenth century, colloidal gold was commonly used in the United States as the basis of the cure for dipsomania (an uncontrollable craving for alcoholic beverages). Since then, traditional uses have included treatments for arthritis, burns, skin ulcers, and various types of punctures, as well as use in certain nerve-end operations. The rural Chinese believe in the restorative powers of gold to this day; they cook their rice with a gold coin in the pot.

Though colloidal gold doesn't have the same germicidal/antibiotic action as colloidal silver, it can have a tremendous balancing and harmonizing effect on the physical body, particularly with regard to unstable mental/emotional states such as sorrow, fear, despair, anguish, frustration, melancholy, depression, and suicidal tendencies—ailments commonly associated with the heart—and even seasonal affective disorder (SAD). Gold directly affects the rhythmic, balancing, and healing activities of the heart, and helps improve blood circulation.

It's also highly beneficial to the digestive system and to sluggish organs, especially the brain, and has been used to help rejuvenate the glands, stimulate the nerves, and release nervous pressure. Used alternately with silver, gold helps build strong natural defenses against disease, and promotes renewed vitality and longevity.

Aurum™ (Latin for gold).[46] A brand of colloidal gold, is an all-natural mineral supplement composed of minute particles of gold that have been electromagnetically charged and suspended in deionized water. It is flavorless and nontoxic.

Oxygen (O_2). Oxygen,[47] which all animals and plants need to survive, is obtained through respiration as well as by eating fresh raw fruits and vegetables (which contain hydrogen peroxide, converted to stabilized oxygen by the body). Stabilized oxygen comes in a powdered form that speeds digestion, facilitates removal of diseased and dying cells, and cleanses the system by oxidizing fecal matter without harming the mucous membranes or the lining of the intestines.

Pat McKay suggests we provide ourselves and our cats with supplemental oxygen, on a regular or occasional basis, just as we would with vitamins.[48] It has proven effective in her nutrition practice in the treatment of many serious feline illnesses.

The brand I use is PuriZone by Best Friends. Give your cat somewhere between $1/16$ and $1/4$ tsp., depending on the animal's size and health, once daily for a few days.[49] Ascorbic acid (vitamin C) facilitates the action of O_2, so I add a pinch (about $1/16$ tsp.) of Bio-C to $1/4$ tsp. O_2 and about 1cc distilled water. You may administer this orally (with an eye dropper or a syringe), or mix it into a tiny raw meatball or a little chicken baby food as a treat. When O_2 is mixed with food or water, its action lasts only about twenty minutes, so be sure the mixture is consumed immediately.

Pat McKay says that if your cat has a creamy stool, which may look like anything from mashed potatoes to pea soup, it's time to cut back on the dosage (amount and frequency) of supplemental oxygen.[50] Such a soft stool differs from diarrhea in that O_2 does not cause a loss of electrolytes, vital fluids, or nutrients. The stool probably becomes liquid in order to facilitate a deep cleansing of the lining of the colon. If you see little hard black balls in your cat's litter box, this is old fecal matter, which may have been in the colon for weeks, months, or even years (mucus and worms may be eliminated also). Pat says all these things are healthy signs of progress.

DMG. Many experts recommend the supplemental use of DMG (N, N-Dimethylglycine) in our cats' diets. Extensive research in the United States has demonstrated that this nutrient may enhance health and well-being. Though DMG is not a vitamin or mineral and is not essential for the prevention of a deficiency disease, it does have an essential role in optimizing the metabolic workings of the body and countering the consequences of stress. When working in conjunction with vitamins, minerals, and other cofactors, DMG neutralizes many of the wear-and-tear phenomena caused by physical and/or mental stress, including such degenerative diseases as arthritis, diabetes, heart disease, and even cancer, which are caused not by the lack of a specific nutrient but by the body's inability to cope with or adapt constructively to stress.

DMG was first recognized as being a component of the metabolic pathway of the cell in 1941, but its true importance to optimum health and sustained physical output wasn't discovered until decades later. A normal, physiologically active substance found in such foods as cereal grains, seeds, and meats, it has a wide range of beneficial effects on the body. DMG has been found to:

- Enhance the immune response system, the body's natural defense mechanism against disease.[51]
- Enhance oxygen utilization and to retard the buildup of lactic acid in the muscles.
- Reduce elevated cholesterol and triglyceride levels, and help normalize high blood pressure.
- Assist detoxification of the body and improve the function of such organs as the liver, pancreas, and adrenals.
- Help the body normalize blood glucose levels, and sustain high energy levels and improved mental acuity.

J. W. Meduski, M.D., Ph.D., has completed extensive evaluations of DMG and has found it to be an extremely safe nutrient, even when fed at very high levels. Dr. Meduski has also shown that laboratory animals taking DMG may enhance their oxygen uptake ability when the environment is low in oxygen.[52]

I include DMG in my cats' regime when they are stressed or ill. Many nutrition experts recommend administering DMG by dropper directly into the cat's mouth, but a few of my cats have thrown up when I've used this method. However, when I mix it with their food, they don't even know it's there.

Dr. Chambreau suggests giving DMG only to sick cats, which may truly need such nutritional support, rather than administering it as a basic supplement. Remember, follow your own holistic practitioner's advice on the use of all supplements mentioned in this section.

Standardized Grapefruit Extract. Standardized grapefruit extract, in its liquid concentrate form, is an essential product. *However, please exercise caution when using this extract. Never use it full strength! Keep away from eyes and sensitive areas. If accidental contact occurs, flush with water for ten minutes. Irritation is temporary, but may last up to forty-eight hours.*

As previously mentioned, the citricidal action in standardized grapefruit extract sterilizes meat (see How to Prevent Contamination and Spoilage, page 90), ridding it of many harmful microscopic organisms.[53] It may also be used internally and topically, as follows:

All-purpose cleaner: Add 30 to 60 drops to a 32 oz. pump sprayer filled with water. Use on all surfaces where cats eat or where raw meat is handled.

Cutting board cleaner: Use as a spray or apply 10 to 20 drops to cutting board, and work into the surface with a wet sponge or dishcloth. Leave on for 30 minutes, then rinse with water. Keep cats away during this process.

Dish-cleaning additive: Add 15 to 30 drops to sink dishwashing water, or to automatic dishwasher with dishwasher detergent, or to final rinse of either. You may add a few drops directly to dishwashing liquid.

Sink wash: Add 30 or more drops to a sink full of cold water and briefly soak vegetables, fruit, meat, or poultry.

Spray wash: Add 20 or more drops to a 32 oz. spray bottle of water. Spray on vegetables, fruit, meat, or poultry.

Shampoo: Add one drop to 1 oz. of shampoo then add 10 ozs. of catalyst-altered water (see Pure Water, page 92) or distilled water. Shampoo as usual. Leave on two minutes and rinse with water.

Skin Treatment: Add two drops to 2 oz. aloe vera juice or distilled water, and apply topically three to four times daily. This is an excellent treatment for ringworm and other skin problems.

Dental, ear, and nose wash: One drop in 2 oz. purified water or aloe vera juice as a dental and gum swab. Apply with a cotton swab, gauze, or finger brush and massage gums. The same formula may be used to gently cleanse ears; use a cotton swab to apply, but be careful not to go past the outer ear, or you may cause inflammation or infection or puncture the eardrum! Clean nostrils with a dilution of one drop standardized grapefruit extract to 8 oz. water or aloe vera juice, using a cotton swab or cotton ball to apply. Remember, keep away from eyes.

Water Purification (internal use): One drop in 8 oz. purified water, poured into drinking bowl. If this is too strong, add more water to your cat's taste. This also provides an antioxidant boost.

Chapter Five

Natural Remedies

DETOXIFICATION

AS YOU begin to make changes in your cat's diet and environment, and work with natural healing substances and holistic therapies—such as herbs, supplements, homeopathy, nosodes, flower essences, acupuncture, and aromatherapy—needed to remove the residue and effects of drugs, vaccines, anaesthesia, cortisone, chemicals, and any other infective agents, the animal will go through detoxification. In this natural part of the healing process, things often get worse before they get better; you experience a big step forward and then a small step backward, as health and balance are restored.

Paraphrased below, Dr. John Fudens's notes will give you an idea of what many of his patients have endured in the process of getting cleansed and well, a positive but sometimes painful experience. Dr. Fudens uses a detox program at the beginning of treating any animal, in order to clear the residues and harmful effects of all drugs, vaccines, chemicals, and other toxins that accumulate in the body from living in modern society and being exposed to the conventional medical treatment.

Again, one of the cornerstones of holistic medicine is the emphasis on symptoms being the immune system's way of expressing weakness and crying out for help. Absorption and accumulation of toxins damage the immune system, which must then work harder to protect the body and keep it functioning normally. Eventually, the immune system becomes over-whelmed, and various problems and symptoms develop that cause us to seek medical or veterinary treatment. In order to return the immune system to its normal, healthy state, the sub-stances that caused the difficulty must first be removed. This is what detoxification is all about.

Dr. Fudens tailors his detox program to the individual being treated. Each instance of previous contamination and accumula-tion of toxins is addressed as the immune system is repaired. Through the use of all-natural therapies such as diet, supple-ments, homeopathy, herbs, and glandular extracts, the various toxins are released by the cells and eliminated through the ears, eyes, skin, and respiratory and excretory systems. As a result, all or most of the symptoms suppressed by conventional drugs and treatment return.

But don't be surprised or alarmed if your cat's symptoms return or even worsen during detox. As long as her energy and vitality increase, the program is working. Whatever discharge or drainage you see is the result of the body cleansing itself and thus becoming healthier.

For example, a cat with a skin condition is treated with cor-tisone, which only suppresses the symptom and harms the immune system. When this cat undergoes detoxification, the residue of cortisone is removed from her system and the skin rash returns. However, if detoxification is continued, eventually the rash goes away by itself, as the actual imbalance that originally caused the rash, such as improper diet, has been corrected.

Sometimes additional holistic therapy is needed to continue to rebuild the immune system and body, directing special attention to certain areas. But holistic therapy works very poorly or not at all in a badly contaminated body. So the detox program must come first, in order for the animal to derive maximum benefit from further treatment.

Detoxification may be implemented in various degrees in order to maintain control of the process and prevent further damage to the body. To promote good health, a fast (see Fasting in chapter 4, "Nutrition") and/or detox program should be carried out periodically under strict holistic veterinary guidance.

As with all other healing therapies, this process must be done gently so as to avoid dehydration or undue stress. For example, detox that causes a softened stool (the consistency of mashed potatoes) is a gentle cleanse, whereas diarrhea (brown or yellow water) may cause the patient to become dehydrated. Stay in close touch with your practitioner so he can be sure your cat's electrolytes and fluids stay balanced.

But what if the cat is already suffering from something as serious as cancer? To most people cancer is synonymous with death, but it's actually a symptom of our toxic modern lifestyle. Dr. Fudens calls it a "disease of the mind, emotions, and spirit . . . expressed on the physical body level . . . the way the spirit deals with its problems.

"Carcinogens, stresses from virus, bacteria, pollutants, drugs, vaccinations, chemicals, radiation, and poor nutrition all play a part in creating the toxic and suppressed immune system that allows abnormal mutant cells to grow and organize into . . . cancers," Dr. Fudens continues. "But there also exists an ongoing aberrated negative force or energy in the family involving the pet and the person(s) the pet is bonded to. The negative force of energy is best described as a form of mental turmoil that leaves the person(s) paralyzed or helpless in controlling their lives, low self-esteem, anger, hostility, guilt, resentment toward life and others, lack of communication . . . feelings of mistrust and the lack of love and respect towards self and others. . . . Combined with the physical stresses and contaminants listed previously, our pet companions can very easily be overwhelmed . . . and thus a fertile breeding ground for cancer occurs.

"It is their unhealthy, unwell attitude towards life, on all levels, that allows a cancerous process to develop. This negative force is stronger than surgery, drugs, and radiation, which is why, for the most part, these treatments do not work. Holistic therapies work by changing the negative energy or force into positive energy, allowing the immune system to repair and rebuild itself. This includes addressing the mental turmoil in the pet's environment to reduce that stress and strain. Animals . . . help heal us. They take away the negative energy or force, absorb it, neutralize it or become overwhelmed by it and get sick. They can show us how sick we truly are. Our pets are mirrors as to what is going on in and around us in this so-called modern society."[1]

Dr. Fudens recommends, as do all the holistic practitioners with whom I consult, that we start by changing the diet from commercial foods and any junk food or snacks to one with fresh, natural, and nutritious ingredients. Feeding the fresh food diet to your cat is the beginning of a full detoxification program that may consist of one or several of the natural remedies and therapies described in this and the following chapters.

As I've said throughout, please don't attempt to treat your animal without the guidance of a holistic veterinarian. The health of our animals is very precious, and we owe it to them to treat them with competent medical attention.[2]

DEHYDRATION AND FLUID THERAPY

IF YOUR cat, which eats normally and drinks water occasionally, suddenly stops doing either, take his temperature to be sure he's not running a fever. The normal range for a cat is about 100° to 102°F rectally; Dr. Chambreau considers 101.5° normal, and anything higher a fever. Don't get concerned if the temperature is a bit below this but still above 100°. If your cat has a fever, call your holistic veterinarian or natural health practitioner as soon as possible.

Dehydration in a cat is extremely dangerous. You can check to see if your cat is becoming dehydrated by gently lifting the skin at the nape of the neck. If the skin doesn't slide back normally when you release it, the cat may need subcutaneous fluids (this condition may also occur with rapid weight loss or in elderly cats). Your veterinarian can teach you how to do this and sell you the equipment you need in order to administer the fluids yourself. Anitra Frazier's book *The New Natural Cat* contains an excellent description of the procedure. This simple therapy may save your cat's life; at the least, it's possibly the single most important thing you yourself can do to help him through an illness or a crisis (see chapter 4 for information on force-feeding.)

HERBS

THE SUBJECT of herbs, like so many of the healing therapies addressed in this book, cannot be covered in depth in one chapter. So I've tried to share with you some of the highlights of this fascinating field. Herbal medicine is very powerful. As with homeopathy, I don't recommend self-diagnosis, but rather, working with a holistic veterinarian or an herbal practitioner who can guide you responsibly.

I have many herb books in my personal library—among them, *The Complete Medicinal Herb: A Practical Guide to the Healing Properties of Herbs with More Than 250 Remedies for Common Ailments* by Penelope Ody, *Herbally Yours* by Penny Royal, and *Today's Herbal Health* by Louise Tenney[3]—and I use them often for reference. You may also work with companies that specialize in herbs, as I do. I like having a network of experts to consult with.

Ody gives us a wonderful historical look at the ancient Egyptians, Greeks, and Romans, and the Arab world. Influenced by the cultures that came before us, healing systems all over the world today embrace herbalism. The Indians embrace Aryuvedic medicine, which links the microcosm to the cosmos; they commonly include herbal remedies in their medical practices. Tibetans, whose medicine was under the control of the lamas and therefore closely linked to their religion, carefully coordinated the harvesting of herbs to coincide with helpful astrological influences. Swiss alchemist Paracelsus subscribed to the doctrine of signatures, which used the outward appearance of a plant to give healers an indication of what it could cure (nutmeg and walnuts were supposed to resemble the brain when they were cracked open, and thus were thought to improve mental abilities).

The Chinese view disease as a sign of disharmony within the whole person. Herbs have been crucial to Chinese medical practitioners since about 2,500 B.C.. Many of their formulas go back thousands of years, handed down through the generations in herbal dynasties. The five elements in Chinese herbal medicine—wood, water, metal, earth, and fire—form a network of relationships. Each element represents a season, a taste, an emotion, and parts of the body (for examples, fire represents summer, bitter taste, joy, and the heart, small intestine, tongue, and blood vessels). The forces of yang and yin (see chapter 8), and qi (or chi) complement the basic model of the five elements, yang and yin representing balance, and qi, vital energy.

Herbalists use the bark, berries, bulbs, flowers, fruit, gum, hips, hulls, leaves, roots, root bark, seeds, tops, and the whole plant—all according to tradition or recipe. It's important to remember that nearly all medicines are based on the active ingredient of some herb. The salicylic acid in aspirin was isolated from white willow bark, cortisone from yucca, digitalis from foxglove, and valium from valerian root.[4]

Herbs are often sold individually, but most work better in combination. There is a synergy that is created when they are combined. Most herbs shouldn't be given over long periods of time. I recommend that most medicinal herbs not be used longer than two to three weeks because the body seems to build up a tolerance and they cease to be effective.

Now let's examine the various forms used to administer herbs. Remember, always use purified or spring water when preparing your herbs.

Decoction. A tea made from roots and bark. Gently boil 1 tbsp. of cut herb or 1 tsp. powdered herb in 8 oz. water for 30 minutes, then let stand for 10 minutes.

Infusion. A tea made from leaves or blossoms. Boil 8 oz. water and remove from heat. Add 1 tsp. powdered herb, cover, and steep 10 minutes.[5]

Extract.[6] A liquid solvent into which a principal ingredient of herbal powders have been dissolved. Herbal powders are put through a process of cold extraction—cold percolation of the herbs with suitable solvents for each herb, such as alcohol, water, grape brandy, or apple cider vinegar, singly or in combination—which causes the herbs to render their nutrients. Extracts are in liquid form, which makes them easy to assimilate. These formulations are excellent for cats, as they may be further diluted in water when necessary.

Tincture. An extraction of herbs in vinegar or alcohol.

Oil of Herbs. An extraction of herbs in an oil base.

Fomentation. A cloth soaked in and wrung from a hot infusion or decoction, and applied to an affected area.

Poultice. A moist, hot herb pack applied topically (more effective than fomentation). When using fresh herbs, crush and bruise them. If powdered, mix with mineral water to form a thick paste. Spread on clean cloth and cover affected area. *Never reuse—always make a fresh one as they lose their potency.*

If you're a do-it-yourself kind of person, you may whip up many brews in your own kitchen. I don't pretend to be an herbalist, but look to others whom I can trust to properly harvest and prepare food-grade and medicinal herbs.[7]

In addition to fresh herbs and grasses (see "Nutrition"), I use extracts and tinctures, both internally and externally. I sometimes also employ *solarization* to prepare herbs, adding the contents of 1 herbal capsule to 2 to 4 ozs. of water, straining it through cheesecloth or a coffee filter, placing the liquid in a clear glass container outside in the sunshine for a few hours, then further diluting the mixture in water (one drop to 1 ounce of water), and shaking it. You may administer this dilution by eye dropper or mix it with a little food.

I've found the following mixture to be a powerful immune booster: 1 or 2 drops each of the herbal tinctures echinacea (an herb prescribed for blood purification and as a detoxifier to increase resistance to infection) and goldenseal, 1 or 2 drops of Kyolic garlic, and a few drops of water. When I suspect an upper respiratory problem, I give a drop of this mixture in an eye dropper three to four times daily, at different intervals from the homeopathic remedy that I may be using.

Herbal Combination Formulas

THE FOLLOWING sampling of combination herbal formulas includes the herbs most commonly used for various conditions that may trouble cats from time to time. These combinations have been suggested by several herbal experts, but are not intended as medical advice. Please consult your holistic practitioner prior to experimenting with any medicinal herbs. As always, proceed with caution. (See Resources for further information about brand-name supplements.)

You may find prepared combinations utilizing several of these herbs on the shelves of your health food store; however, remember that the dosage for cats is slightly less than that suggested for infants or very young children. I generally recommend using one drop of an extract in 1 oz. water. Use equal portions of the herbs you choose to combine, unless your practitioner suggests otherwise. There may be many more possibilities, so check with your holistic veterinarian or herbal consultant prior to administering the substances listed.

For allergies, upper respiratory problems, or sinusitis combine:

Goldenseal. Natural antibiotic-like herb for congested membranes; reduces swelling, helps clean system.

Lobelia. Stimulates, removes obstructions (acts as an expectorant), relieves spasms.

Capsicum. Relieves congestion, disinfects, acts synergistically to increase power of other herbs.

Parsley. Increases resistance to infection.

Marshmallow. Helps remove mucus from lungs.

Chaparral. Tones system.

Burdock. Purifies blood.

Helpful hints: Simplify diet (for example, for food allergies feed raw ground lamb, cooked barley flakes, zucchini); make changes weekly, one food at a time, and be certain to include vitamins A, B-complex, and C with bioflavinoids (rutin and hesperidin), zinc, bonemeal for calcium (1 to 2 tbsp. per pound of meat) in each meal. Help build up pollen immunity by including Kyolic aged garlic and tiny amounts of bee pollen. Use trace mineral products such as montmorillonite clay, Super Blue-Green Algae to boost the overall immune response, and include alfalfa sprouts regularly.

For lung problems:

Comfrey. Soothes respiratory system.

Fenugreek. Helps soften hardened mucus.

Helpful Hints: Give vitamins A, B-complex, B_6, C with bioflavinoids and rutin, D, and E, in a high-potency multivitamin/

mineral supplement including folic acid, which helps strengthen lungs. Barley water helps relieve bronchial spasms. Offer lots of Kyolic garlic, and honey (if your cats enjoy it, in herbal teas served lukewarm). Foods high in potassium—dandelion greens, celery, string beans, brussels sprouts, and even melons—are excellent choices. Run a warm-mist vaporizer with eucalyptus oil daily for two to three hours, but don't leave it unattended and make sure the air circulates freely. This treatment should be subtle, as cats' sense of smell is much more sensitive than ours. If eyes become irritated, discontinue eucalyptus oil.

For heart and circulation problems or fatigue combine:

Hawthorne. Strengthens heart.

Capsicum. Facilitates the action of other herbs on the heart.

Garlic. Natural antibiotic and immune stimulant.

Helpful hints: Give cold-pressed oils (including wheat germ oil), vitamin E at least once weekly (400 IU), and whole grains, which contain B-complex. Food process sweet potatoes, celery, carrots, and parsley, strain and include with raw meat and serve as a broth; excellent for fasting days.

For digestive upsets, irritable colon, or diarrhea combine:

Comfrey. Soothes lower bowel.

Marshmallow. Contains mucilage, which aids bowel.

Slippery elm. Soothes, draws out impurities, heals, acts as a buffer against irritation.

Ginger. Relieves gas, settles stomach.

Wild yam. Relaxes stomach muscles, acts as sedative on bowel.

Lobelia. Relaxant, removes obstructions from bowel, heals.

Helpful hints: Vitamins A, E, and B-complex, cold-pressed oils (including wheat germ oil), acidophilus, sweet potatoes, yogurt, comfrey, kelp, brown rice, sprouts, and whole wheat bread are all good dietary inclusions. For diarrhea, fast the cat for twenty-four hours to let the system rest and repair. Provide fresh purified water at all times, and consider fluid therapy, as cats become dehydrated rapidly when dealing with diarrhea. Administer fluids with an oral syringe or have your veterinarian administer subcutaneous fluids (my veterinarian taught me how to do this myself and I purchased the necessary equipment from him). I keep Pedialyte on hand to use instead of or mixed with purified water 50/50. Return to solid food when diarrhea stops, but make it simple (raw sterilized chicken, vegetables, and grains) for a day or so. Follow basic fresh food recipe (see page 70, in chapter 4, "Nutrition") but puree in your blender.

For blood purifying, cleansing, eczema, ringworm, or cancer combine:

Pau d'arco. Natural antibiotic, antifungal.

Licorice. Supplies energy, natural expectorant.

Red Clover. Tonic.

Sarsaparilla. Cleanses, stimulates body defenses.

Cascara sagrada. Effective laxative.

Oregon grape. Tonic for all glands.

Chaparral. Deep cleansing, fights bacteria.

Buckthorn. Calms gastrointestinal tract.

Prickly ash. Increases circulation.

Peach. Contains healing properties.

Stillingia. Removes toxic waste.

Helpful hints: Be sure food is fresh. Millet, buckwheat and barley are excellent grains. Give sprouts and sprout supplements such as Biogenetics Bioguard or Vitality and Feline Balance twice daily. Full vitamin/mineral supplements (MinerAll Plus), as well as

Pycnogenol (^{1}/$_2$ to one 20 mg tablet per pound of body weight daily) and 400 units vitamin E once weekly. Lecithin, kelp, parsley, carrots, and celery, as well as lots of Kyolic garlic, chard, beet greens. It is imperative to work with a holistic practitioner for cancer cases. Many recommend kombucha tea for its cleansing action (see Supplements section in chapter 4, "Nutrition").

For worms and other parasites combine:

Pumpkin Seeds. Expels tapeworms.

Garlic. Makes the digestive tract inhospitable to parasites.

Black Walnut. Oxygenates blood to kill parasites.

Helpful Hints: Once again, feed the fresh food diet, including raw or cooked pumpkin (food processed to a mulch), which will greatly help expel worms. Garlic is antibiotic in its effect, and fresh raw vegetables keep the colon healthy, creating an environment unfriendly to parasites. Be sure to keep environment free of fleas, through which cats may contract tapeworms. A clean, healthy natural diet is the kind of preventive medicine I like best. Check with your holistic veterinarian regarding treatment for parasites. Dr. Richard Pitcairn has several natural ways to go about this.

For liver problems combine:

Red beet. Nutritious for liver.

Dandelion. Stimulates liver.

Parsley. Cleans out toxic waste.

Horsetail. Builds, tones body.

Liverwort. Helps heal damaged liver.

Birch. Helps cleanse blood.

Lobelia. Removes obstructions from body.

Blessed thistle. General tonic to system.

Angelica. Helps eliminate toxins in liver and spleen.

Chamomile. Helps cleanse toxins from liver.

Gentian. Stimulates liver.

Goldenrod. Stimulates circulation. **Or instead combine:**

Barberry. Causes bile to flow more freely.

Ginger. Stimulant.

Cramp bark. Good for congestion and hardening of liver.

Fennel. Helps move waste material out of body.

Peppermint. Cleans and strengthens entire body.

Wild yam. Good for hardening and blockages of liver.

Catnip. Strengthens liver and gall bladder.

Helpful Hints: Give vitamins A, B-complex, B_6, B_{12}, C, D, E, and K, as well as magnesium, zinc, sulphur, choline, inositol, methionine, and Pycnogenol. Vegetables—including cauliflower and collards with $1/2$ tsp. nutmeg—are extremely important. Try dandelion tea mixed into food, along with watercress and parsley. Avoid eggs, cream, butter, and all cooked oils and fats (cooked meat is greasy, so I recommend using only fresh raw meat; see chapter 4, "Nutrition").

For kidney, bladder, or urinary tract problems combine:

Goldenseal. Helps kidneys eliminate toxins.

Juniper. Antiseptic to kidneys.

Uva Ursi. Strengthens urinary tract.

Parsley. Nutritional to kidneys.

Ginger. Cleanses kidneys.

Marshmallow. Soothing to urinary tract.

Lobelia. Helps clear obstructions.

Helpful hints: Lecithin and vitamin E help purify kidneys. Some cats enjoy melons, such as watermelon or cantaloupe. Feed watercress, asparagus, celery, and parsley. Include zinc and high potency vitamin/mineral supplements, antioxidants, and Pycnogenol.

For strengthening, stimulating, and cleansing the glands combine:

Kelp. Contains iodine, which strengthens glands.

Dandelion. Stimulates glands, increases activity of liver.

Alfalfa. Increases glandular secretions. **Or instead combine:**

Lobelia. Removes obstructions in system.

Mullein. Calms nerves.

Helpful hints: Glandular supplements are also helpful; check with a holistic veterinarian or feline nutritionist for specific suggestions. Feed raw meats and organ meats (liver, kidneys, heart—one part organ to five parts muscle), alfalfa sprouts, avocado, broccoli, parsley, yams, raw nuts and nut butters (almond), cold-pressed olive oil, rye, seeds (pumpkin, sunflower, sesame), brown rice, oatmeal, raisins, as well as high-potency vitamin/mineral supplements, including antioxidants, vitamin E, zinc, and Pycnogenol.

For thyroid and weight problems combine:

Irish moss. Purifies, strengthens cellular structure.

Kelp. Promotes glandular health.

Parsley. Increases resistance.

Watercress. Acts as tonic.

Helpful Hints: Give raw eggs (treated with standardized grapefruit extract; for sterilization technique, see How to Prevent Contamination and Spoilage in chapter 4, "Nutrition"). Iodine is a trace mineral known to be beneficial to the thyroid, and pumpkin and sunflower seeds, sprouts, and yogurt are helpful too, but give yogurt only if your cat tolerates dairy products. Make sure your cat gets lots of exercise.

For nervous disorders combine:

Black cohosh. Is a relaxant.

Capsicum. Helps other herbs get to parts of body that need assistance.

Valerian. Relaxes nerves.

Hops. Contains B vitamins for nerves.

Passionflower. Combines well with valerian.

Chamomile. Calms and soothes.

Helpful hints: Feed whole grains, which are rich in B vitamins; don't forget buckwheat, barley, and millet. Fenugreek and chamomile tea are soothing. Brussels sprouts and cauliflower are excellent. Be sure to supplement diet regularly with trace minerals, such as in MinerAll Plus or AniMinerals; put a few drops in cat's water.

For bone healing combine:

Comfrey. Heals wounds, bones, entire system.

Goldenseal. Natural antibiotic with healing powers, contains vitamins and minerals.

Slippery elm. Draws out impurities.

Aloe vera (unpreserved).[8] Natural detoxifier, removes toxic matter from body, heals and protects.

Helpful hints: Kelp, broccoli, sprouted grains, vegetables high in calcium (such as kale, parsley), seeds (sunflower seeds and almonds are excellent) added to grain mixture. Vitamins A, B-complex, C with bioflavinoids, D, and E, bonemeal, and zinc all aid in healing bones. Also suggested for teeth and calcium deficiency are comfrey, horsetail, oat straw, and lobelia. Include Pycnogenol daily.

For arthritis or inflammation of the joints combine:

Bromelain. Reduces swelling, inflammation.

Yucca. Precursor to synthetic cortisone.

Comfrey. Cleans, purifies system.

Alfalfa. Contains alkaloid for pain, nutrients for body strength.

Black cohosh. Relieves pain, irritation, acid condition of blood.

Yarrow. Cleans blood, helps regulate liver.

Capsicum. Catalyst for other herbs.

Chaparral. Dissolves uric acid.

Lobelia. Relaxant.

Burdock. Reduces swelling.

Centaury. Good for muscular rheumatism.

Helpful hints: Emphasize raw chicken and turkey in diet. The fiber in whole grains helps cats keep from getting constipated. Add chlorophyll extract to food or drinking water, just enough to make water light green. Use a pinch of fresh parsley in food. Include lots of sprouts, and be sure wheatgrass is always available to nibble on. Vitamin C is a must in each meal, at least 1 tsp. of Bio-C (1,000 mg., plus 500 mg. of bioflavinoids), as well as a B-complex supplement in liquid or capsule form (see Supplements, page 95). For vitamin A, feed raw liver or cod liver oil occasionally (liver no more than once a week). Consider a weekly fast (see Fasting in chapter 4, "Nutrition") on raw meat broth and pure water. Be sure to exercise your cat.

For skin and coat problems combine:

Alfalfa. Contains trace minerals, which benefit skin and coat.

Aloe vera. Contains allantoin, which has healing properties.

Burdock. Good for burns and wounds.

Chaparral. For sores and wounds.

Goldenseal. Helps stop itching.

Helpful hints: The fresh food diet (see chapter 4, "Nutrition") is the best approach to improving skin and coat. Cold-pressed oils, including wheat germ, cod liver (occasionally), and flaxseed oil, are excellent, as well as vitamin E once a week (400 IU).

Garlic taken internally helps heal all skin sores. Run a humidifier to moisten dry air. Bathe (therapeutic bath in gentle herbal shampoo, such as Woolly 'n Wild's Pure Comfort aloe vera juice, followed by their Comfort Spray) and brush cat regularly. If your cat is very uncomfortable, spray aloe vera juice on him or dab the hot spots with cotton saturated with aloe vera juice. Try touch and massage therapy (see chapter 6, "Hands-on Healing").

For eye problems combine:

Goldenseal. Natural antibiotic.

Bayberry. High in vitamin C.

Eyebright. Strengthens immunity to eye complaints.

Helpful hints: Bathe eyes in sterile saline solution (or to 1 oz. saline, add one drop eyebright). Also use homeopathic *Similasan*, Formula 1 for irritation and Formula 2 for allergies. Vegetables good for strengthening eyes are leeks, broccoli, cabbage, carrots, turnips, collards, and watercress. Pycnogenol has also proved helpful for conditions of the eyes. Use Silverloid™ colloidal silver, one drop in each eye, two to three times daily for problems such as conjunctivitis.

For birthing, pregnancy, estrus (heat cycles) combine:

Red raspberry. Strengthens uterus, regulates uterus during delivery, prevents hemorrhage, reduces false labor pains.

Blessed thistle. Helps promote flow of milk, eliminates mucus congestion.

False unicorn. Strengthens ovaries, overall tonic for system, rich in trace minerals.

Black cohosh. Helps in uterine disorders.

Pennyroyal. Useful just before delivery.

Hops. Reduces problems associated with heat cycles, can reduce male sexual tension.

Helpful hints: Sprinkle a pinch of hops over food to reduce anxiety in both male and female breeding cats. Increase bone-meal from 1 or 2 tbsp. to 3 or 4 tbsp. per pound of meat. Omit aloe vera juice from fresh food recipe during first trimester of pregnancy. Include MinerAll Plus and Bio-C daily. Add contents of one red raspberry capsule to each meal in last trimester of pregnancy. Keep *caulophyllum* 30C (homeopathic) on hand for difficult labor (administer once weekly in last three weeks of pregnancy if your practitioner agrees). Urtica urens 30C can help bring on milk, if needed. Female cats usually love a little yogurt during pregnancy. Be sure all is ready for queen by sixty-first day. Feed her as often as she wants, and give her lots of love and support. Try not to let her get too rambunctious prior to birthing. During labor, give caulophyllum 30C every 15 to 30 minutes to keep contractions strong. Give one dose after last kitten to help cleanse after birth.

For fasting combine:

Raw meat broth and vegetable broth with a pinch each of one or more of the following herbs as seasonings:

Licorice. Good for strength and quick energy, nourishes glands, inhibits growth of harmful viruses.

Hawthorne. Burns up excess fat, strengthens heart, helps insomnia, calms nervous system.

Fennel. Internal anesthetic, relieves gas, cramps, and mucus accumulation.

Beet. Stimulates and cleans liver, strengthens system.

Helpful hints: Fasting is extremely cleansing, but is not intended for the chronically ill, older cats, or young kittens. Don't eat or cook in front of the cat—fast with them.[9] Provide pure water and broth at intervals throughout the day. Begin by feeding breakfast, substituting broth for dinner, then feeding a simple breakfast the following morning. Broth may be fed by syringe.

I have included here only some of the many herbs and combinations used in healing. Again, you may explore one of the books recommended in this chapter or try some of the many preparations available at your health food store. Talk to the salespeople—they're usually a wellspring of information.

Again, a word of warning. Medicinal herbs are exactly that—medicine. Please consult and work closely with a holistic veterinarian, someone who treats the whole animal. Many of the associations listed in the Resources section will help you find practitioners in your area or who will work with you by phone.

HOMEOPATHY

DEEPAK CHOPRA, M.D., tells us that "quantum healing" is the ability of one mode of consciousness (the mind) to spontaneously correct the mistakes of another (the body).[10] When in crisis, the human body, as well as that of the feline, speaks to us through its symptomatic picture.

Allopathic, or conventional, medicine applies the Law of Opposites to the treatment of disease: the medicine is different from the disease. In other words, the medication prescribed by the doctor or veterinarian acts against the patient's symptoms (as described by such names as *anti*biotic, *anti-inflammatory*, and so on). Allopathic drugs act in such a way that they suppress symptoms, but in themselves, they don't necessarily cure disease. The bodies of both humans and animals take action to heal themselves.

Homeopathy uses exactly the opposite approach, using remedies which are based on the Law of Similars. When used appropriately, homeopathy works with the body, not against it, promoting actual cure, not suppressing symptoms. Symptoms are the banners of our immune system, manifestations of our attempt to heal ourselves, so we need to honor them, not rush to eradicate them. They are our windows to the internal process. Homeopathic remedies act in the same way as the natural defense reactions of the body. The remedy stimulates the immune system, enabling it to complete the job it was already trying to do. Homeopathy may also aid in ameliorating behavior problems (such as poor litter box habits, scratching, spraying, or fighting).

For me, homeopathy is a wonderful method for treating feline imbalances because cats are subtle creatures that live in the moment. When they don't feel well, they often hide or don't wish to be fussed with. Homeopathic remedies are easy to administer, and they give the body a gentle yet powerful nudge to help heal itself.

After numerous visits to your allopathic veterinarian, when your cat has received vaccinations for every conceivable disease, and antibiotics and steroids for every infection or skin irritation, you may begin to explore alternative medical treatment. Through homeopathy, which most conventional veterinarians know nothing about, a real cure to most chronic diseases can be achieved where allopathic medicine provides only a quick, and often temporary, fix.

If your cat has undergone long-term allopathic drug therapy, homeopathy may not work immediately, with persistence it may help restore the cat's health in many difficult cases where conventional veterinarians might recommend euthanasia. It's at such traumatic times that homeopathic veterinarians are asked to perform miracles, and many have done exactly that. When very ill animals are treated with homeopathy, they may not be cured, or even palliated; but in the process of attempting a cure, they may feel better for a while and will usually die on their own, without any need for euthanasia. However, you don't have to wait until hope is all but lost—take your cat to a homeopathic veterinarian now.

The History of Homeopathy

HOMEOPATHY was developed by Samuel Hahnemann in the late eighteenth century. At that time, people were being treated with poisonous substances to "get the bad out of them" by making them vomit, have diarrhea, sweat, salivate, and bleed. Many died from these treatments.

Hahnemann felt such practices were barbaric and stopped practicing medicine. While making a living translating books, he came across William Cullen's write-up on the action of *Cinchona officinalis*, the herb used to make quinine for the treatment of malaria. Hahnemann disagreed with Cullen's conclusions and, to prove his point, took a small amount of the bark himself. He developed symptoms of malaria lasting a few hours. Hahnemann repeated the experiment several times, each time developing symptoms that went away by the next day. (He was a healthy man to start with, or this wouldn't have worked).

From this research Hahnemann developed the Law of Similars, a concept that had been considered since ancient times by such men of science as Galen, Hippocrates, and especially Paracelsus. When an individual (human or animal) is made ill in a particular way by being exposed to a substance, that individual may also be cured by being treated with the same substance.

For example, bee venom (*Apis mellifica*) causes pinkish-red swelling in healthy individuals. Symptoms are often of sudden onset, are accompanied by itching and burning, and are relieved by the application of cold water. At the same time, the person isn't thirsty, may be restless, and may be better if he doesn't lie down. In homeopathic dilutions, bee venom improves or cures itchy, burning eruptions that come on suddenly and are relieved by cold compresses, especially when the individual is less thirsty than usual.

The eruption doesn't have to have been caused by a bee sting in order for bee venom to be effective as a remedy. It may have been caused by sunburn, hypersensitivity to food, vaccinations, or drugs. As well, this remedy is often prescribed for burning during urination and cystitis (bladder inflammation).

Hahnemann believed that the vital forces of the body respond to the energy of the remedy. The Theory of Vitalism, which states that our spirit (or soul) creates the physical substance of our bodies—predates our current biochemical understanding of life by thousands of years. Therapeutic touch and the spiritual aspects of disease and healing aren't new or foreign territory to even the most conservative doctors of internal medicine.

No one has yet been able to explain how homeopathy works, though Hahnemann did *provings* for each of the more than two thousand remedies used with humans (fewer than fifty are generally given to cats), that is, he gave each remedy to healthy people and meticulously recorded every change they underwent. Animal lovers will appreciate that Hahnemann did all his testing and research on human subjects only. However, homeopathic veterinarians have found that the symptoms the remedies produced in people correspond to symptoms in all types of animals, so our cats may now reap the benefits of this work.

How a Disease Runs Its Course

IN HOMEOPATHY, a cure is obtained by giving the substance whose experimental symptoms in healthy individuals are most similar to the patient's own symptoms. Since this therapy is based on an individual's total symptomatic picture, you must learn the characteristics of each remedy as well as observe carefully all the symptoms your cat is now exhibiting and has exhibited in the past, as well as her general characteristics. For example: First you sense an energetic imbalance. Your cat seems to be getting sick; there aren't any symptoms, but you just know something's starting.

Then there are functional changes. For instance, she's going frequently to the litter box, but there's no straining and the urinalysis is normal. If the disturbance is treated right away, even severe symptoms may resolve quickly or be avoided; however, your conventional veterinarian may not be able to pinpoint the problem.[11]

If the disturbance remains untreated, you'll see inflammatory changes; the body trying its hardest to rebalance itself. At this stage the cat is sick—fever, redness, swellings. Any conventional veterinarian will have some "anti" medications to treat a patient in this condition.

Finally, the body tries to ward off the problem by moving into pathology: thickened bladder wall; bladder stones; thick, hairless skin; distorted nails; fluid accumulation in abdomen or chest; thickened lung or bronchial tissues; and so on. Once this stage has been reached, it takes longer to effect a cure, and the cat must go back through the stages: inflammatory, functional, and energetic imbalance. This is why it often looks as if the cat is getting worse before it gets better.

Working with Homeopathy

A CURE in homeopathy is more than just making the symptoms go away, which can happen with many kinds of treatments. Rather, it's when the symptoms go away and stay away permanently; the cat feels, and is, healthy in every respect (none of the symptoms of latent disease listed earlier). She may still get minor ailments, but she recovers from them with very little or no treatment. When a cat is given an appropriate remedy, you'll often see an immediate mental and emotional response of contentment, even though the final "physical" cure may take much longer. A very rough rule of thumb is that it takes one month to heal for every year of illness.

It's important to understand that homeopathy is not herbal medicine. Rather, it utilizes medicines derived from plant, mineral, and animal sources. Just because a medicine is derived from plants doesn't mean it shouldn't be handled with caution. We must drop the stereotypical notion that if synthetic medicine is dangerous, plant-based medicine is mild in its action. Since homeopathy is powerful enough to cure, it's also powerful enough to do harm.

It's difficult for the newcomer to homeopathy to fully grasp the idea that selecting a remedy in haste could cause an aggravation or palliate the symptoms (suppress them, as allopathic drugs do). If you work this way, you aren't practicing traditional homeopathy, or even good holistic medicine.

It's always best to work with a homeopathic practitioner, as selecting the right remedy in the right potency and waiting before represcribing is not as easy as it might seem. I'm now able to treat simple things myself, but I always consult with my practitioner to be sure I'm on the right track before I administer a homeopathic remedy. You can't lose by deferring to those with more experience.

However, beware—not every homeopath is competent. Regardless of which practitioner or healing modality you choose, you must always be responsible for observing what's happening to your animal companion. You'll learn in this chapter how to tell if your cat is responding well to your practitioner's prescriptions. I recommend that, when you begin to treat your cat homeopathically, you keep a journal, noting observations and remedies along with the date, time of day, and even weather conditions or related stress. The homeopath lists all symptoms present now and all that have occurred in the past, as well as all characteristics that make the individual special and unique. The homeopath asks about every body system and what makes each symptom better or worse. He looks for changes in symptom pictures and tries to discover a cause for the changes (for example, symptoms started after the cat's human companions divorced).

In prescribing homeopathic remedies, the smallest things are important. How does your cat react to situations, people, other animals, noise, and other stimuli? Does she seek warmth under your covers or lie on top of the bed? Does she catch the breeze in a window, lie on the carpet or cool, hard surfaces? How much water does she drink? Does she like dry, soft, or soupy foods? How does she interact with other cats in the house? Is she the boss or the low cat on the totem pole?

Once the homeopath has this complete picture, a list is made of characteristic symptoms (those symptoms that aren't normally associated with the disease). For example, everyone with the flu feels tired and achy, but not everyone gets better from being consoled, worse from exposure to an open window, or better from having only cold drinks. These uniquenesses are what homeopaths look for.

Then the homeopath looks up the most important and unique symptoms (and this takes experienced judgment) in a *repertory* (such as by Kent, Kunzli, or Murphy, to name but a few of the most often used repertories). The repertory lists millions of symptoms, along with recommended remedies known to help each symptom. By cross-referencing the important symptoms, the homeopath comes up with the two to five best potential remedies.

Then he studies a *materia medica* (a book containing in-depth descriptions of the remedies) to compare his choices. *Materia medica* range from very small books (by Boericke, MacLeod, Day, and many others), in which the authors have put down their interpretation of how the remedies act, to multivolume versions (by authors such as Hering, Clarke, Allen, and Hahnemann) that list the specific symptoms that occurred in the provings. The more comprehensive *materia medica* are more useful in the treatment of animals.

I find my knowledge of the astrological signs helps me with the use of homeopathy, as personality traits are extremely important in selecting the appropriate remedy. Please refer to chapter 8, "Astromedicine for Your Cat," for further information on the astromedical approach.[12]

References and Materials

I HAVE on hand George Macleod's *Cats: Homeopathic Remedies,* as well as his *Veterinary Materia Medica and Clinical Repertory; Your Healthy Cat* by H. G. Wolff; *The Homeopathic Treatment of Small Animals—Principles & Practice* by Christopher E. Day; *The Science Of Homeopathy* by George Vithoulkas; Boericke's *Materia Medica and Repertory;* and repertories by Kunzli, Murphy, and Kent. *The Family Guide to Homeopathy* by Alain Horvilleur, M.D., helps me understand the role of homeopathy in the treatment of human problems.

Christina Chambreau, D.V.M., cautions that MacLeod's and Wolff's books are organized from an allopathic standpoint (that is, they advise on the best remedies to treat particular problems or diseases), so if you use their books, you'll have trouble standing back and treating your animal holistically. Christopher Day, on the other hand, takes a deep treatment approach in his book.

Dr. Pitcairn has many tapes on homeopathy, which are available through his office, and there are tapes available through the annual conferences of the American Holistic Veterinary Medical Association (AHVMA) and the National Center for Homeopathy (NCH). Look through the publications list in the Resource section for more suggested reading.

Homeopathic kits for home use are available, which contain remedies for common symptoms. Dr. Chambreau also teaches a wonderful veterinary homeopathy course and has made a video entitled "Homeopathic First Aid for Pets," in which she guides people new to homeopathy in the use of six common remedies for simple problems. She reminds us, however, that it's best to create health by preventive homeopathic care. Moreover, homeopathy may not be able to cure your cat if you continue to vaccinate and to feed a poor diet.

Homeopathics can be difficult to find in the United States, unlike in Europe, where homeopathic pharmacies seem to out-number conventional drugstores. However, more and more places (even regular pharmacies) are beginning to carry homeo-pathic remedies, as the alternative health care movement sweeps the country. Always beware of combination remedies, however. See the Resources section at the back of this book for more information about books, tapes, courses, and supplies.[13]

Cure, Palliation, and Suppression

AS DR. CHAMBREAU explains, there are four possible outcomes of any treatment—complete cure, partial cure, palliation, and suppression—whether you use allopathic medicine, homeopathy, herbs, acupuncture, or any other intervention. These outcomes are described below.

When the correct curative homeopathic remedy is given, the energy field of the body immediately starts to react to the medicine (this is why it's best to give single doses even of the lower potencies). At first we see the primary response (the drug response) to the remedy, which may be an overall feeling better and/or lessening of symptoms, or perhaps we can't discern any changes, but we get a sense that, energetically, things are better.

Then, three to five days after the remedy has been given, if the cat has been sick for a while or has been treated over the years—or only minutes to hours with more superficial or newly contracted diseases—we see a reaction, possibly the current symptoms getting worse, older symptoms returning, new symp-toms arising. This is a good sign, the energy of the body starting to heal itself. One clue that this is a good aggravation—and not just a response to a wrong remedy—is that, even given these symptoms, we feel the cat is better, we're picking up on her improving energy.

At this point, we must wait and not use another homeopathic remedy. We can make our cats more comfortable with other gentle treatments, such as massage, herbs, flower remedies, and Reiki, but not homeopathy, acupuncture, or conventional medicines. Certain herbs, such as mint and other strongly aromatic substances, can counteract homeopathy. Check with your homeopath for any contraindications of other substances.

Finally, the symptoms slowly start lessening. Again, the length of time needed for a cure is proportional to the depth of an illness and the amount of prior inappropriate treatment received (whether allopathic, homeopathic, herbal, or other). Cures take time and patience, and often requires several remedies over years' time. It's best to start with the parents and then treat the offspring deeply. Finally, in three to four generations (with fresh food and no vaccines, of course), we have very healthy cats that never need treating.

The second outcome is toward a cure, but not all the way there yet.

The third outcome, a very common one, is that the symptoms go away almost immediately (even if they've been present or recurring for years). This makes us happy because the cat has, for instance, stopped itching or stopped crying when urinating. But then the symptoms come back. So we think, okay, let's give another dose of that remedy or herb, or drug—and again the symptoms go away. But then they return, so we try another remedy or drug. And on and on.

This is palliation, the need to keep giving something to keep the symptoms away. The cat just keeps getting sicker, at the deeper, energetic level. Work with your homeopathic practitioner to be sure this is not happening.

The fourth outcome is suppression. Again, we're relieved when the symptoms go away immediately with treatment, in this scenario they don't reappear. But we notice that the cat is less friendly or more aggressive, or a few months later he comes down with hepatitis or another more serious disease. The symptoms have gone, but the cat has gotten sick at a deeper level. It's like plugging the outlet of a volcano: it gets hotter and hotter inside until it explodes at a deeper, more dangerous level.

Modern (allopathic) medicines are very good at palliating and suppressing. Homeopathy (as well as other natural therapies) may produce any of these outcomes—curing (complete or partial), palliating, and suppressing—so you must be the judge of how your cat is responding to the remedy. If you feel that symptoms are going away too fast (as mentioned, a minimum of one month is needed for each year of disease) or recurring too often, talk to your homeopath. If she can't convince you that your cat is moving toward a cure, get a second opinion.

Dr. Chambreau shared the following case with me: "A nine-year-old cat named Baby had been getting steroid injections every six weeks to keep her symptoms of feline endocrine alopecia [licking all the hair off her belly, creating big, raw, open areas there] from getting worse. Her owner stopped the vaccinations, started all five of her cats on a raw diet [it took one year to switch completely], and, with homeopathic remedies, Baby was cured. It took nine months of her belly being worse than ever, and four or five different remedies given progressively before she stopped the licking. That was five years ago. She has never licked her belly again. I have never had to treat her for anything else. She self-cured an upper respiratory problem and a fever/lethargy problem. She is now fourteen years old and acts like a five-year-old."[14]

My Celina also had a severe alopecia problem, which occurred after a vaccination. At the site of her vaccine (the nape of her neck), she suddenly displayed a small, round bald patch. She seemed perfectly normal except that, out of the blue, she'd twitch or jerk, and then stop and lick herself and twitch some more. I treated the irritation topically and administered homeopathic remedies according to her symptoms, but she continued to lick herself until she was bare all across her chest and shoulders. Her temperature was normal. She ate, played, and slept well.

The symptom that led my practitioner to her remedy was the twitching, something like St. Vitus' dance, that Celina would break into. She got worse before she got better. I continued to treat her topically with colloidal silver and aloe vera juice laced with a drop of standardized grapefruit extract. Over time, the hair grew back, and she was cured. Now her coat is beautiful, and she no longer does that twitchy little dance.

Homeopathy is tailored specifically to each individual. If one remedy doesn't produce the cure after an appropriate period, your homeopathic practitioner may try another one. Often, as I've said, an aggravation occurs (the crisis point of the disease), and this is extremely trying, of course, to both us and our cats. Patience is the keynote. We're so used to the quick fix we get from drugs.

It was extremely difficult for me to see my first litter of kittens, which were vaccinated with the typical feline series (rhino, calici, distemper), come down with the very upper respiratory disease from which they were supposedly being protected. The impulse to rush them to the nearest emergency facility (where, inevitably, they were given more drugs), was overwhelming. The symptoms went away, only to return later on in much more severe form. I battled long and hard to cure these babies holistically. We must learn to trust that our bodies have the ability to heal themselves if we work with them.

Again, a word of caution. I don't advocate amateur diagnosis. A responsible practitioner should always be consulted. Remember, many symptoms require immediate attention by a qualified emergency veterinarian. It's far better to be safe than sorry. However, you have every right to explain to an allopathic veterinarian that you're working with a homeopathic veterinary practitioner who needs to be consulted prior to (or as soon as possible after) any drug therapy or medical procedure.

Dr. Chambreau says emergency allopathic care is rarely a problem if you call your holistic practitioner as soon as possible. If your cat develops a life-threatening asthma attack on Saturday, steroids may be life-saving, a reasonable intervention until you can reach your homeopath on Monday. But it could be a problem if you panic during a healing crisis with a cat already under homeopathic care, and get allopathic treatment or give a homeopathic remedy on your own. It is difficult to know what requires emergency treatment and what is an acceptable level of crisis reaction. Only you can make that decision.

Many caring conventional veterinarians will welcome your search for another way to heal your cat. Others may be threatened by new approaches, or feel they're not appropriate. Just be honest and, if you can, enroll them as your partner in healing.

Dr. Chambreau suggests telling your allopathic veterinarian that you value and need their expertise in examination and diagnosis, but don't want them to administer drugs or vaccinations. Dr. Chambreau doesn't recommend using homeopathic remedies along with allopathic drugs, but feels that all other therapies in this book may be used compatibly until you find a homeopathic practitioner.[15]

How Homeopathic Remedies Are Prepared and How They Work

ORIGINALLY, though Samuel Hahnemann gave small amounts of his remedies in their crude form to his patients, they got very sick before they were cured. He decided to dilute the remedies, in order to see if they'd be gentler in their action. Indeed, the dilutions worked just as curatively, but didn't cause such severe aggravations. Homeopaths following Hahnemann diluted the remedies further, finding appropriate dilutions for each case. James Kent taught that the simillimum (curative medicine) is the right remedy at the right potency. This is the concept of the minimal dose.

Today homeopathic remedies are prepared according to specific guidelines found in the *Homeopathic Pharmacopoeia of the United States,* which follow the instructions given by Hahnemann in his book *The Organon.*[16] If possible, an alcoholic tincture is made (some substances are not soluble in alcohol and are prepared differently). Dilution and succussion (shaking) of the tincture produce a *potentized* homeopathic remedy.

The following notation is used to denote the level of dilution: One drop of the mother tincture diluted with nine drops of alcohol (or other solvent) creates a potency of *1X* (as in *X,* the Roman numeral for ten). Similarly, 1 drop of the mother tincture diluted with 99 drops of alcohol creates a potency of 1C (as in *C*, the Roman numeral for 100); dilution with 999 drops creates a potency of 1M (as in *M*, the Roman numeral for 1,000). Potencies range from 1C to MM (100,000C).

By the time a potency of 12C is reached, the dilution is beyond Avogadro's number (6.023×10^{23}) which in physical chemistry means that not one molecule of the original substance remains in the dilution; therefore, nothing poisonous or toxic is left, no matter what the remedy has been made from. For instance, the nosode Lyssin,[17] which I recommend giving after rabies vaccinations, is made from rabid dog saliva, but 30C dose is even more dilute than a 12C, so it contains not even a single molecule of the toxic saliva. Think of the remedy as if it contained the spirit, the energy or ghost, of the original substance.

It's important to know that, paradoxically, the more dilute the remedy, the more powerful it is. At the lower potencies you're dealing with a dilute solution of the physical substance, but as the potency increases, you're dealing with an increasingly strong energy of that substance. Thus, potencies lower than 30C can be given one to three times a day for a week or so. Higher potencies should only be given one time (except in emergencies), and then the cat needs to be given time to react to the remedy. This may take a week, or it may take six to twelve months. The remedy is only repeated when there is no change in symptoms for a few days to a few weeks, depending on their severity.

Homeopathic remedies are made from a wide variety of substances, from innocuous herbs such as chamomile to known poisons such as hemlock. But as mentioned, even the most toxic substance is safe to ingest in submolecular dilution. Poison ivy, agaricus, aloe, leopard's bane, arsenic, nightshade, blister beetle, oyster shell, Spanish fly, lava from Mount Heckla in Iceland, coral snake, flint, club moss, sulphur, cranberry, salt, aurum, rue, cuttle-fish ink, tissue from dogs with distemper, and tissue from tuber-cular lungs are among the many sources of these remedies.

Cell Salts (The Twelve Tissue Salts of Schuessler)

CELL SALTS are among the homeopathic remedies listed in *materia medicas*. Wilhelm Heinrich Schuessler, a nineteenth-century physician, physiological chemist, and physicist, saw that when the cells of the body were reduced to their basic elements, there were twelve integral salts. Thus, he deduced that illness reflected an imbalance of these twelve cell salts. He felt balance could be restored to the body using only these twelve remedies from among hundreds of homeopathics.[18]

Each of the twelve cell salts serves to stimulate the body in a certain way. They include:

Calcarea flourica (calcium fluoride)
Calcarea phosphorica (calcium phosphate)
Calcarea sulphurica (calcium sulfate)
Ferrum phosphoricum (iron phosphate)
Kali muriaticum (potassium chloride)
Kali phosphoricum (potassium phosphate)
Kali sulphuricum (potassium sulfate)
Magnesia phosphorica (magnesium phosphate)
Natrum muriaticum (sodium chloride)
Natrum phosphoricum (sodium phosphate)
Natrum sulphuricum (sodium sulfate)
Silicea (silica)

How to Select a Potency and Administer a Homeopathic Remedy

THE CHALLENGE facing homeopaths is not only the selection of the appropriate remedy, but the determination of the optimum potency from a wide range of possibilities. H. G. Wolff, D.V.M., recommends that you keep on hand a homeopathic kit (see Resources) for emergencies (6X dosage).[19] When a different potency is required, it may be purchased from a homeopathic pharmacy either in person or by mail, if a prescription isn't required (see Resources).

Dr. Wolff cautions that just reading a book does not make a homeopathic practitioner out of you. Homeopathy is more complex than you may at first think. So don't take chances with your precious cat's life. Join a homeopathy study group and be supported by your lay peers; if there isn't one in your area, consider starting one yourself. And always work with a practitioner well versed in small animal homeopathy, either in person or on the phone, to select the right remedy, potency, and schedule of administration.

Remember, homeopathics stimulate the immune response; if symptoms disappear, there is no need to repeat the remedy. If your cat curls up and takes a nap after her dosage, this is a good sign that the correct remedy has been chosen, says Dr. Wolff. When the illness is acute, you may administer two to three doses a day for several days; some remedies may be administered every hour for up to five or six hours.

Remedies are available in pellets, tablets, and granules. The dosage is the same for humans as for animals; the size of the animal isn't important:

1 dose = 1 tablet

or 5-10 granules (tiny, poppy-like seeds)

or 3 pellets (#20 or #35)

The potency selected and how frequently it's given is of primary importance. If your cat doesn't swallow a complete dose (i.e., exactly 3 pellets), don't worry, he'll still get the benefit. All vials of homeopathic remedies indicate a recommended quantity and frequency. Remember that this is a requirement of the Food and Drug Administration (FDA), rather than an absolute, so work with your homeopath to determine a proper schedule of dosage.

Though the FDA requires an expiration date on all pharmaceutical containers, homeopathic remedies don't seem to lose their effectiveness unless you store them improperly, so please don't throw remedies away if they've "expired." Remedies even a hundred years old have been used successfully! Just make sure to store your remedies in a special corner far from sunlight, heat, microwaves, and disinfecting agents. Also, strongly aromatic substances, such as perfumes, camphor, chamomile, mint, tea tree oil, coffee, garlic, and even powerful herbs such as goldenseal and echinacea may neutralize the effects of homeopathics and even antidote a homeopathic action if they are included in your cat's food.

As much as possible, try to avoid touching the remedy with your hands, as you may have the residue of chlorine (from tap water) or other strong substances on your skin, which will deactivate the remedy. Or you yourself may be susceptible to the remedy and accidentally absorb it.

Dr. Chambreau recommends that pellets not be pushed down the throat, as cats don't react well to this indignity. Instead, crush the pellet, tablet, or granules in a folded index card, then open the cat's mouth just enough to pour the powder in, using the folded card as a funnel. (Homeopathic remedies are administered orally because the mouth contains such a large number of nerve endings.)[20]

It's best that the cat not have a taste of food in his mouth when you administer a remedy, so if giving only one dose, before bedtime might be the best time. I usually give my cats their dosage upon arising, on an empty stomach (thirty minutes before a meal or one hour after is the general rule). Your practitioner may suggest that certain remedies be administered at specific times of the day for greater effectiveness (see Ideal Schedule chart, page 175).

If necessary, the remedy may be given in milk or cream, since that's the medium of the pellets, tablets, and granules. If you can't get your cat to take the remedy any other way, it's okay to put it in his food. As a last resort, mix it with some baby food chicken or raw hamburger. This isn't ideal, but it's better than not administering the dosage. However, if the remedy then doesn't work, you're left with the question of whether it was the wrong remedy or it was inactivated by the food.

I find it easier to dissolve the remedy in water and administer it with an eye dropper. You may make up a liquid remedy as follows: Add the prescribed number of pellets or tablets to 1 oz. distilled water in a sterile amber dosage bottle. Shake bottle vigorously 1 to 2 minutes, or until the remedy has dissolved completely.

Also available are tinctures such as calendula (marigold) or euphrasia (eyebright), which are recommended for eye inflammations and conjunctivitis and which should never be used undiluted. For eye baths start with 1 drop of tincture in 1 oz. boiled or distilled water in a sterile dropper bottle; if this is too strong, dilute it even further.

Anitra Frazier recommends shaking or tapping the bottle against your hand several times when diluting tinctures in water or saline.[21] I use ten seconds as my guideline for succussion (shaking). Remember to be very cautious about anything you administer to the eyes; it must be sterile.

I especially like euphrasia as an eyedrop; mix 1 drop into 1 oz. sterile saline solution. I use this to cleanse the nasal passages as well, as it helps cats suffering with nasal and sinus conditions smell their food or broth. For this purpose, I also like colloidal silver (see Supplements, in chapter 4, "Nutrition"), which I use prior to mealtime and as a cleansing and healing treatment. The homeopathic *Similisan* formulas are excellent as eyedrops as well (Formula 1 for red and irritated eyes, Formula 2 for allergies).

The following *materia medica* and minirepertory are for general purposes and information only. I don't advocate working without an experienced homeopathic practitioner. Remember that every remedy listed here may be used for many different conditions—again, homeopathy treats the whole individual, not the problem. Each being presents a different picture, so if your cat has an abscess, you'll need help from an expert to find the proper remedy. For example, if *Carbo vegetabilis, Aconite,* or *Hepar sulphuris* fits the patient's total symptomatic picture, they'll treat an abscess better than, say, *Silicea,* which doesn't fit the picture, even though *Silicea* is another remedy used for abscesses. See how tricky this is?

Materia Medica

THE FOLLOWING, in my personal experience, are excellent remedies to have on hand for emergencies or for convenience when teleconsulting with your homeopathic practitioner. Each remedy is listed by its full Latin name, although each also has an abbreviated name (for instance, *Aconitum napellus* is commonly referred to as *Aconite; Cinchona officionalis* is known as *China*, as it is the source of quinine).

I keep these remedies and many more on hand for my personal use as well as for my cats. I prefer the lower potencies (6X to 30C), and recommend starting low (6X) for chronic disease, and working up from there; acute disease may require higher potencies. Always consult your practitioner before administering remedies; for pregnant and lactating cats, it's wise to consult several holistic veterinarians.

I generally use a 30C potency unless otherwise indicated. You will note that I also recommend decreasing the dosage with improvement. During an acute stage or crisis you may need to repeat the dosage. When something is chronic, sometimes one dosage will be sufficient.

Aconitum napellus. For early stages of feverish conditions of sudden onset associated with chills: high temperature, dry skin, anxiety, intense thirst, agitation. Ailments due to fear or fright. Prior to surgery. Dosage: 3 pellets every 1–2 hours; decrease frequency with improvement.

Allium cepa. For what appears to be a head cold or upper-respiratory infection with acrid, watery nasal discharge, mild tearing of the eyes, and sneezing. Symptoms producing laryngeal discomfort; cat may even sound hoarse. Dosage: 3 pellets every 1–2 hours; decrease frequency with improvement.

Alumina. For conditions affecting mucous membranes. Constipation with inertia of the rectum. Dryness (skin, nose, cough, and so on) is the characteristic of this remedy. Dosage: 3 pellets twice a day.

Antimonium crudum. Produces strong action on stomach and skin, producing symptoms that are aggravated by heat. Also for nausea and vomiting after excess intake of food with white tongue. Dosage: 3 pellets 3 times a day.

Antimonium tartaricum. For respiratory discomfort and excess mucus. There could be a rattling in the chest and/or shortness of breath, and an accumulation of mucus in the chest, associated with little expectoration and a desire for frequent sips of cold water. Could also show lack of thirst. Eyes may be covered with mucus in pneumonic stages. Dosage: 3 pellets 2 times a day.

Apis mellifica. For stings and bites that usually feel better with cold applications. Also for irritated skin or tissue that's pinkish and puffy but when pressed, looks whitish. A guiding symptom is intolerance of heat around eyes and ankles. Also useful for conditions of throat where the tissues seem full of water (edema). For stings and bites, remove stinger and wash well. Dosage: 3 pellets every 1/2 hour for 6 doses.

Argentum nitricum. For eye conditions. Produces irritating effect on mucous membranes and free-flowing mucopurient discharge. Dosage: 3 pellets 3 times a day; decrease frequency with improvement.

Arnica montana. Helps relieve discomfort of mild trauma (accidental injuries). Reduces shock and helps control bleeding. Helps relieve bruising. Excellent before and after surgery. Also excellent during pregnancy at regular intervals. Dosage: 3 pellets immediately, then 3 pellets every 1/2 hour; decrease frequency with improvement. See also Creams and Ointments, page 170.

Arsenicum album. For gastric disturbances, diarrhea, and vomiting, or if bad food is the expected cause. Cat is anxious, restless, feels weak and cold, and has a strong desire for small amounts of water. Good remedy for colibacillosis or coccidiosis, also upper respiratory problems and pneumonia if symptoms become worse toward midnight. Dosage: 3 pellets 2–3 times a day.

Baptisia tinctoria. For low-grade fevers and muscular lethargy. Secretions are offensive, and gums become ulcerated and discolored. Tonsils are red, and stool tends to be dysenteric. Could be useful in feline enteritis. Dosage: 3 pellets every hour; decrease frequency with improvement.

Belladonna. For feverish inflammatory conditions that appear violently, and in which symptoms progress rapidly. Condition causes a state of excitement and active congestion. Cat has a full, bounding pulse, and dilation of pupils, cannot tolerate bright light, and experiences painful swallowing. Take temperature frequently to monitor and give fluid therapy above 104.5° F or if skin is slack on back of neck and slides back into place very slowly when lifted and released. Dosage: 3 pellets every 2 hours; decrease frequency with improvement.

Bryonia. For upper respiratory symptoms and pleurisy. Rheumatism of the joints with inflammation. Cat is worse from movement, wants to lie still. Dosage: 3 pellets 3 times a day.

Cantharis. For severe rash with intense itching of skin. Cystitis with blood. I personally recommend caution with this remedy for cats, as aggravation may occur. Dosage: 3 pellets 2–4 times a day.

Carbo vegetabilis. For lack of resistance to infection and/or conditions that develop slowly where a general lack of vitality is present. Coldness of body surface; may help raise a below-normal temperature. Dosage: 3 pellets 1 time and check temperature.

Caulophyllum. For difficulties at parturition with breeding females. For uterus disability, which may be accompanied by fever and thirst. Tendency to retain afterbirth with accompanying bleeding. May revive labor pains and has been used in place of Pituitrin injections. Especially helpful in establishing normal pregnancy in those who've had miscarriages. Dosage: 3 pellets for three to four doses.

Chamomilla. For teething and accompanying gum irritation, pain, mild fever, and diarrhea. Condition improved by motion. Dosage: 3 pellets 3 times a day.

Cinchona officinalis. For conditions characterized by a draining of fluids associated with a general weakness, bleeding, and diarrhea. Dosage; 3 pellets every 10 minutes for bleeding and after each bowel movement for diarrhea; decrease frequency with improvement.

Cocculus indicus. Mainly for motion or travel sickness with tendency to vomiting. Dosage: For travel sickness, 3 pellets 1 hour before trip and then every hour. as needed; decrease frequency with improvement. For general malaise from travel; 3 pellets in the evening once you've arrived at your destination.

Colocynthis. When diarrhea is yellowish and forcibly expelled. Aggravation occurs after eating or drinking. Dosage: 3 pellets at time of discomfort.

Cuprum metallicum. For occasional sudden severe cramps. Muscles contract and show twitching. Also for fits and convulsions that take an epileptic form. Head is drawn to one side. Dosage: 3 pellets every hour; decrease frequency with improvement.

Euphrasia officinalis. Mild inflammation of eyes and tearing. Principally, conjunctivitis and corneal ulcerations. Dosage: 3 pellets three to four times a day. As an eyedrop: one drop of mother tincture in 1 oz. sterile saline solution. One drop in each eye 3–4 times daily.

Ferrum phosphoricum. This cell salt, like *Aconitum*, may be used in early stages of throat inflammations and pulmonary congestion. Also if hemorrhages are present. Dosage: 3 pellets 3–4 times a day.

Gelsemium sempervirens. For conditions that produce weakness and muscle tremors. Dosage: 3 pellets 4 times a day; decrease frequency with improvement.

Hepar sulphuris calcareum: For conditions showing extreme sensitivity to touch indicating acute pain. Also for upper respiratory problems with purulent discharge. Dosage: 3 pellets 3–4 times a day; decrease frequency with improvement.

Hypericum perforatum. For lacerated wounds with damage to nerve endings. To give relief of pain caused by injury to spine. Injured part usually feels worse if moved. Dosage: 3 pellets every hour; decrease frequency with improvement.

Ignatia amara. For cat that seems unhappy, which could be caused by either excitement or emotions (fright, grief, or disappointment). Also for indigestion or motion sickness. Dosage: 3 pellets in the morning; decrease frequency with improvement.

Ipecacuanha. For persistent vomiting or diarrhea usually caused by diet. Dosage: 3 pellets every 15 minutes; decrease frequency with improvement.

Kali bichromicum. For runny nose, discomfort, and pressure at base of nose. Nasal discharge is yellow-green and viscous, and may form a crust. Sinusitis, presence of thick, sticky, stringy mucus. Could be useful in bronchopneumonia. Dosage: 3 pellets 4 times a day.

Ledum palustre. To give relief from pain caused by minor puncture wounds from sharp pointed instruments such as teeth, claws, or bee stings. Excellent following surgery or for insect bites. Affected parts are generally cold to the touch and feel better after cold applications. Dosage: 3 pellets every 15 minutes;

decrease frequency with improvement. See also Creams and Ointments, page 170.

Lycopodium clavatum. For flatulence with distension of abdomen under navel, gastric symptoms that increase in the evening (4:00 P.M.–8:00 P.M.), and right-sided symptoms. Dosage: 3 pellets 1 time daily for 3 days.

Magnesia phosphorica. For cramps, such as uterine spasms, and leg and foot cramps; acts on muscles that cramp or go into spasm; effective for symptoms that are improved by heat, pressure, massage, and exertion. Dosage: 3 pellets every 15 minutes; decrease frequency with improvement.

Mercurius solubilis. For spongy, sore gums; sore throat; mild fever; thirst; shivering; and excess salivation associated with a cold, thick, coated tongue. May be useful in acute stomatitis (inflammation of gums). Dosage: 3 pellets every hour; decrease frequency with improvement.

Nux vomica. For intestinal discomfort, abdominal pain, diarrhea, indigestion, travel sickness, congestion. Stools are usually hard. Dosage: 3 pellets every hour; decrease frequency with improvement.

Phosphorus. One of the most important remedies in homeopathy. For dry, hard, racking cough with fever that develops rather quickly from a cold settling in the chest. Has an effect on eye situations. Cat craves cold food and water. Dosage: For nosebleeds, 3 pellets at time of bleeding; don't repeat. For other indications, 3 pellets 3 times daily.

Pulsatilla. Recommended when there is a creamy, bland, thick, yellow nasal or vaginal discharge. Cat is better with cool air, cold food, and water. Dosage: 3 pellets 3 times daily.

Pyrogenium. For fever with weak, thready pulse. Dosage: 3 pellets (200C potency) 1 time or as directed.

Rhus toxicodendron. Pains from joint conditions such as rheumatism, neuritis, and achy flu-like symptoms that are worse when cat is inactive and much better when active. Cold applications make symptoms worse; heat or warm compresses make them better. Also for skin eruptions looking like eczema or herpes, and so forth. Dosage: 3 pellets every 6 hours.

Ruta graveolens. Facilitates labor by increasing tone of uterus, and for injury characterized by a sore area near where the tendon is attached to the bone. Excellent following the use of Arnica for the muscles. Most symptoms are worse when cat is lying down. Dosage: 3 pellets 3 times a day or until improved.

Silicea. For feline acne, fibrous growths, minor skin eruptions and abscesses, and chronic sinusitis. Also for certain cases of renal insufficiency. Dosage: 3 pellets 2 times a day until improved.

Spongia tosta. Thyroid gland becomes enlarged. Lymph system also involved. Used as a heart remedy. Dosage: 3 pellets every 6 hrs.

Sulphur. Has a wide range of action, among them skin conditions such as ringworm★ and mange. Also aids action of other remedies. Dosage: 3 pellets the first day symptoms appear; decrease with improvement or cessation of symptoms.

Staphysagria. Postoperative remedy, reduces trauma and helps heal wounds. To reduce desire to spray in males after neutering the dosage is 6C, 3 times daily for seven days.

Symphytum officinale. Hastens union of bone in fractures. Helps relieve pain and promotes healing of injured tissues, especially those injured by a blunt object. May be used with Arnica. Also used for symptoms relating to the eyes. Dosage: 3 pellets 3-4 times a day.

★The nosode *cobacillinum* has also been found to be effective for ringworm, 200C once weekly until you see improvement.

Thuja. Used (along with *Sulphur*) to clear the effects of vaccinations. Dr. Pitcairn recommends a course of this remedy prior to administering nosodes to clear vaccinations. Dosage: 6X *Sulphur* 2 times daily for 7 days; 6X *Thuja* 2 times daily for 7 days. Repeat for an additional fourteen days.

Urtica urens. Helps queens to increase milk supply and later on to dry it up. Dosage: To bring milk in, 3 pellets (30C) 3 times a day. To dry up milk supply, 3 pellets (6X) 3 times a day.

Ustillago maydis. For alopecia and dry coat. The remedy has an affinity for genital organs of both sexes, also for male spraying. Dosage: 200C 3 times per week for 4 weeks.

Veratrum album. Vomiting associated with painful, watery diarrhea and cramps alternating with extreme exhaustion and cold sweats. Chills extend from head to feet, limbs are cold. Cat craves cold water, which is then vomited. Dosage: 3 pellets 2–4 times a day.

Also keep on hand:

Mother Tincture

Calendula officinalis tincture. For mild burns, insect bites, and superficial skin irritations. Dosage: a few drops in wet compress 2-3 times a day.

Creams and Ointments

Arnica montana cream. Stimulates healing of wounds and bruises, also for spasms. Dosage: 2–3 applications a day.

Calendula officinalis cream. For mild burns, insect bites, and superficial skin irritations. Dosage: 2–3 applications a day.

Ledum palustre ointment. For punctures, bites, and stings. Dosage: 3–4 applications a day.

Warning: As with any drug, when your cat is pregnant or nursing, seek the advice of a holistic veterinarian or practitioner before using any of these remedies. If symptoms persist or worsen for more than 3 days, consult your practitioner. Keep these and all medications out of the reach of children and animals.

MINIREPERTORY
(ORGANIZED BY SYMPTOM)

Note: Please consult a homeopathic practitioner prior to administration of remedies.

Abscesses	Silicea
Abdominal distension associated with gas	Carbo vegetabilis
Anxiety	Aconitum napellus
Bee sting	Apis mellifica
Bleeding gums	Phosphorus
Boils	Hepar sulphuris
Boils (grouped, recurring, red)	Sulphur
Bruising	Arnica montana
Burns (mild and dry)	Calendula tincture/cream
Colds (high temperature of sudden onset, strong thirst)	Aconitum napellus
Colds (of the head with acrid, watery discharge and tearing)	Allium cepa
Colds (sudden onset with redness and rapid pulse)	Belladonna
Constipation	Alumina
Cough (dry, hard with fever)	Phosphorus
Cough (dry, hacking, croupy)	Spongia tosta
Cough (croupy, early stages)	Hepar sulphuris
Diarrhea (dietary indiscretion)	Ipecacuanha
Diarrhea (with cadaverous smell)	Arsenicum album
Deficient milk	Urtica urens (30C—lower dosages dry up milk.)
Eruptions (recurring, burning, itching)	Sulphur
Exhaustion (emotional cause)	Ignatia amara
Eyes (inflammation, tearing)	Euphrasia officinalis
Fever (sudden onset with rapid pulse)	Belladonna

Flatulence (bloating under the navel, worse in evening)	Lycopodium clavatum
Gas	Carbo vegetabilis
Gastric upset	Pulsatilla
Grief	Ignatia amara
Indigestion	Nux vomica
Indigestion (with gas)	Carbo vegetabilis
Injury (sore area located where tendon connects to bone)	Ruta graveolens
Insect bites (topical applications)	Calendula tincture/cream or Ledum ointment
Insect bites (improved by cold)	Apis mellifica
Insect bites	Ledum palustre
Leg cramps (sudden, severe)	Cuprum metallicum
Leg cramps (improved by heat, massage, pressure, exertion)	Magnesia phosphorica
Motion sickness	Ignatia amara or Cocculus indicus
Nasal discharge (bland, yellow, creamy)	Pulsatilla
Nasal discharge (yellow-green, viscous)	Kali bichromicum
Nausea	Ipecacuanha
Nervousness before an event (such as cat show)	Gelsemium sempervirens or Aconite
Pregnancy (stimulate uterus)	Caulophyllum
Puncture wounds (superficial)	Ledum palustre
Pyometra (bland, creamy yellow vaginal discharge)	Pulsatilla
Pain over kidneys (with depression and vaginal discharge)	Helonias
Rash (skin)	Arsenicum album
Rheumatism (joints)	Bryonia
Runny nose	Kali bichromicum
Sinusitis (thick, sticky)	Kali bichromicum
Skin rash (sudden onset)	Arsenicum album

Sprain	Arnica montana
Spraying (after neutering) or territorial behavior	Staphysagria or Ustillago maydis
Strain (overexertion)	Arnica montana or Rhus toxicodendron
Surgery	Arnica montana alternated with Hypericum
Teething	Chamomilla
Throat (sore)	Belladonna
Trauma (general, minor)	Arnica montana
Vaccinosis	Thuja or Sulphur
Vaginal discharge (yellow, creamy, bland)	Pulsatilla
Vomiting (nausea/indigestion caused by diet)	Ipecacuanha or Nux vomica

IDEAL SCHEDULE OF 69 OF THE MOST
COMMON REMEDIES[22]

Note: This schedule suggests the time of day each remedy is most effective; not all homeopathic practitioners feel the time of day is pertinent. (+/-) indicate remedies without a precise schedule because of different hours of aggravation. Remedies with asterisks are those that Dr. Pitcairn finds most useful for treating chronic disease (underlying energy imbalance).

Aconitum	12 P.M.-6 P.M.
Alumina	12 P.M.
Antimonium crudum	6 A.M.-4 P.M.(+-)
Antimonium tartaricum	6 A.M.-4P.M.
Apis mellifica	4 P.M.-6 A.M.
Argentum metallicum	6 P.M.-6 A.M.
* Argentum nitricum	6 A.M.-6 P.M.(+-)
* Arnica	12 P.M.-6 P.M.
* Arsenicum album	6 A.M.(+-), -7P.M.
* Aurum metallicum	12 P.M.-4 P.M.
Baryta carbonica	12 P.M.-4 P.M.
* Belladonna	6 A.M.-12 P.M.
Bryonia alba	12 P.M.-6 P.M.
* Calcarea carbonica	12 P.M.-6 P.M.
Calcarea phosphorica	4 P.M.-6 P.M.
Calcarea silicata	6 A.M.-6 P.M.
Carbon animal	12 P.M.-6 P.M.
* Carbon vegetal	12 P.M.-6 P.M.(+-)
Causticum	12 P.M.-6 P.M.
Chamomilla	12 P.M.-6 P.M.
China	6 P.M.-7 P.M.
Coffea tosta	12 P.M.-7 P.M.
Colchicum	6 A.M..-4 P.M.
Colocynthis	6 A.M.-4 P.M.
* Conium maculatum	12 P.M.-4 P.M.
Crotalus horridus	6 A.M.-7 P.M.
Digitalis	4 P.M.-6 P.M.
Drosera	12 P.M.-7 P.M.
Dulcamara	6 A.M.(+-)-12 P.M., 8 P.M.-12 P.M.
Ferrum metallicum	4 P.M.-6 P.M.

Gelsemium	12 P.M.-12 A.M.
* Graphites	12 P.M.-6 P.M.
* Hepar	12 P.M.-6 P.M.
Hyoscamium	6 A.M.-6 P.M.
Ignatia	6 P.M.-12 A.M.
Iodum	6 A.M.-6 P.M.
Ipecacuanha	6 A.M.-6 P.M.
Kali Bichromicum	12 P.M.-4 P.M.
* Lachesis	12 P.M.-6 P.M.
Ledum palustre	6 A.M.-4 P.M.
Lilium tigrinum	6 A.M.-4 P.M.
* Lycopodium	6 A.M.-12 P.M.
Medorrhinum	6 A.M.-8 P.M. (+-)
* Mercurius solubilis	6 A.M.(+-)-6 P.M.(+-)
* Natrum muriaticum	4 P.M.-6 A.M.(+-)
* Nitric acidum	12 P.M.-4 P.M.
Nux moschata	12 P.M.-6 P.M..
*Nux vomica	12 P.M.(+-)-12 A.M. (+-)
Phosphoric acidum	12 P.M.-4 P.M.
* Phosphorus	12 P.M.-6 P.M.(+-)
Phytolacca	12 P.M.-7 P.M..
Platina	12 P.M.-4 P.M..
Plumbum	6 A.M.-6 P.M.
Podophyllum	12 P.M.-12 A.M.
* Psorinum	12 P.M.-6 P.M.
* Pulsatilla	6 A.M.-5 P.M.(-+)
* Rhus toxicodendron	6 A.M.-12 A.M.(-+)
* Sepia	6 A.M.-12 P.M.(-+)
* Silica	6 A.M.-12 P.M.(+-)
Spigelia	12 P.M.-7 P.M.
Spongia tosta	6 A.M.-6 P.M.
* Staphisagria	12 P.M.-7 P.M.
Stramomium	12 P.M.-6 P.M..
* Sulphur	12 P.M.-6 P.M.(+-)
Syphilinum	6 A.M.-6 P.M.
* Thuja	6 A.M.-12 P.M.(+-), 4 P.M.-12A.M.(+-)
Tuberculinum	12 P.M.-12 A.M.
* Veratrum album	12 P.M.-6 A.M.
Zincum metallicum	6 A.M.-4 P.M.(+-)

FLOWER REMEDIES

UNLIKE dangerous antidepressants and tranquilizers, which only mask emotional distress, flower remedies act as gentle catalysts to alleviate underlying causes of stress and restore emotional balance. Flower remedies are absolutely benign in their action and may therefore be safely prescribed for humans, animals, and even plants. The subtlety of this therapy makes it especially well suited to the profound emotional nature of our feline companions.

Note that flower essences are not herbal remedies. Herbs possess powerful medicinal qualities, and should not be dealt with lightly (see Herbs, page 128). Herbal extracts may be made from flowers such as chamomile and goldenseal; however, flower essences are merely the life force collected from the energy field, or aura, of plants.[23]

To make these remedies (and you may make your own—see below), the flowers of wild plants, bushes, and trees are picked at dawn, at the height of their vitality, submerged in water, and solarized (exposed to sunlight) for a few hours. The resulting liquid is diluted and strengthened several times.[24]

The History of Flower Remedies

THE CONCEPT of flower essences dates back to the ancient alchemists, who felt the morning dew was sacred. They utilized this early form of flower therapy in their healing practices. Flower remedies have been used for centuries in India and China, in Australia by aboriginals, and in Europe in the sixteenth century by the master physician and alchemist Paracelsus.

However, the first formal research and development of flower essences is attributed to Dr. Edward Bach (1886–1936), an acclaimed twentieth-century British physician, bacteriologist, and homeopath.

I was introduced to the Bach flower remedies at a cat show in Los Angeles. At the time, my cat Chloe seemed to be having difficulty adjusting to the addition of other cats in our home, and I wondered if she might be happier going to a new home, where she could be an "only child" again. Chloe didn't seem ill, just angry, tense, and aggressive toward the other cats and me. A volunteer from a local animal adoption center suggested I go to the nearest health food store and purchase a bottle of Rescue Remedy, which had been used extensively at the shelter, with great success. I'm sure Chloe would still rather she were my only cat, but with a little help from Rescue Remedy, she's doing fine. She rarely even needs it anymore.

Rescue Remedy is a combination of five of the thirty-eight flower remedies developed by the late Dr. Bach. While practicing medicine, Dr. Bach had observed that his patients' states of mind were directly related to their physical ills. In 1930 he gave up his lucrative medical practice and research, dedicating his life to studying the relationship between the mind and the onset and progression of disease.

Dr. Bach noticed that inharmonious states of mind such as fear, loneliness, depression, hopelessness, and boredom not only inhibited our natural ability to heal ourselves but were actually the primary cause of disease itself. He believed the only way to truly cure illness was to address its underlying emotional causes, a view diametrically opposed to that of traditional medicine, which treats symptoms.

After many years of researching the healing properties of flowering plants, Dr. Bach developed thirty-eight natural remedies to alleviate every negative emotional state he identified; in addition, he created the combination formula Rescue Remedy, intended for immediate action in emergency situations. Today these remedies are world renowned for their effectiveness.[25]

The Flower Remedies Handbook: Emotional Healing and Growth with Bach and Other Flower Essences by Donna Cunningham describes several other prominent sources for flower remedies, including Flower Essence Services (FES). Working with North American plant species, FES has created more than seventy well-documented essences, and many more are being developed.[26]

Christina Chambreau, D.V.M., highly recommends the flower essences produced by Molly Sheehan's Green Hope Farm. Sheehan's Emergency Trauma Solution may be taken in situations of sudden trauma (just like Rescue Remedy), and she claims this remedy was even used to help keep the electrical system of the farm from shutting down.

Recognizing the importance of animals in our lives, Sheehan has also developed Animal Emergency Care, a fine-tuned version of the original emergency formula.[27] Ellon USA (an American company that distributes flower remedies) receives correspondence reporting wonderful results with the use of flower remedies on cats, dogs, birds, tropical fish, horses, cattle, snakes, and even African rhinoceroses and elephants. Some people include flower remedies in the water they use on their special plants.

No one can dispute the genius of Dr. Bach's pioneering contribution; his work has touched the lives of countless health practitioners and individuals throughout the world. However, though many of his followers believe his thirty-eight remedies are the only viable ones, other pioneers continue to expand the repertory, offering us a vast array to choose from.

How to Use Flower Essences

As you explore the flower remedies, it's important to remember that Dr. Bach believed that negative thoughts and feelings poison the system, bringing about ill health and unhappiness, and hindering treatment and recovery. Everyone of us experiences negativity from time to time, but some people are better able to deal with it and thus bring their systems and minds back into harmony.

Flower Remedies Handbook by Donna Cunningham includes affirmations to be spoken aloud when using flower remedies. We cat lovers may speak these words while administering the remedies to our cats. Being the highly sensitive creatures they are, cats react even to subtle changes in their environment, including changes in the moods of their human companions. Since our animal friends often suffer from the same stresses that affect us, I usually take the same remedy I give my cats, saying "We embrace our feelings and deal with them openly," or whatever seems appropriate in the moment.

Especially when obvious medical problems are ruled out as the cause, flower remedies assist the cats suffering from the ill effects of stress, which we all know lead to disease. In fact, many behavioral problems are a sign of physical illness. So check with your holistic veterinarian, who may recommend a complete workup, including but not limited to a fecal (stool) test and complete blood panel, in order to rule out (or, if necessary, treat) any pathological problems.

Bach flower remedies may be used to complement the treatment recommended by your holistic practitioner, as they seem to act as a catalyst for healing. Many homeopaths recommend their use, since they don't, as herbal formulas sometimes do, usually interfere with homeopathic treatment. However, some practitioners may believe otherwise, so it's best to ask. You may wish to contact a certified flower essence consultant for a personalized program.[28]

Administering flower remedies couldn't be easier. Vigorously shake the dosage bottle vertically, in increments of eight shakes (twenty-four is a good number) to energize the remedy. Then simply add a few drops of the concentrate to the cat's drinking water (two drops of remedy per ounce of purified or spring water). With Rescue Remedy, mix two to four drops of the concentrate into the cat's food, or place two drops of the remedy on the tip of the cat's nose or ears (so they'll lick it off) or administer it orally, but dilute it with spring water first.[29] You may fill a spray bottle and atomize the air with appropriate remedies, too.

Ideally, flower remedies are given four times a day. In cases of extreme stress, they may be given as often as every half-hour, and Rescue Remedy every five to eight minutes in times of crisis until you see improvement. If there is no improvement or symptoms worsen, seek advice from your holistic veterinarian.

You may use up to a maximum of six remedies including Rescue Remedy (even though it's a combination, it counts as one when mixed with others). Make up and store the combinations you deem appropriate for your cat; I use 1 ounce amber dosage bottles with glass droppers.[30] With these combinations I usually administer half a dropper's worth at a time, orally. Afterward, be sure to rinse the dropper in warm water because the dropper may have touched the animal's tongue, and you don't want to risk contaminating the remainder of the formula.

When the remedies are given in food or water, there's no need to worry about their effect on your other animals. If another animal (or human, for that matter) doesn't need the remedy, it will have no effect, so all your animals may share the same bowls freely. To ensure potency, always prepare the remedy-enhanced food or water fresh daily. To preserve flower essences, keep the bottle in the refrigerator or mix an ounce of remedy with a teaspoon of vegetable glycerine.

Before you begin using flower remedies, remember to look at yourself and your cats as objectively as possible. It's important to know which of their behaviors are normal. Many times human beings accuse animals of being spiteful or vindictive when they behave in ways we don't like, but this is often only our own inability to understand animal behavior.

For instance, it's natural for kittens to bite and scratch, not a sign of mean-spiritedness. But since such natural behaviors aren't acceptable to us, we must find gentle ways to discourage them, or rather, to channel their normal behaviors into acceptable outlets. With positive reinforcement (see Nonverbal Communication in chapter 2, "Interacting with Your Cat"). This way a kitten soon learns to uses its toys and scratching post instead. The flower remedies Chestnut Bud and Walnut can help this transition.

You can obtain a self-help guide to the flower remedies (designed for human use) through Ellon USA (see Resources). As you read the descriptions for each essence, compare the behaviors listed to those of your cat, and then read the feline interpretations below.[31] You'll soon get the hang of it.

See what combinations you come up with both for yourself and your cats. Use a little poetic license as you interpret the descriptions, and explore the numerous other flower essence companies, which are making major breakthroughs in this exciting field.

The Remedies and Their Uses with Cats

Agrimony. For animals suffering from skin irritations, feral cats that cannot adjust to captivity, and restlessness at night when you'd rather the cat slept.

Aspen. For the "fraidy-cat," that slinks from safe place to safe place and startles easily at any sound, even nonthreatening ones (if this condition was brought about by trauma or abuse in the past, use Star of Bethlehem; when in doubt, use both). Give Aspen during intense storms or after earthquakes, or to a kenneled or sheltered animal that senses impending harm. Aspen may actually help reveal to your cat what it's actually afraid of, so she can learn to deal with her own fear.

Beech. For cats with little tolerance for other animals or certain people. Effective with Walnut to assist in keeping peace between two cats who are always fighting. For the cat that is intolerant of a new relationship in the house, and the cat that sprays on the belongings of his owner's newfound mate. For the cat that always seems irritated. Also good for picky eaters.

Centaury. For the quiet, submissive cat that doesn't stand up for himself, allows himself to be abused by a dog, a child, or another cat. Increases will to live when fighting an illness or during the hard delivery of a kitten.

Cerato. For flighty, inattentive animals. Valuable during shows or training sessions, when cat's ability to be undistracted and to relate to your requests is required. Excellent for anxiety and related problems, such as feline eating disorders, especially during pregnancy.

Cherry Plum (one of the ingredients in Rescue Remedy). For the cat that loses control, becomes wild, angry, and vicious when provoked. In competition situations, when the cat is stressed by strange people, the smell of other cats, and unfamiliar noises. For cat that doesn't travel well. For retaining control during heat cycles and/or mating (for both sexes); good for pregnant queens that seem unusually stressed. In situations where the cat could lose bladder and/or bowel control. Also for the cat that constantly chews himself or chases his own tail. For allergies to grasses, and to help cats stay away from biting at stitches after surgery.

Chestnut Bud. Used to break bad habits, or during training sessions, to increase memory retention and a keen sense of awareness. Helps cats learn lessons necessary for us to coexist (such as not to scratch the couch).

Chicory. For the extremely affectionate cat, which may be possessive and jealous, wanting always to be near you, to be held, petted, and fussed over. For the mother cat overly possessive with her litter, especially when it's time for her kittens to leave home. For the cat that thinks she owns the house or tries to get attention in negative ways.

Clematis (one of the ingredients in Rescue Remedy). When the cat appears stunned or experiences unusual, prolonged patterns of sleep, beyond the typical catnap. To help while regaining consciousness following surgery or an accident. In conjunction with Rescue Remedy, helps newborn kittens wake up and breathe. Give them one drop every few minutes on tips of ears or nose.

Crabapple. This remedy is especially cleansing during or after any illness, rash, open wound, worming, or flea infestation. Used to detoxify and heal. For cat with a poor self-image, that cowers during shows, or cat previously abused or abandoned.

Elm. For the cat that must change location, go to the groomer, or be subjected to too many people at a time (a show or guests and relatives).

Gentian. For setbacks of any kind (as when the cat gets worse before it gets better during the course of an illness, arthritis symptoms, rehabilitation from surgery, the ill effects of a stillborn kitten). Helps to give cats an inner fortitude to deal with whatever comes their way.

Gorse. For apathy, depression, and despair, when the cat refuses to eat or to improve. When battling cancer, a critical injury, or surgery.

Heather. For the center-of-attention cat, the cat that annoys or is a pest, or the cat that cries when left alone. For the cat left at a kennel or in a shelter, wanting attention from everyone.

Holly. For the cat showing signs of temper. When there's a need for more love. Especially good for abused or neglected cats that may need to be quarantined, or rescued cats at the shelter or the veterinarian's office. Helps nourish the heart, and release jealousy and anger.

Honeysuckle. Helps cats stop sulking after change or loss of loved one. For the cat that has been chased to exhaustion by a dog, a child, or another cat. After a long birthing experience; for the mother caring for her young after a cesarean section. For the cat that has lost too much blood or whose vital signs are low. Before selling a cat or kitten, when moving to a new home, or when the cat must be hospitalized or placed in a kennel.

Hornbeam. For fatigue. The strengthening remedy, helpful in assisting the runt of the litter or building up any sickly animal.

Impatiens (one of the ingredients in Rescue Remedy). For the cat that gets agitated by too much excitement, or overly anxious at mealtimes or before a cat show. Also for the cat in pain.

Larch. For cats low in the cat hierarchy of the household, or the runt of the litter. Also for the cat with low self-esteem.

Increases confidence before a show, so he can hold his head high.

Mimulus. For fear of particular things or circumstances, such as thunderstorms, vacuum cleaners, trips to the veterinarian, or visits by small children. Also for deep fears, such as fear of starving, strangers, abandonment. When fear turns to terror, use Rock Rose or Rescue Remedy. For illnesses that don't respond to treatment, such as postinfluenza.

Mustard. For the depressed cat, complicated by hormonal changes (such as kitten coming into heat for the first time, or the stud discovering girls). During pregnancy, if depression is noticeable, or if the cat is cantankerous during heat. Use on cranky, older cats that like to be alone and get obnoxious when approached.

Oak. For last weeks of pregnancy, when the cat feels overburdened. For long chronic illness, especially if the cat begins to struggle. To rebuild strength after harsh living conditions, starvation, or abuse. For loss of elimination functions and/or loss of control of limbs or muscles.

Olive. For exhaustion following a long ordeal or long-term pain. For elderly cats that become exhausted easily. For the cat plagued by stressed adrenals or allergies. For caged cats that exhaust themselves to get out.

Pine. For the cat given away or left behind. In competition, for the cat that never makes it to the finals though she's show quality. For the cat that looks guilty whenever their human companion is upset, even though it wasn't the cat's fault.

Red Chestnut. For the cat that constantly watches out the window when their human companion is late coming home. For the mother worrying over her kittens.

Rescue Remedy (a combination of Star of Bethlehem, Rock Rose, Impatiens, Clematis, and Cherry Plum). For any kind of trauma. Be sure to take it yourself; if you're calmer, it helps your cat. In the case of an accident, see your veterinarian immediately; however, Rescue Remedy can help you through the trauma of getting the cat to the veterinarian's office. Used on pregnant queens, on car trips, for boarding, during long absences from home, before and after surgery, or whenever the cat experiences unusual stress. Also, it can stop a seizure very quickly.[32] Often used as a last resort, with remarkable results—I always reach for it first. I use Rescue Remedy or 5 Flowers Remedy[33] during travel to and from cat shows, and often just before going to the ring for judging.

Rock Rose (one of the ingredients in Rescue Remedy). For cats that experience panic or terror. After an accident, injury, or other terrifying event.

Rock Water. For increased joint flexibility. For picky, inflexible eaters.

Scleranthus. For the cat with equilibrium problems or neurological confusion, as in some kinds of seizures, with complications to one side (such as with stroke or partial paralysis).

Star of Bethlehem (one of the ingredients in Rescue Remedy). For all trauma. Loss of loved one, trauma after injury or abuse, birthing difficulties, intense heat or cold. Use to comfort those left behind in a kennel. For the ill or injured cat that must be hospitalized and is deprived of his human companion's comfort.

Sweet Chestnut. For the high strung cat, at its wit's end. For the cat forced to remain in tiny kennel or carrier. To prevent burn out in show cats, or any time the cat needs endurance or energy.

Vervain. For intense, hyperactive, or for the very high-strung cat.

Vine. For the "boss cat," that thinks he's in charge ("top cat"), the strong-willed cat that rules with claws rather than velvet paws. To boost the self-esteem of the "undercat."

Walnut. Helpful through any changes, including weaning and heat cycles. Eases adjustment to houseguests, holidays, or a new home. Protects against pollutants and pollens from grasses. For the very sensitive cat that is easily disturbed.

Water Violet. Constitutional remedy for most cats, helps them keep their instinct for solitude in balance with the enjoyment of interactions with people and other animals in their environment. Also for grief, loneliness, and lack of joy.

Wild Oat. For the bored cat that doesn't feel useful anymore, the cat retired from shows, movies, or TV. For the cat that chews curtains or furniture out of boredom. For competitions, where the cat needs to have a strong desire to win.

Wild Rose. For cats to remain happy and content when you bring a new kitten home. For the older, grouchy cat, or the cat placed in a cage during a cat show.

Willow. For resentment, the cat that ignores you when you come home because you left it alone all day, or the show cat that punishes you by urinating on the bed (check for health problems, too, with this behavior) for not taking him to shows anymore or not paying attention to him, or the cat that chews up your electrical cords.

Flower remedies, as mentioned above, often work well in combination. Use your intuition to come up with mixtures that are right for your cat. Here are a few ideas: Aspen, Star of

Bethlehem, and Larch may be used singly or in combination with shelter or stray animals that have been abused or neglected; Aspen and Larch for fear and mistrust, Star of Bethlehem for grief and trauma. Try combining Red Clover, a great calmer for group hysteria (such as cat shows), with Rescue Remedy or 5 Flowers. If travel is traumatic for your cat and motion sickness often accompanies it, withhold food and water for at least one hour before departure, and give Rescue Remedy (or 5 Flowers) and/or Scleranthus. Use Crabapple, Olive, and Rescue Remedy together or separately for cats with upper respiratory infections. They're also good to use after spaying, neutering, or during and after bouts of fever.

The Australian Bush Flower Essences (see Resources) include a wonderful remedy called Kapok Bush. This is supportive for those who get easily discouraged and give up. Borage, by FES, gives us cheer and courage in facing up to challenges—healing ourselves and assisting the healing of our companion animals is indeed challenging.

Consultant Yolanda LaCombe recommends several of the healing herbs and FES remedies for cats, among them Mariposa Lily for the motherly cat that needs to mellow out, Queen Anne's Lace for cats that have had a trauma to the head (you may suspect abuse in their past), Manzanita for anorexic cats, and Red Clover for calming in tense situations. I combine all of these with Water Violet and 5 Flowers, and dose myself and the cats as soon as we arrive at cat shows.

I've started carrying my flower reference books with me to shows, as I'm always being asked what makes my cats so centered and able to handle this unusual stress.[34] If you consider that each cat is an individual being made of the same "stuff" we are, it isn't any wonder that, when we observe their personalities and traits, we can prescribe flower essences for them as easily as we can for ourselves.

How to Make Your Own Flower Essences

IN *Natural Healing for Dogs and Cats,* Diane Stein tells us how easy it is to become a do-it-yourself maker of flower essences.[35] You'll need a clear glass bowl, free of design, which can hold up to 12 ounces of water. Stein suggests using distilled or spring water; I prefer spring water with flower essences as well as with gem elixirs (see Crystals in chapter 7, "Other Healing Approaches"). You'll also need stainless-steel tweezers, several amber glass dropper bottles sterilized in boiling water, a glass funnel, some labels for the bottles, and brandy (as a preservative).

Place your bowl outside on the soil or grass, next to your desired flowers. Fill the bowl with spring water. Pick blossoms or petals from the healthiest plants; use the tweezers, not your fingers, for picking, so as not to contaminate the essence with whatever may be on your hands. Cover the surface of the water with the flowers or petals. Organically raised flowers or wildflowers are best; don't use flowers treated with chemical pesticides.

Pick only one kind of flower at a time; it's okay to select from different plants and colors, just stick with a single species (such as only roses) in your bowl. However, if you can only obtain a single flower, this is fine too.

Leave the water and flowers in the sunshine for three hours. If you begin in the early morning, while the dew is still on the petals, you may need to solarize longer. Spring and summer are the best seasons; pick a cloud-free day for best results.

Fill your sterile dosage bottles halfway with brandy. With your tweezers (again, no fingers, please; you may also use a leaf from the same plant, or even a crystal), remove the flowers and any debris from the water. Add the water to bottles containing the brandy, filling them to the neck, sealing, and labeling them. It's a good idea to include the date. You may even label them with the phase of the moon or astrological sign under which they were prepared.[36]

If you're making more than one flower essence, wash your hands before proceeding to the next flower. In fact, it's a good idea to wash your hands before preparing or administering any treatment. Try to use unscented soap, as aromatic materials may interfere with the potency of flower essences and homeopathics.

You now have a mother tincture. Potentize your essences by *succussing* (shaking) or hitting the bottle against the heel of your hand in increments of eight shakes or taps.

For everyday use add two drops of the mother tincture to another dropper bottle filled with equal amounts of spring water and brandy. Another way to dilute the remedy is to mix one ounce spring water, two drops potentized flower essence, and one teaspoon brandy; or substitute one teaspoon vegetable glycerine for the brandy, if you wish to avoid the alcohol altogether.

Now you may use your homemade essences just as you would those you buy at the health food store (see administration instructions above).

Nature and the Higher Self

FOR A lesson in communing with the nature spirits, or devas, I recommend reading *Behaving As If the God in All Life Mattered* by Machaelle Small Wright, one of my favorite authors; her *Flower*

Essences and *Nature Healing Conings for Animals* are also excellent resources.[37] One of Wright's Perelandra Essences is comfrey, which is used to repair soul damage occurring in the present or in a past lifetime.

Wright and other spiritual writers have awakened in me a confidence that each one of us is blessed with an ability to contact our higher selves. This higher self can in turn be in touch with another person's or animal's higher self, and thus be a party to healing. I've found that, even if I feed the perfect diet, select an array of herbal and homeopathic remedies, use every kind of supplement imaginable, and even pray for an animal friend to be healed, unless I release myself to the laws of nature, healing will be thwarted every step of the way.

AROMATHERAPY

SCENT IS a powerful component in holistic health care for cats. The subtle use of aromatherapy can enhance all of our healing therapies, especially for cats, whose sense of smell is so much more complex and acute than our own. Their olfactory ability is the result of evolution: the acuteness of their senses allowed cats to survive predators and other dangers in the wilderness.

The history of the use of scent by humans dates back to the ancient Egyptians. Symbolic representations of incense appear on the walls of Egyptian tombs and temples, author Scott Cunningham tells us in *Magical Aromatherapy*. The Egyptians had such a high regard for scent that they traded valuable commodities such as gold for fragrant substances, and used them in medicine, food preparation and presentation, and the rituals of religion, magic, and even their journeys to the afterlife.

The Greeks anointed their deceased with essential oils, burned incense on altars, and lavished their bodies with expensive fragrances. They also believed that the fresh scents rising from living plants maintained physical health, constructing their homes so rooms would open out onto herb gardens surrounded by flowering plants. They inhaled specific perfumes to heal various ailments, such as quince or white violet for stomach upsets, grape leaves to help clear the head, and roses to relieve headaches.

The American Indians, through centuries of trial and error, developed uses for fragrant plant materials in every aspect of their daily lives, from food, medicine, and tools, to personal adornment and toys.

The Hawaiians traditionally used and still use fragrances, especially scented coconut oil, maile, hale, and pukiawe, which was burned by the kahuna, or witch doctor, who chanted and prayed while it fumed.

Humans use aromatherapy to stimulate the immune system and promote healing, typically employing essential oils, the distilled or expressed product of aromatic plant materials, for this purpose. These aromatic essences have many desirable qualities, ranging from antibacterial and antiviral to antispasmodic.

Some are reported to have diuretic properties (promoting the production and excretion of urine), are vasodilators or vasoconstrictors (widening or narrowing blood vessels, respectively), and act on the adrenals, ovaries, and thyroid. Others aid in digestion or are beneficial in treating infection, modifying immune response, and balancing moods and emotions, according to Kurt Schnaubelt, director of the Pacific Institute of Aromatherapy.[38]

Scott Cunningham describes the utilization of scent in three different forms:[39]

Fresh plants. Contain large amounts of energy in their flowers, twigs, and leaves. Grow your own or buy them at health food stores, farmer's markets, and organic nurseries.[40] If you do plant your own garden, please observe organic principles, and never let the cats sniff plants sprayed with synthetic pesticides.

Dried herbs. Ideal because the essential oils haven't evaporated during the drying process. Check local herb shops for a lovely variety or peruse the shelves of your health food store for both herbs and spices.[41]

Essential oils. Volatile aromatic substances that naturally occur within specific plants, such as rose and garlic, giving them their pungent odor. These can be purchased at most health food stores.[42]

How do cats react to scent? An adult cat (over the age of seven months) will retract his upper lip to expose his teeth while approaching, sniffing, and licking feline urine; this is known as the Flehmen response. He'll flick the tip of his tongue repeatedly against his palate behind the upper incisor teeth, then lift his head, open his mouth, and lick his nose. This transfers the urine to the *vomeronasal organ* (a sense organ located between mouth and nasal cavity above the hard palate, also known as Jacobson's organ). In this way the cat can identify the sex of the animal that produced the urine.

The female in estrus (heat) has a unique component, valoric acid, in her vaginal secretions, which makes her restless and induces a searching reaction. Exposure to this scent may trigger other females to come into season. As you can see, cats naturally use a kind of aromatherapy in their own social hierarchy.

The essential oils most frequently used in pet care are eucalyptus, tea tree, lavender, citronella, rosemary, pennyroyal, cedarwood, chamomile, cinnamon, tangerine, patchouli, mint, lemon, terebinth, thyme, and sage. These may be used to mask odors; help with exhaustion, fatigue, birthing, and weight loss; to treat anemia, anorexia, abscesses, coryza (common cold), fractures, sprains, and poisoning; to control fleas and other pests; and for many other conditions.

For cats suffering from an upper respiratory virus, Dr. Joanne Stefanatos mixes equal parts eucalyptus oil (a well-known respiratory stimulant) and diluted catalyst altered water (CAW; see Pure Water, in chapter 4, "Nutrition"), and places this in the infuser cup of a vaporizer. Patients inhale the fumes for the first twenty-four to forty-eight hours of their stay at her hospital, after which they can usually breathe better and smell their food, and they begin eating, so they are permitted to leave the hospital. Dr. Stefanatos suggests continuing this therapy at home. I use a diffuser or a vaporizer.

For the same purpose, Nelly Grosjean, author of *Veterinary Aromatherapy*, suggests using the following blend of essential oils in an aromatic diffuser: 20 ml eucalyptus, 10 ml pine, 5 ml tea tree, and 2 ml thyme; she also feels eucalyptus is fine on its own.[43]

Don't forget to dilute the eucalyptus oil in water if you use a vaporizer, as used straight it may irritate your cat's sensitive eyes. And never use essential oils to massage your cat or apply them directly to any part of the cat's body, Grosjean warns, as their sensitive skin cannot tolerate it.

Dr. Stefanatos uses oil of lemon to sedate a fever. For tonification she suggests rosemary, peppermint, sage, or thyme. Essential oils of sage and lavender can be used to stimulate a diuretic response; Dr. Stefanatos suggests administering them in a nebulizer or diffuser for two to eight hours. For gastrointestinal problems, she uses basil, chamomile, thyme, and peppermint. Oil of bane helps speed restoration of health after the course of many diseases.

For excessive heat cycling, false pregnancy, and swollen mammary glands, oil of sage is recommended. Grosjean suggests an infusion of, hydrosol[44] of sage, or an infusion of verbena added to the queen's food three to four days prior to labor. Dr. Stefanatos believes oil of cloves may prevent the need for a caesarean section. For heat as well as asthma problems, Dr. Stefanatos prescribes oil of cinnamon at bedtime. I also use it for diarrhea.

For abscesses Grosjean suggests a poultice of cabbage leaves (crush large outer layers first) or of clay, followed by cleaning with compresses and several drops of lavender. She also recommends clay poultices to promote healing of wounds.[45] Grosjean suggests sprinkling mint leaves or lavender seed into the cat's bed for flea problems.

Although not technically a component of aromatherapy, catnip is perhaps the first herb or scent we think of in relation to cats. It contains the chemical nepetalactone, which produces a behavior that closely resembles that of a female in heat, though it doesn't have sexual side effects. Nepetalactone is not a pheromone but a hallucinogen, inducing pleasurable sensations and stimulating playful behavior.[46] The catnip response appears to be inherited.

At cat shows I often use catnip to amuse my cats, as well as to block the smell of other cats. A whiff of bay rum or vanilla extract applied to a cotton pad prior to a ring appearance is helpful as well. Basil, calendula, chamomile, sage, and rosemary are also scents that seem to attract cats. My cats are fascinated by the potpourri I have placed strategically throughout the house. You too may buy or assemble little bags of herbs, dried flowers, fruits, seeds, pods, and so on, and lace them now and then with essential oils.

Try the following oils and combinations to assist in a variety of circumstances:

- To enhance beauty: *rose, catnip*
- For comfort: *calendula*
- For courage: *sweet pea, yarrow*
- To relieve depression: *jasmine*
- For psychic dreams: *jasmine, calendula, mimosa*
- For stilling emotions: *costmary*
- For happiness: *apple, bergamot, orange, neroli, sweet pea, water lily*
- For healing: *clove, coriander, cypress, eucalyptus, myrrh, melon, niaouli, palmarosa, pine, sandalwood, spearmint*
- For maintaining health: *carnation, eucalyptus, garlic, lavender, lemon, melon, pine*
- For longevity: *fennel, rosemary*
- For love: *carnation, jasmine, lilac, rose, vanilla, water lily (and many more)*
- For magical energy: *nutmeg, orange, vanilla*
- For meditation: *myrrh, sandalwood, chamomile*
- To improve memory and impart wisdom: *sage*
- For peace: *chamomile, gardenia, rose*
- For physical energy: *cinnamon, lemon, nutmeg*
- For sleep and calming: *chamomile, hyacinth, jasmine, lavender*

Certain aromas are also associated with the days of the week, the seasons, and the lunar cycles, as well as the four elements:

Earth: cypress, honeysuckle, lilac, mimosa, oakmoss, patchouli, tonka, tulip, vetiver

Air: bergamot, calendula, carnation, cumin, nutmeg, rosemary

Water: apple, chamomile, freesia, gardenia, hyacinth, jasmine, myrrh, plumeria, rose, sandalwood, vanilla

Fire: bergamot, calendula, coriander, frankincense, ginger, lime, nutmeg, orange, rosemary, saffron

Essential oils may be utilized by placing one to three drops on a cotton ball or clean cotton handkerchief. Place wherever you feel the need for scent. You may also use an aromatic diffuser or a potpourri simmerer to diffuse essential oils through the air.

Grosjean recommends the use of the aromatic diffuser not only to help us benefit from the fragrance of essential oils, but also to protect against microbes and pollution. She feels that the regular use of the diffuser regenerates, cleanses, ionizes, enriches, and revitalizes the air we breathe.[47]

Another means of distributing scent is to bring distilled or purified water to a boil in a nonmetallic pot, pour the water into a large heatproof bowl, and add a few drops of an essential oil or fresh herb while you visualize pictures (such as your cat restored to glowing health or in harmony with your family).

Cut fresh flowers before sunrise (except jasmine and tuberose, which should be cut at night); when you buy flowers from a florist, they've probably been cut before sunrise. Place freshly cut flowers in fresh water. Your cats will probably smell them even before you do. My Romeo loves roses. Valentine's Day is his favorite day of the year!

Whatever form of aromatherapy you use, remember to practice nonverbal communication through visualization and affirmations as you and your cat inhale the aroma; according to Scott Cunningham, this is the key to the power of aromatherapy. Remember to focus on positive images, as they are the only form of communication cats understand (see Nonverbal Communication in chapter 2, "Interacting with Your Cat").[48]

Never use synthetic scents. Just like synthetic food (canned and dry) and synthetic vitamins and minerals, synthetic oils are missing "life energy" and so should never be used in veterinary aromatherapy. The "real stuff" comes from living things, and thus has a direct link with the earth, a subtle energy that can't be duplicated in a laboratory. The energies of these plant materials merge with our own and those of our cats to support healing. For example, genuine rose oil envelops us in scent and guides us through a field of flowers, just like the aroma of fresh roses. A synthetic rose oil contains nothing living; it would probably give you a headache and repel your cat.

Keep essential oils away from strong light, heat, air, and moisture. Never let any living thing drink them. Watch for allergic reactions, and be sure the cats and children don't have direct access to the oils. And take care with your choice of houseplants, as some are poisonous to cats, who may nibble on them if the scent is attractive.

Diane Stein provides this list of common plants that are poisonous to cats as well as humans (so be certain to keep them out of reach of children too!): bittersweet (bark, leaves and seeds), dumb cane (including berries), poison hemlock, ivy (English and Baltic), jimson weed, thorn apple, marigold, marsh marigold, hemp, mistletoe, oleander (all parts), philodendron, poinsettia, poison ivy, potato (unripe tubers and sprouts from tubers), rhubarb (leaf blades).[49] Poisoning symptoms include vomiting, diarrhea, convulsions, coma, dizziness, loss of muscular control and coordination, disordered vision, intense thirst, rapid pulse, swelling of mouth and throat, and itching, redness, and blistering of skin.

Hands-on Healing

THIS CHAPTER describes a number of hands-on therapeutic interventions normally associated with human healing but also beneficial to cats. Its purpose is to explore the various options that exist and help you find practitioners who may be of service to you. Know that, regardless of what modalities you choose, if you approach your companion animal with honor and respect, the therapy will most likely be welcome. Remember to consult your holistic veterinarian before embarking on any course of treatment.

For further information about any of the treatments described here, see the Resources section at the back of this book.

CHIROPRACTIC

FOR AT least a hundred years, humankind has been helped by chiropractic therapy, even though the profession has been maligned and discriminated against by the American Medical Association (AMA), many of whose member physicians believe alternative therapies are practiced by "quacks" and are not based on scientific principles. Since alternative health care is perceived to be a threat to allopathic doctors' income, it's in their best financial interests, along with those of the pharmaceutical companies, to discourage us from seeking alternatives. Most physicians and veterinarians opposed to chiropractic have no direct experience with it.

Chiropractic is another method that treats the whole being. Dr. Chambreau says this modality is one of the best ways to help an animal being treated homeopathically. Applying chiropractic to cats is not such a strange idea, since they have many of the same musculoskeletal problems people do. A chiropractor trained in animal anatomy can work effectively to restore healthy function to your cat.

Sharon Willoughby, D.V.M., enrolled in chiropractic school and learned some information she felt had been missing from the veterinary repertoire: "When a cat's vertebrae [the bones that protect the spinal cord] are out of alignment, they keep the spinal cord from sending certain nerve impulses to the rest of the body. When some of the vital parts of the cat's body get cut off from these impulses, the cat can become ill. He can be in intense pain. He can have difficulty moving."[1] The chiropractor works to realign the vertebrae by applying gentle force to specific vertebrae or joints in the spine, tail, knees, shoulders, and other areas of the body. "When a cat's vertebrae are out of alignment, the joint caps stretch. The surrounding muscles may go into a spasm. These things can be very painful," she states.[2]

If you notice your cat persistently chewing at a spot, perhaps on her chest or back, she may be trying to tell you something about her physical state. You may think you're dealing with an attitude problem, but when cats hurt, they have very limited means of communicating their pain to us.

The basic principle of chiropractic, whether for people or animals, is to work with the peripheral nerves at the root level, which is where the nerves exit between the vertebrae. The nerves are very sensitive to pressure there, and the spine can get sprained just like any joint. A misalignment, or *subluxation*, between two vertebrae puts pressure on the nerve root, thus interfering with its function. This pinched nerve is usually accompanied by pain, but may also cause a functional problem.

Chiropractic may also be used to treat certain internal disorders. Dr. Willoughby cautions that chiropractic is most helpful when an internal disorder has just begun. In very advanced cases, it's not usually as effective.

Chiropractic isn't the correct treatment for fractures, infectious diseases, abscesses, or blocked urinary tracts. It's best to have a veterinarian examine the cat before employing chiropractic therapy. Often, X-rays are needed to determine whether a fracture is present or if there's some other reason the cat should not be adjusted by a chiropractor.

Veterinary schools don't teach chiropractic, and chiropractic schools teach how to work on people, not animals. In 1989, in order to fill this gap, Dr. Willoughby started the American Veterinary Chiropractic Association (AVCA). A 100-hour course in animal chiropractic is available to both veterinarians and chiropractors. After certification, practitioners may take postgraduate courses. In 1991, twenty AVCA-certified practitioners were accredited in the United States, with another forty working toward accreditation.

Because chiropractic is a very sophisticated science, it's best to find a practitioner who's AVCA certified and trained in adjusting small animals. An unqualified practitioner may inadvertently do great harm to the feline skeletal system, which is quite delicate. A thrust at the wrong angle could injure the joints permanently.

Prior to making an adjustment, the chiropractor needs to observe how the animal stands, moves its head, walks, and turns, as well as how it behaves or reacts, in order to determine where soreness occurs. Sometimes, the practitioner must work on parts of the body that are already painful to the touch. Dr. Willoughby teaches her clients how to massage their cat at home between visits, so the animal will be more relaxed during the next treatment and she may more easily make her adjustments.

Network Chiropractic

CREATED by Donald Epstein, D.C., in New York, network chiropractic pulls together the various approaches to this modality. I was first introduced to it by Mark Haverkos, D.V.M., who spent six years with the Hopi Indians as their veterinarian. In addition to network chiropractic, he also practices homeopathy, acupuncture, and herbal medicine. In 1993, he demonstrated his network chiropractic techniques at the American Holistic Veterinary Medical Association (AHVMA) Conference.

As we become aware of our body, says Dr. Haverkos, we begin to realize that all its parts are related, that they're all part of a single system. Rather than viewing a body as something that needs to be fixed (a view held by conventional medicine), network chiropractic aims to make all the particles of the body remember that they're relatives and deserve a loving relationship with each other.

Dr. Haverkos learned from the Indians that everything happens for a reason. Animals do the best they can each moment to adapt to whatever conditions prevail, and their current physical state reflects these conditions. Just as the Indians know that less is more, so do practitioners of network chiropractic. They don't need a heavy hand, but simply a specific intent, so the body can make positive use of the energy offered.

If a chiropractor simply tries to force the spine into "normal" alignment (the problem with traditional chiropractic), it will quickly revert to misalignment. Network chiropractic seeks to discover why the bones are aligned the way they are, and to release some of the chaos that caused the misalignment so the body can move on to another level.

Dr. Haverkos asks animals' permission to work on them before he begins, rather than imposing himself on them. This request need not be in words. He feels words aren't our highest form of interaction, as we've learned from working with nonverbal communication (see chapter 2, "Interacting with Your Cat"). When Dr. Haverkos begins a treatment, he feels himself "resonating" energetically and spiritually with his patient. He can actually sense, in his own body, what he does to the animal.

Certain manipulations provoke particular emotional responses. Though we think of animals as being present in the moment, their spines may tell a different story. For example, an abused animal (perhaps one rescued from a shelter) may have been dishonored by a human being at some time, and thus, on an energetic level, be stuck in the past. During a network treatment, emotions associated with such mistreatment may come up and be released.

Cats respond very quickly to this kind of therapy.

Dr. Haverkos does nearly all his adjustments on standing animals. As he feels down the spine, he asks the animal how she feels, does she feel heat or a sticking sensation, for example. He palpates the musculature and asks himself, "Does it feel smooth or rubbery?" He advises practitioners not to think too much, but rather, just to feel.

Even if you can't find a network chiropractor to do this astounding work, you yourself can learn to "resonate" with your animal, making it your intention to facilitate her well-being. Gently feel your cat's muscle tone. Watch the way she moves and how she looks at you as you go over her body. Watch her breath—it should have a nice, rhythmic flow. If it catches somewhere, there's a blockage, a residue from the past. Trust your senses. Such observation may give you insight into her homeopathic type, and so may lead to the appropriate remedy. Or you may feel she needs acupuncture or some other intervention.

ACUPUNCTURE

ACUPUNCTURE, a technique that stimulates specific points in the body in order to rectify imbalances, originated some two thousand years ago in China.[3] According to legend, thousands of years ago someone noticed that lame war horses, when wounded by arrows in certain spots, would stop limping (another legend tells a similar tale about humans). The same spots were stimulated in other lame horses, and they also stopped limping.

After the energy pathways of the body were discovered and mapped, it was concluded that any disruption of the energy flow, qi (or chi), caused disease. The placement of small needles along exact points on these pathways was found to enhance the flow of *qi* and promote a state of health. So, in essence, acupuncture is simply another means to help the body heal itself.

Originally, stone needles were used. Today acupuncturists may choose from among metal needles, heat, pressure, massage, electrical stimulation, injections, magnets, gold beads, lasers, or any combination of these methods to stimulate a point.

Human and veterinary acupuncture began separately, using different charts. The human charts showed a system of interconnected pathways (meridians and collaterals) through which flows the energy of the body. Hundreds of acupuncture points are spread throughout these pathways.

Identification of animal meridians was less complete, and their points were usually given different names from human ones, even when the location and function seemed identical. Charts were developed primarily for farm animals, especially the horse, chicken, pig, and water buffalo. Today in China, though cats and dogs are treated with acupuncture, the emphasis is still on farm animals.[4]

Approved by the American Veterinary Medical Association, acupuncture was ruled a valid method of treatment in 1989. Many holistic veterinarians are now embracing this technique in their practices. In order to become a certified veterinary acupuncturist, a practitioner must complete a year-long training course accredited by the International Veterinary Acupuncture Society (see Resources).

Richard Pitcairn, D.V.M. speaks positively about acupuncture and oriental medicine, and has several colleagues who practice it enthusiastically. He tells us that the Chinese advocate the holistic approach as a means of preventing disease. They resort to acupuncture and herbs when their preferred methods—meditation, exercise, and massage—have proven insufficient.

Although acupuncture, like western medicine, may be used to treat symptoms alone, the best approach is to correct the underlying imbalances that have created the conditions fostering specific diseases. Therefore, most contemporary acupuncturists emphasize a total approach to health, include in their practice advice on the use of food, herbs, and the like.

"The basic theory behind this comprehensive system," says Dr. Pitcairn, "is that the fundamental energy fields that compromise the body (as well as all aspects of the universe), manifest two poles which are actually expressions of one whole. One pole, yang, is described as being positive. The other, yin, is seen as disruptive, expanded and negative. An individual's health depends on the proper balance between these two extremes."[5]

As John Ihor Basko, D.V.M., "reaches deeper levels of mastery, he often discovers that the more you know, the more you don't know. . . . Oriental medicine comes from [the insight] that ultimately we don't know how the body works, and nature cannot be explained by the mind. You can't always go by the recipe." Dr. Basko sometimes gets a hunch to put a needle in a certain point without knowing why, then later will read about it and discover the ways in which it was appropriate. Ultimately, any improvement seems to owe itself to a rebalancing of the entire body and mind.[6]

As with homeopathy, it's important to glean as much information about the cat's general habits, attitude, background, and family life. Placement of the needles may be determined according to such factors as the personality and characteristics of the cat, the time of day the problem occurs, and the kind of weather that makes it worse.

During the physical exam, the anatomy of the cat is examined, as are acupuncture points along the backbone. A specific point may be tender or painful when a cat has a problem with organs or meridians associated with that point. Some veterinary acupuncturists, including Dr. Nancy Scanlan, D.V.M., use traditional tests such as blood panels, X-rays, and stool tests to help them assess the animal's condition.

Animal acupuncture is used to treat arthritis, spinal and disc problems, kidney disorders, metabolic imbalances, aging disorders, cataracts, asthma, and allergic dermatitis. It's helpful in unblocking obstructed urethras in unneutered male cats, may be used during surgical emergencies for shock and respiratory arrest, in treating infertility, and to build immune response. Have your acupuncturist show you how to needle the emergency rescue point; nonbreathing kittens can sometimes be resuscitated this way.

Acupuncture has also been used as an anesthetic; studies have shown that endorphins and enkephalins (pain relievers produced naturally by the body) are released when certain acupuncture points are stimulated. However, restraining a cat anesthetized by this means is problematic.

Relief is often experienced after only one acupuncture treatment, but it usually takes at least three visits before dramatic results are seen. The most difficult thing about acupuncture, as with homeopathy, is that some cats may get worse before they get better. But once through the crisis, their improvement may be quite dramatic and enduring. Says Diane Stein, "In veterinary use, the method is described as giving successful cures in seventy to seventy-five percent of animal cases, many of them listed as incurable by standard veterinary medicine."[7]

You may wonder how your cat will tolerate acupuncture. Many holistic veterinarians report that cats that resist treatment at the first session often prove extremely cooperative in subsequent visits. Many times the cat will let the practitioner know where it hurts and then purr throughout the treatment. If your cat resists acupuncture, please don't force her to be needled. Try just one point and come back another day.

In the experience of Jeanne Demyan, D.V.M., cats generally don't tolerate traditional needling, which requires the patient to sit still for fifteen minutes, while needles are placed and twirled.[8] So she uses a variation called "aquapuncture," in which she injects small quantities of liquid, usually a solution of vitamin B_{12}, at the therapeutic points. She also often administers a homeopathic dose of Aconitum to settle the cat down for its physical exam.[9]

Note that acupuncture may interfere with homeopathy, and the two therapies aren't often used together. If your cat is being treated with a homeopathic remedy, ask your practitioner to tell you what other therapies are complementary.

I wish more conventional veterinarians were open to referring their patients to alternative practitioners when their own methods fail. Many use steroids to rescue animals from acute or life-threatening episodes, but the practice gets out of hand when they prescribe these powerful drugs routinely for chronic conditions. Steroids are known to lead to the loss of normal function in the adrenal glands, which regulate so many body processes essential for a long and healthy life. Furthermore, these substances don't cure; they merely get rid of symptoms. However, cats that have long suffered with chronic disease such as arthritis, often get safe relief through acupuncture, especially if nutrition and other holistic treatments are included in the healing regimen.

THERAPEUTIC TOUCH

THERAPEUTIC TOUCH (T-Touch) therapy, a method devised
by Linda Tellington-Jones, is a type of nonverbal communication
through cellular memory. The practitioner speaks to the cellular
intelligence in her hands, which in turn speaks to the cells in the
body. When working on animals, simply by placing our hands
on the body and moving them in a circular manner, we create a
kind of kinesthetic (sensory) interspecies communication.
Tellington-Jones addresses the issues surrounding Therapeutic
Touch in her books, articles, and videotapes (see Resources).

Many holistic veterinarians employ Therapeutic Touch to
calm and soothe their patients prior to therapy. Circular touch
(generally clockwise) is done gently all over the body. This
method also gives the caregiver valuable information concerning
the cat's state of being. Moreover, the circular method provides
the animal with all four types of brain waves (alpha, theta, beta,
and delta[10]). Dr. Chambreau feels this method supports animals
under homeopathic treatment, and she has heard of excellent
results with behavioral problems as well as severe physical problems. Tellington-Jones cannot explain scientifically how Therapeutic Touch works; nevertheless, it does work.

She initially studied the Feldenkreis Method, which opens
new neurological pathways to the brain through the use of non-
habitual movements.[11] Tellington-Jones then developed her own
techniques based on Feldenkreis's work, beginning with the
concept that every cell in the body knows its function. The use
of the circular movement when done with respect, increases the
speed of healing at the cellular level.

Animals may actually be born with habitual holding patterns, but even the most resistant animals respond to this

technique and learn to release stuck energy. Tellington-Jones has even been successful in changing an animal's self-image and increasing its self-confidence.

Allow your hands to find their own way as they communicate with the cells of your animal companion. Try to tune into her breathing and her response to your touch. You may find your own breathing falls into sync with your cat's. The caregiver need not do anything more than concentrate on making the circles and on sensing the animal's response. And, as always, approach your cat with respect.

I imagine the face of a clock as I touch my cat. Begin at six o'clock and gently push the skin clockwise all the way around, past six and finish at nine. At nine o'clock, I pause and begin again in another spot. It's important to maintain a constant pressure and close the circles. I use my middle three fingers and make $1\frac{1}{4}$ circles at each spot, then I move on and repeat. I rest my thumb and fourth finger (pinkie) against the cat's body to steady my hand.

At the beginning of each session, the speed of your circles should be about one per second. As you feel your cat entering a state of bodily listening, slow down to one circle per two seconds.

Don't do the same area twice and don't connect three circles in row (which we all tend to do initially). Remember to lift your fingers as you close each circle and begin again. You may also use your left hand. Tellington-Jones has found her right to be more effective, but she has trained herself to use both hands.

She calls this circular touch, which generates an energetic release, the "clouded leopard touch." The circular motion seems to imprint on the animal's cells more than simple petting or stroking, which although loving and beneficial, doesn't seem to activate the cellular awareness in the same way.

Tellington-Jones also does little butterfly motions, a kind of touch-and-lift maneuver. Remember, nothing is gained through force. This healing technique enables people and animals to release fear and replace it with trust. Experiment to find the optimal pressure; it may vary from very light, with just one finger, to somewhat heavier, using the entire hand. Be gentler, of course, in areas where the animal feels pain. You shouldn't get tired doing this; it should benefit you as much as your animal companion.

Tellington-Jones suggests we stroke our cat's ears. Many of us do this instinctively. Like most major breakthroughs, this technique is so simple that you may be doing it without even knowing you're healing. However, it becomes even more effective when you do it with intent.

Let your fingers lead you, but don't forget the ears. It's often the best place to start. Work the area of the muzzle and move inside the mouth (working the gums calms the fight-or-flight mechanism). Also work the hindquarters and neck. Do short sessions (fifteen minutes is fine) on a daily basis.

When using Therapeutic Touch we become focused and grounded and thus focus and ground our animals, rather than just offering a few strokes while we think about what we've got to do next in our day. When we are fully present, our cats allow us to connect with them in a profound way, so much deeper than words. Touch is basic to both our species and theirs, and may even extend life.

A Therapeutic Touch video for cats is available (see Resources), and courses are offered frequently around the country.

REIKI
Universal Life Force Energy

PROFOUND healing may result from the power of touch. Reiki, which uses this power, is the channeling of energy in the form of a pure white light through an individual who has been initiated in this method. Reiki originated in Tibet thousands of years ago, and its history may be traced through India, Egypt, Ephesus, Greece, Rome, China, and Japan to the United States.

The difference between Therapeutic Touch and Reiki is that Reiki isn't dependent on the energy clarity or the healing ability of the practitioner, who is only a conduit for the flow of pure white light. Thus, no negative energy may be absorbed by the healer or transferred from the healer. In Therapeutic Touch the intensity and effectiveness of the healing varies with the state of the healer; moreover, the healer needs protection from negative forces and energies, and should center and focus meditatively when engaging in this work.

The Reiki initiation involves a series of four "attunements," which activate and set the energy path in the initiated individual; this energy path remains active for life. It runs from the crown chakra of the individual through their chakra system and ultimately his hands. Whenever an initiated individual touches anything alive, the Reiki energy automatically flows through his hands, with no effort or expenditure of energy on his part.

Three levels are available. First-degree Reiki activates the healing energy so it flows when anything is physically touched. Second-degree Reiki activates the energy so it flows when certain symbols are activated by the Reiki practitioner, who can activate healing at a distance, without physically being present; the practice of second-degree Reiki heightens the power of the energy tenfold. Third-degree Reiki activates the healing energy that sets the Reiki pathways in another individual, allowing the Reiki master to initiate others.

The Reiki method may be used on plants, animals, people, babies and elders, even on mechanical things such as cars and computers. It has been shown to be effective in the treatment of anything from mild imbalances to life-threatening illnesses. You may learn more about this modality by reading *The Reiki Handbook: A Manual for Students and Therapists of the Usui Shiko Ryoho System of Healing* or by contacting Eleanor Haspel-Portner, Ph.D. (see Resources), who initiated me into Reiki.

Dr. Portner, also a psychologist and an accomplished astrologer, felt I'd be able to make good use of this healing therapy in my work with cats. During my initiation, one of her own cats became very vocal, jumped into my lap, and nudged me. I saw in my mind's eye (or through my third eye) a pyramid with a white light coming up and out through the top of my head, and then great bursts of purple, magenta, and rose. My body went from cold to warm and my hands felt energized. That evening I read the material Dr. Portner had given me and practiced on one of my kittens, which had injured her ankle slightly by jumping down from the cat tree. Within a day she was healed.

Dr. Portner told me the story of her introduction to Reiki. After the first attunement, she was instructed to do the first four Reiki positions on herself at home that night. When she awoke the next morning, she noted that she could see without her glasses, which she wears for very severe myopia. After the second attunement, her perfect vision lasted an even longer time.

Dr. Portner (by then a Reiki master) and her family worked on their cat Tippy, which had a highly malignant tumor, from a distance while he was in surgery and in the days following. Much to the surgeon's surprise Tippy recovered, with amazing speed and without any negative effects. Dr. Portner's elderly cat Noble was near death and being overloaded with fluids by his veterinarians. The family did round-the-clock Reiki on him, sustaining him until they could find a veterinarian able to intervene. Within twenty-four hours, he was stable and proceeded to recover.

In recent times, many factions have developed in the Reiki organization. Be careful in your choice of practitioners, since not all individuals who claim to teach Reiki have the keys to do the attunements, and some people who claim to teach Reiki don't even realize that a specific attunement process is required to set the energy path. If you have a desire to learn Reiki first hand, check holistic publications for lectures or seminars being conducted near you.

MASSAGE THERAPY

PET MASSAGE techniques are described in both *The Magic of Massage* by Ouida West (one section) and *The Healing Touch* by Michael Fox (the entire book). Fox suggests we work in the following sequence: feet and paws, legs, abdomen (when my pregnant queens are in labor, I use the same effleurage movement—little butterfly circles on the belly—that I learned in my own Lamaze natural childbirth classes), torso, spine, and neck, head, and ears. Since touch seems to be such an important conduit in the human/animal bond, it's no wonder that it can be an important healing element.

Summing Up Touch

TOUCH THERAPY of any kind is also an excellent way to help us get closer and strengthen the bonds with our cats. But never force your cat to accept any hands-on work (see also chapter 7, "Other Healing Approaches")—let him tell you how much is okay with him, and for how long.

Here's what many touch therapists recommend. Hold your hands, if your cat will allow it, on any one of the seven chakras or a painful spot. See if you can let positive healing energy flow from you via your right hand into your cat, and let any negative or painful energy flow from the cat into your left hand. (If you are more comfortable using the opposite hands, this is fine too.) Then—and this is very important for your self-care as a healer—shake your hands to release any negative energy from your body. Let the cat rest comfortably and utilize this healing in her own way.

Chapter Seven

Other Healing Approaches

VETERINARY ENERGY MEDICINE

A CHANGE in energy precedes a change in structure. As we understand more and more about the workings of the body, medicine will be increasingly energy based, instead of relying on drugs and surgery, Dr. Joanne Stefanatos believes.[1] Robert Becker, M.D., and Strom Nordenstrom have demonstrated that electrons flow through the body in complex circuits at the cellular level, and that changes in the flow of electrons occur in many disease conditions. Likewise, Kirlian photography presents evidence that a halo, or aura, of energy surrounds every living thing, and that disruptions in that aura may be associated with various disorders.

There already exists an electroacupuncture biofeedback instrument that can detect pathological dysfunctions in animals before any physical conditions or symptoms arise. Using such technology, veterinarians will be able to recognize potential danger signs, pinpointing and eliminating disease-producing toxins from the body long before they can become destructive. Most agree that when this form of medicine is readily available, we'll look back on invasive procedures such as surgery and vaccinations as if they were techniques of the Dark Ages. Until then, our only alternative is to think constantly about prevention.

Below I've described some of the modalities that apply principles of energy to healing. See the Resources section at the back of this book for further information about these techniques. As always, consult your holistic veterinarian before implementing any therapy.

LIGHT AND COLOR HEALING

THE HISTORY of light and color healing is both extensive and impressive. Records found in the pyramids revealed that the Egyptians used colors in healing with great success. The Rosicrucian Society has used color therapy since the fifteenth century. Edward D. Babbitt, author of *The Principles of Light and Color*, told of the many values of color healing nearly a century ago; noted spiritualist Edgar Cayce also wrote of its benefits. Over two dozen significant twentieth-century works have expounded on this therapy.

Einstein proved that light is an electromagnetic phenomenon, and that color is a manifestation of the vibration of light waves at distinct and measurable frequencies; each color has its own frequency. White light contains all colors, as seen in a rainbow or prism. The primary colors of white light are red, blue, and green; the secondary colors are yellow (a combination of red and green), cyan (green plus blue), and magenta (red plus blue). See chapter 8, "Astrology," for the correlation of colors to the sun signs of the zodiac.

An *aura*, or energy field, surrounds each living thing. The colors of an aura vary depending upon the condition of the being. A deficiency of vitamins and minerals, for example, would cause deficiencies in aura colors. Vitamins themselves possess color: vitamin A is yellow, B vitamins are orange and red, vitamin C is lemon yellow, vitamin D is violet, vitamin E is scarlet and magenta, and vitamin K is indigo. In addition, each *chakra*, or energy center, in the body has its own frequency, color, and harmonic note. Cats and dogs, like humans, have seven chakras, each of which corresponds to a color (see Auras and Chakras, page 223).

Joanne Stefanatos, D.V.M., refers to light as waveforms or pockets of energy cells (*photons*, particles that travel at the speed of light). Light carries information; sunlight carries all the wave lengths of the color spectrum, including infrared and ultraviolet, which are not visible to the human eye. The sun's rays are absorbed by the aura of the body and, through the chakras, penetrate the body itself. At the cellular level, DNA traps light within the water molecules of an organism. Thus, sunlight resonates within the body to create glowing health.[2]

Though many practitioners may not be aware of it, all healing systems depend on the chemical reaction in the body that produces color and brings about a change in body function. Stanley Burroughs, author of *Healing for the Age of Enlightenment,* tells us that a human burn victim or someone running a high fever has a surplus of red, which relates to the element hydrogen. When a blue light (related to oxygen) is projected, the two elements combine, producing water—in this case perspiration. Thus, blue is apparently cooling; it lowers the fever and cools the burn.[3] However, when color is integrated into the body through medications (generally allopathic), there's a danger of side effects in functions such as digestion, ingestion, and oxidation.

How can you use color therapy at home with your animal? Dr. Stefanatos suggests you surround him with color in the form of bedding, blankets, collars (you might even use little colored kerchiefs for whimsy, if he'll tolerate it), or harnesses. Through the use of color, you can introduce energy that assists in the elimination of waste and congestion. Color, many healers feel, can also repair many forms of damage done by illness and injury.

By wrapping a jug of water in red plastic wrap and leaving it in the sunshine for about twelve hours, you can create energized water, which Dr. Stefanatos says will boost the immune system and acts as a blood builder. Other colors produce different effects. Green-energized water stabilizes energy, yellow treats constipation problems. Note that the water doesn't actually turn colors; it is merely energized by color.

Dr. Stefanatos uses colored utility lights to treat her animal patients, clipping the appropriately colored light onto the animal's cage and running it as often as she deems necessary. She uses only Dura Test Vita light bulbs at her hospital, as they provide the full spectrum visible light along with UVA rays; these bulbs may be purchased, along with a compatible holder, at hardware stores and some health food stores.

If your cat has a painful area, Dr. Stefanatos suggests you use the color green on the area for ten minutes, followed by the color red, which stimulates the immune system and decreases pain. You can use pieces of colored fabric to make a kind of color compress.

For stress, Dr. Stefanatos suggests the use of blue, which stimulates the pituitary gland and decreases anxiety, over the sixth chakra (at the brow, or third eye). A cool color, as mentioned, blue also reduces nerve paralysis, and may be used to treat mange, eye problems, or an itchy rash (hot spots). Blue light also helps cats sleep.

I provide color therapy for my cats by giving them cuddle beds in the appropriate colors. A wonderful seamstress, my mother, Helene Yarnall, makes colored slipcovers for the beds which I change as needed. She also designs the exhibition cage curtains for my show cats, selecting colors that both soothe the animals and show them off.

As you can see, color is very important to our well-being and healing, as well as those of our animals. In addition to being beneficial, color therapy has no harmful side effects.

THE AURA AND CHAKRAS OF A CAT

THE AURA is made up of four bodies (see page 225): the physical body (and, just above it, the etheric double), the emotional body, the mental body (two layers, higher and lower), and the spiritual body (three layers, higher, middle, and lower). Dr. Stefanatos explains that the chakras are aligned along a spiral column in the etheric double, and energy is absorbed from the surrounding air and brought through the chakras into the physical body.

The ancient clairvoyants saw the seven major chakras as spinning wheels of light (chakra means "wheel" in Sanskrit). The various spiritual schools have different systems of identification for the chakras, but a widely accepted version identifies seven major chakras, beginning with the first, or root, chakra, located at the base of the spine; and moving up the body to the seventh, or crown, chakra, located a few inches above the top of the head. (There are also five minor chakras, at the hands and feet/paws and the hollow at the base of the skull, where the brain meets the spine.) A color is associated with each chakra.

First chakra (root/base of spine): Red stimulates the immune system by building up the blood and detoxifying it. This color fights tumors, builds the blood, has an antiviral effect, and relates to the reproductive system and the procreative imperative to survive. Cats with feline leukemia and compromised immune systems should be surrounded by the color red as much as possible.

Second chakra (chi/below navel): Orange is an appetite stimulant and a lung builder. It depresses the parathyroid glands, and stimulates the thyroid as well as the mammary glands in the production of milk. The qi (chi) emanates from this chakra.

Third chakra (solar plexus): Yellow stimulates the gastrointestinal system and helps keep hormones in balance. It's also beneficial for the liver, gallbladder, kidneys, and for diabetes and hard chronic tumors. The fear/fight/flight mechanism originates here.

Fourth chakra (heart): Green stabilizes energy and is a bronchiodilator. It's beneficial in the treatment of infections. Many believe that love emanates from the heart chakra.

Fifth chakra (throat): Turquoise (blue/green) aids in the healing of third-degree burns, scratches, sores, and infections. It's beneficial for all fevers that respond quickly when used in conjunction with holistic remedies. Turquoise soothes irritations, inflammations, and itching. It helps induce sleep, and should follow green in treating all infections. It is known as the chakra of self-expression.

Sixth chakra (third eye/brow): Indigo worn around the neck helps stabilize the thyroid if an animal has a hyperthyroid condition. The brow chakra is best known for providing living things with intuition and instinct.

Seventh chakra (crown/above head): Violet increases the white blood cell count, stimulates the spleen, and is a color for high spiritual attainment in humans.

A Cat's Aura

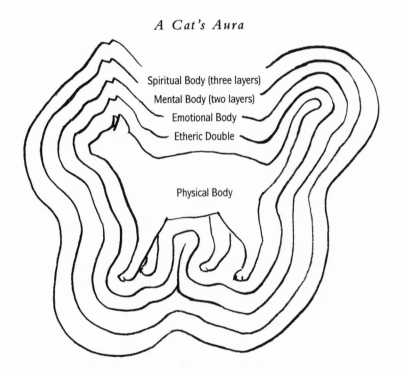

The etheric double is the nearest nonphysical level.

The Major Chakras and Their Colors

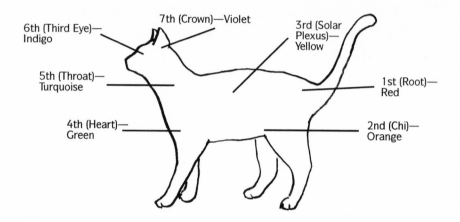

6th (Third Eye)—Indigo

7th (Crown)—Violet

3rd (Solar Plexus)—Yellow

5th (Throat)—Turquoise

1st (Root)—Red

4th (Heart)—Green

2nd (Chi)—Orange

CRYSTALS AND HEALING

MANY OF us have browsed through crystal shops at one time or another. But what actually are crystals? Basically, they're solidified substances created when water combines with an element under certain conditions of pressure, temperature, and energy.

Sand (silicon) combined with water, forms quartz (silicon dioxide). Quartz amplifies, transforms, stores, focuses, and transfers energy. This crystal has the ability to vibrate at precise rates, making it invaluable in the manufacture of modern timepieces.

If quartz is squeezed, it generates electricity. When an electrical current is sent through it, it swells; alternating currents cause quartz to swell and shrink, an action that, when done rapidly, becomes oscillation. Quartz vibrates at specific rates based on the shapes into which it's cut, and transforms electricity into waves that can be broadcast, such as radio and television signals. A bit of quartz crystal in a microcircuit increases an electrical signal; this is how microphones and all audiovisual equipment evolved.

Quartz is also used to transmit information within computers, thin slices storing large amounts of data in memory. Quartz focuses energy in lasers, and helps astronomers measure distances in seconds. It can burn through a steel wall as readily as it assists in delicate eye surgery.

Dael, author of *The Crystal Book,* explains that crystals have piezoelectric properties[4] (that is, they can produce a small electric current when mechanical stress is applied to them). Since the body is electromagnetic in nature, it responds to crystal therapy. Crystals don't interact directly with the physical body, but rather with the fundamental energy system that creates and supports the body, and connects it with the mind and emotions. The physical body exists only by virtue of energy; we get energy from food, water, air, and the earth itself. In conjunction with the mind, crystals can create functional changes that manifest in the physical body.

Healing can be viewed as getting energy back into the cells of the ailing being when something has been blocking the flow of energy into those cells. When energy is brought back, new and healthy cells form, and the patient becomes well.

Pain is a signal from the cells to the brain that something is wrong in the body. When painkillers coat the nerve pathways and thus block communication from the cells, the brain doesn't receive the distress signal and therefore doesn't know anything's wrong. So it doesn't send the necessary healing energy to the cells, and the condition worsens.

Unlike painkillers, crystals actually feed energy to the cells, which can then repair themselves and turn off the pain signal once it isn't needed anymore. Quartz crystals oscillate at the same frequency as the RNA and DNA in human beings and animals, says Dr. Stefanatos, as their geometric structure is the same.

The Shapes and Sizes of Crystals

TUMBLED or polished stones seem to open up and increase energy.

Crystal balls disperse energy in all directions. Egg-shaped stones are excellent for scanning auras; just point the small end toward the body. Some practitioners use the egg shape in acupressure.

Collect several crystals in different sizes and shapes. Listen to your heart as you select them. But please don't use your own crystals on your cat—get special crystals for use on other beings.

Varieties of Healing Crystals

IT'S IMPORTANT to use only quartz crystals. Dael lists clear quartz, smoky quartz, and green quartz as the most effective for the physical body—clear as an overall energizer, smoky for grounding, and green to interact with the endocrine glands for balance and harmony.

Rose quartz (pink) and citrine work on the emotional body. Rose quartz balances the loving emotions of the upper four chakras (heart, throat, third eye, and crown). Natural citrine (light orange to brown) balances the emotions of the lower three chakras (root, chi, and solar plexus). Tumbled golden citrine stimulates the crown chakra.

Amethyst (purple) is the spiritual stone, and it charges or transmutes lower energies into higher, more spiritual levels. It's also used in healing.

Any of these stones may be made into an amulet and suspended from your cat's collar. When worn point down over the heart chakra, they have a grounding effect. The stone may even be inscribed with the cat's name and/or your phone number. It may be cut to a special shape, such as a heart, a cross, a star, or an angel. Before wearing them, be sure to wash stones in soap and water, then place them in salt water for seven days. And don't forget to program your stones with loving thoughts and emotions.

Using Crystals to Help Your Cat

TO DO an aura scan, Dael writes, gently assist your cat to lie on her right side. Hold the crystal point down between the thumb and the first three fingers. Start at the top of the cat's head (or seventh chakra), about an inch away from the body. You are now within your cat's aura. As soon as you feel heat and some tingling emanating from the cat, move the crystal over the body from chakra to chakra, ending at the root chakra and, finally, the tip of the tail. The entire process can be done without actually touching the cat.

When you feel or sense something (coolness, resistance, more tingling, or just a hunch), stop at that place and make a counterclockwise movement around the center of the disturbance. Keep circling in this way until the crystal feels heavy. Move your hand down to make contact with the body and touch the point of the crystal gently to the center of your circle.

Keep going over the body and making these corrections. When you reach each of the four paws, sweep from the head to the paw as if you were smoothing the coat. This aligns the energy of the aura into a smooth, even pattern.

Then turn the cat over and repeat the entire process on the left side. Once you've opened the chakras by this means, close them again by imagining a zipper at the cat's rear paws. Just pretend to pull the zipper all the way up to the top of the head. The cat should be relaxed and even sleepy, with a feeling of balance and well-being restored.

Diane Stein tells an amazing story about her fourteen-year-old poodle, Duffy, which had been diagnosed with a grade-3 heart murmur on the left side. Stein had tried homeopathy and acupuncture, and reached what she describes as a plateau. A recent blood profile on Duffy had showed an elevation of certain heart muscle enzymes, which indicated damage. The dog was clearly not improving.

Stein placed a quartz crystal pendant around the dog's neck at the thymus gland and applied smooth tumbled quartz crystals to the dog's halter, one crystal over each heart valve (the right and the left) and one each at the top and bottom of the chest, forming a double pyramid encircling the heart chakra. Six days later, Duffy's cough subsided, her murmur disappeared, and her blood tests showed normal heart enzyme levels. Stein continued to monitor the dog, which (at the time Stein wrote her book) still showed no sign of the condition that had ailed her.[5]

Please note that Stein placed four crystals in the shape of a pyramid around the heart chakra on the inside of the halter.[6] The pyramidal design is appropriate to healing, as it focuses energy in a tight beam through the apex, or top, of the pyramid. Quartz grows in a spiral pattern, causing energy to flow out of it in the same pattern. When pyramid and spiral are combined, energy flows in a tight spiral beam, which may be focused very easily. If you took two Kirlian photographs of an animal, one as is and another with the animal wearing a halter with crystals, you'd see that its aura had increased fivefold.

You may create a kind of gem elixir by placing a clean gem in spring water in the sun for two or three hours. The solarized water is then charged with its own energy, the color of the stone, and the full-spectrum electromagnetic energy of sunlight.

You may also energize your cat's food by placing a crystal underneath the food bowl. Dr. Stefanatos energizes a feline patient by placing a crystal at each corner of the cat's bed, under the bedding, with the base of the crystal toward outside air and the point toward the cat. She feels this stimulates the immune system.

You don't need to believe that crystal therapy works in order for it to have an effect; however, a positive belief system does provide a supportive atmosphere. Dael suggests that belief consists of getting out of the way of what you want to accomplish. Regardless of what you believe, it goes without saying that you want both you and your animal companion to lead a happy, healthy life.

If one of my cats or kittens isn't feeling well, there's very little I wouldn't try in order to assist her in healing. I recently slipped crystals under the bedding of three queens during the birthing of their kittens. They produced thirteen live births out of thirteen. I'll never know if the crystals helped, but you can bet I'll do it again!

HEALING WITH SOUND

THE VERY same noises—squabbling children, barking dogs, lawn mowers, traffic, television—that bombard us from the moment we awake also bombard our cats, but it sounds three times louder to them![7] Humans may learn techniques of stress control—meditation, relaxation—and tap into their own inner resources to find a moment of peace and relaxation.

Cats must deal with it in their own way. Their immune system, like ours, can breakdown amid the many unnatural influences of modern life. And soothing sounds can enhance their feeling of well-being, just as it does ours. The simple act of listening to music or other healing sounds may therapeutically augment other healing therapies.

The ancient Greeks were actually among the first to develop the idea of music as a healing entity. Zithers were played at mealtime to aid digestion. Artistotle thought flutes aroused strong emotions, leading to a cathartic release. The ancients no doubt regarded music as a type of psychotherapy that affected the body through the soul. Henry Sigerist wrote that Greek physicians restored physical balance with medicine, and mental balance with music.[8] Today it's known that some kinds of sound help integrate the functions of the left and right hemispheres of the brain.

The late John Craige, D.V.M., wrote that there's nothing in the universe of real substance. Even the most solid piece of rock consists of an arrangement of energy. All energy (whether in the smallest subatomic particle or the largest heavenly body) is in constant rhythmic motion, such as the cycle of the moon as it revolves around the earth as it revolves around the sun. So it follows that cats have rhythms and harmonies too. Their health depends on their bodies being in harmony with the universe.[9]

Many years ago the engineer Royal Rife, while working with radio wave frequencies, discovered that human cancer patients exhibited disharmonies at certain frequencies. He found that, if he subjected the patients to these frequencies long enough, they came into harmony once again, and many were reported cured.[10]

Dr. Craige obtained a frequency generator and attempted to duplicate Rife's work, using a dowsing rod (see The Dowsing Rod and the Pendulum, page 241) to verify that cancer patients were at the frequencies Rife reported. Dr. Craige then tested animal patients with chronic disorders, and found definite reactions at specific frequencies in cats with FelV (feline leukemia virus) and FIP (feline infectious peritonitis). Moreover, the cats seemed to feel better when listening to these specific frequencies.

This is not to say that he effected a cure by this means. Such work on animals is in its infancy, although much has been published on the subject for humans.[11]

Dr. Craige and his wife, Joy Birdsall-Craige, developed several audiotapes they've found effective in treating common feline viruses; skin allergies and severe itching; joint, tendon, and muscle disorders; circulatory and heart conditions; intestinal tract disorders; urinary tract disorders; and immune system weaknesses. When a cat or kitten is convalescing, I place a small tape player nearby and play the Craige tape specific to its condition.

Using his own voice, Wayne Perry, of Signature Sound Works in Los Angeles, has created a tape that covers all the healing frequencies and is quite pleasing to listen to.[12] I had a headache when I entered the meeting room where he was demonstrating the use of his tape, but, as the sound enveloped me, I felt my body release the pain. Perry reports that he has successfully treated many physical and emotional problems with this method. I regularly play his tape for my cats.

Perry has other materials to supplement his tapes, including a correlative healing chart for sound therapy. He has taken the twelve chromatic notes of Western music and keyed them to colors, physical conditions, emotional conditions, the twelve astrological signs, the chakras, the body's hormones, and the elements tied to the chakras and the levels of consciousness.[13]

Perry refers to this practice as the yoga of the celestial sound within.[14] His philosophy is based on the belief that sound, light, and love are the ingredients for balancing and healing any imbalance or disease. The Sufis used sound for healing, and for millennia Tibetan bells, Gregorian chants, and mantras have been among the tools used to achieve spiritual realization.

Perry suggests that the vibration or frequency of each being is related, as with color, to the notes of the scale. If the note of D is missing or overemphasized in the human voice, for example, problems in digestion can arise. We (and perhaps our companion animals) are drawn to those who have our missing notes. Perhaps our cats are *toning*, and we aren't aware of it. With astrology as a guide, I can use Perry's concept to see why I, a Leo, am so drawn to Romeo, my Aquarius cat; or why a Taurus, whose birth note is C-sharp and whose color is orange, could be drawn to his opposite, a Scorpio, whose birth note is G and whose color is blue-green.[15]

We can use the sounds of our everyday life to heal ourselves and our cats. Instead of allowing the barking dog to annoy us or the construction crew down the street to upset us, we can choose to resonate with these sounds or to deflect them, the way martial artists redirect their opponent's force. Hear the sound. Let it come, then replicate it. Instinctively, when my cats make a sound, I imitate it. Then, they usually come to me or repeat the sound, and we have a little dialogue.

I play new-age music often in my home, to alter the mood and expand awareness. My cats especially like recordings of bird calls, which are available from various nature stores and catalogues. A friend sent me a tape entitled "Pet Pops—For Cats" (see Resources); the cats settle down nicely and meow along with this tape when I play it in the car on the way to and from cat shows.

If you prefer a more conventional seventh-chakra stimulus, play some Mozart. One study found that listening to ten minutes of a Mozart piano sonata improved the scores of college students in a test of abstract reasoning. The researchers believe the music stimulated brain cell activity.[16]

Whatever sounds or music you choose is entirely up to you. Just be sure to your cats can enjoy it too. Try recording conversations between you and your cat, to play when you're not home. I've been told that, when I call my own answering machine to leave a message, my cats run to the phone to hear "Mom." Our voices are pleasing to them, but so is the silence, so let them have some quiet time as well.

MAGNETIC THERAPY

THE OLDEST form of physical therapy known to humankind, magnetic therapy dates back to 200 B.C. Paracelsus used magnets to treat jaundice and hernias. Veterinarians Joanne Stefanatos and John Fudens are among the holistic practitioners who use magnetic therapy to treat animals.[17] Dr. Fudens feels that biochemistry has historically overshadowed biophysics and that, as this emphasis shifts, medicine is undergoing rapid change, as such is illustrated by the use of magnets in healing.

A magnet is an object, such as a piece of iron or steel, that is charged with an electromagnetic field and as such possesses the ability to attract certain substances, such as iron. Each magnet has two poles, north (yin/green) and south (yang/red).

Biophysically speaking, magnetic therapy polarizes anions and cations (negatively and positively charged ions), bringing tissue salts from a state of inactivity and stagnation to one of order and alignment. The body is normally neutral in terms of polarity. When magnetic field lines, or lines of force, impact an organism or its various parts, they permeate and repolarize the cells, each of which acts like a microchip or miniature battery. Where injury has depolarized damaged cells, electromagnetic stimulation causes tissue fluids to flow again, as with a recharged battery (see Radionics, page 238). The body can then eliminate waste products; swelling (edema) and congestion are regulated, and cell metabolism reverts to normal.

Animals suffering from afflictions as diverse as arthritis and hyperactivity may benefit from magnetic therapy. The Massachusetts Institute of Technology, and several European universities have found that certain magnetic devices increase blood flow, which may be useful in treating some orthopedic and congenital problems possibly attributable to a lack of blood flow and a disturbance of nerve tissues.

Many practitioners who use magnets believe that exposure to the north pole of a magnet slows down the processes of the body, and also state that it relaxes the body, decreases blood pressure and growth of abnormal cells, treats fractures by decreasing acidity and thus allows bones to heal faster, sedates the nervous system, decreases the growth of bacteria and viruses, decreases inflammation and assists in the healing of burns, and increases the amount of potassium ions in the body. In addition, exposure to north decreases the white blood cell count and increases the red blood cell count, which when done after birth increases the life span by decreasing protein metabolism and thus increasing intelligence (the south pole increases intelligence when used just *before* birth).

The south pole increases cell growth and stimulates the production of endorphins, but it also increases the size of tumors, growth of bacteria and viruses, the amount of sodium in the body, and the level of acidity; if used on a fracture, it increases healing time. Dr. Stefanatos suggests that we never use the south pole to treat cats which have active infections. And don't use the south pole over the head, as it may create abnormal behavior and increase inflammatory reaction in the body by increasing the white blood cells.

In her video "Holistic Pet Care" (see Resources), Dr. Stefanatos demonstrates several ways to use magnetic therapy. However, I don't recommend trying it at home on your cats, unless you've been instructed by an extremely reputable veterinarian trained in this complex science. Magnets are extremely powerful and may be dangerous if used improperly. Dr. Fudens further warns that very ill or toxic animals need to be treated with extreme caution and only for short periods of time.

To treat a burn, Dr. Stefanatos simply holds the north pole of a magnet against the burn. For abnormal behavior, she holds the north pole over the third-eye chakra. She treats cataracts, glaucoma, and kidneys on the verge of renal failure with little stick-on magnets. Dr. Stefanatos also employs magnetism to treat the beds of arthritic cats, which by this means are then able to sleep peacefully and receive therapeutic treatment at the same time. She uses magnets in pairs to treat many other feline conditions.

Dr. Fudens has constructed a magnetic pad for the animal to lie upon, allowing him to treat the whole body at once. He reports having relieved pain and inflammation, stimulated tissues, increased circulation, increased oxygen to the tissues, and facilitated rehabilitation in his animal patients with the use of magnets. Though we can't achieve miracles with magnetic therapy, many benefits may be derived simply by improving cellular function.

RADIONICS AND
INTRINSIC DATA FIELDS (IDF'S)

ORIGINATED by an American physician Albert Abrams in the late nineteenth century, *radionics* is the study of the energy fields and centers of the body, and how they are affected vis-à-vis health and disease.[18] Radionics comprises a holistic approach to healing based on the force fields that govern the function and well-being of the entire body. Its purpose is to help an organism reestablish optimum health. Physics and paraphysics, science and spirituality meet and merge in radionics.

The basic concept behind this practice is that all life forms are submerged in the electromagnetic field of the earth, and that each life form has its own electromagnetic field, which, when distorted enough, results in disease. Furthermore, the electromagnetic field of the earth provides the link between the practitioner and patient during analysis and treatment. It is an ancient axiom that energy follows thought, and thought is transmitted through the energy field of the earth, allowing the practitioner to attune himself to the patient.

Life begins and ends on the cellular level, and each organism, regardless of the size and shape of its cells, is a product of input from its environment. From a radionics viewpoint, the cell—the essential unit of organic structure—is viewed as an electromagnetic resonator capable of emitting and absorbing vibrations. Each cell has its own particular frequency of resonance.

Health is defined as equilibrium in the vibrations of the cells, and disease as the disequilibrium of these vibrations in absorbing, emitting, or transferring energy. Such disequilibrium originates from external causes, such as toxins or microbes. If a harmful external vibration is greater than the normal vibration of the cell, disease and pain result. If the cell can adequately defend and increase its vibration, health returns; if not, the cell dies.

Many factors enter into maintaining the proper cell frequency. Among the more common are proper diet; clean air and water; a stress-free, high-quality lifestyle; and the ability to receive divine light from a higher intelligence. All cells must be fully mineralized and balanced for optimum health and energy. The higher the rate of vibration, the higher the vitality of the cell and, by extension, the higher the being's overall state of health. Violation of these factors doesn't always lead to disease, but if the violations accumulate long enough and the cells continue to be deprived of balanced energy, exhaustion sets in on the cellular level and disease results.

Consider the body as if it were a car battery. If the electrical charge is drawn from the battery faster than the alternator can replace it, and if the battery is not cared for properly with water and sulfuric acid, soon it won't have enough charge to start the car. With a car, we may simply replace the dead battery with a new one. Unfortunately, we can't do this with a human or animal body.

The vibration of a cell may be measured by an oscilloscope or other monitoring devices capable of registering the rate and level of an electrical impulse. Once these vibrations, or patterns of energy, have been measured, therapy can be selected which will raise or lower them to the appropriate level, and thus balance the energy pattern and restore health. Radionics allows detection of potentially serious conditions at an early stage, so therapy may be instituted before the condition manifests through physical symptoms.

As the body is not physically invaded during measurement or treatment, radionics is totally harmless. New Horizons Trust prefers to use the term *Intrinsic Data Fields* (IDF's), as *radionics* sounds similar to something it is not: radiation. IDF's are fields or patterns of information that describe the nature and relationship of particles. Every particle has an IDF associated with it, and the connection between particles is known as an *IDF link*.

For years scientists have written about the probability of telepathic activity among particles. In 1935 Einstein, along with his colleagues Podolsky and Rosen, proposed the quantum mechanics theory known as the "EPR Paradox," which states that when two particles move apart, measuring one will give us information about the other, that is, a telepathic link exists between the particles. They believed this would happen even if the particles were separated by thousands of miles. Their theory was proven valid in tests by physicist John Bell in 1966.

By learning to read IDF's, we may access valuable information about everything in our world, including the proper intake of food and supplements by humans, animals, and plants (including livestock feeding and crop fertilization); it's also useful in problem solving and decision making. Flashes of intuition, such as knowing who's calling before you answer the phone, are apparently the result of IDF's; what we refer to as our "sixth sense" appears to be the ability of the human mind to read and interpret IDF's.

Government and industry have actually used the dowsing rod, an ancient but powerful instrument (see below), to detect IDF's for the purpose of locating wires and tunnels. Sophisticated software and electronic devices such as New Horizons's SE-5, an instrument somewhat like a biofeedback machine, are also available.[19]

THE DOWSING ROD AND
THE PENDULUM

THE EARLIEST dowsing rods (also known as divining rods) were forked wooden sticks used to detect underground water and metal deposits. Those interested in the history and uses of the dowsing rod and the pendulum may want to read *The Diviner's Handbook: A Guide To the Timeless Art of Dowsing* by Tom Graves (see Resources).

Recently, I was privileged to read an unpublished manuscript entitled "Healing Hands: Energy Flow in Treating Disease" by the late John E. Craige, V.M.D. I had consulted with Dr. Craige many times and was intrigued by his diagnostic use of the dowsing rod to detect oscillating energy, whose presence signals metabolic and traumatic disorders, throughout the meridians of the body.

Dr. Craige learned how to use this instrument from Wayne Cook, a famous water dowser. Using a hand-held antenna made of spring steel, with an aluminum handle and a weight on the end, Cook demonstrated his ability to detect the energy flowing through the body. He was able to discharge such oscillations (or interruptions in normal energy flow) by placing his left hand on the affected part of the body and holding the rod in his right hand.

Cook was even able to discharge the oscillations in his own energy flow through a sort of venturi effect, as with our kitchen faucets, where aeration of the water regulates its pressure and flow, thus cutting down on splashing. To relieve a headache, he placed his left hand on his head and discharged the oscillations accumulated there. Cook worked with Dr. Craige at his animal clinic, and soon the veterinarian was practicing with a rod of his own.

The dowsing rod became invaluable to Dr. Craige in understanding and interpreting the wisdom and knowledge hidden in his unconscious mind. "The most logical explanation of [the success of] acupuncture, homeopathy, faith healing, and possibly chiropractic," he wrote, "is that these procedures manipulate the energy flow through the body, allowing normal healing processes to work effectively. The missing link in this theory is how do they work?" He concluded that the discharge of oscillations or blocking energies might explain how all these healing methods work.

Dr. Craige began experimenting with the dowsing rod in conjunction with acupuncture. Whenever he identified an acupuncture meridian with oscillations, he placed acupuncture needles along that meridian. Ultimately, he was able to plot the course of all twenty-six meridians using the dowsing rod. Though he did observe some differences between traditional acupuncture and the results of his research, for the most part his findings confirmed what acupuncturists already believed.

Although Dr. Craige's opinions and methods are somewhat controversial, he had a long and successful track record combining the dowsing rod technique and use of the soft laser with acupuncture. Once, when I visited his clinic, Dr. Craige asked if he could have a look at my throat. By using the dowsing rod he determined that I was just getting over a bout of the flu, and he began treating my throat with the rod until the oscillations stopped. I felt better after this, as did my cat Romeo, stressed from a heavy show schedule, after his treatment.

Tom Graves suggests that dowsing may be beneficial in conjunction with homeopathy after the practitioner checks the description of symptoms. Then a pendulum may be used to find the appropriate remedy in a potential list.

The pendulum should weigh about two ounces and hang from about three inches of string or links. It should swing, rather than bob around, as you hold it between thumb and forefinger. Mine has a little brass hand to hold on one end of the string, and the pendulum itself is a cylindrical gem. You can use a charm or medallion on a chain.

Rather than starting the pendulum at rest as your neutral position, Graves suggests, begin with an oscillation as neutral, that is, swing the pendulum lightly back and forth while you rest your mind on its oscillations, so its line (axis) of swing remains stable.

Two kinds of reaction are significant, a change from oscillation to gyration, either clockwise or counterclockwise; and a change of swing from side-to-side, to back and forth. The change from oscillation to gyration is the usual reaction to an object, such as a food or a remedy. Traditionally, pregnant women have used the swing of a pendulum to predict the sex of their children in utero. In order for this information to be useful, you must preassign values to the direction of gyration or swing. For instance, you might select a back-and-forth swing for "yes" and a side-to-side motion for "no."

Some people place tremendous trust in energetic healing modalities. If you wish to try them yourself, it's best to remain open and see what you think. The dowsing rod, the pendulum, and other esoteric instruments are best left to those with integrity and a lot of experience, but novices may have success if they're willing to learn something new. Again, consult your veterinarian or holistic practitioner before embarking on any new therapy.

Chapter Eight

Astromedicine
for Your Cat

WHY AN astrology chapter in a book about holistic health care for cats? I don't use astrology to chart my daily life or that of my cats, but I'm interested in the signs of the zodiac (the twelve sun signs), and their corresponding personality traits, as they apply to us, our cats, and the special relationship we have with them. Astrology is much more than reading newspaper horoscopes—it can be used as a healing science.

For hundreds of years we've known that the seasons result from changes in the distance and angle of the sun's rays relative to the earth, and that the phases of the moon affect the tides, the planting of crops, even the success of the fisherman. It isn't a big leap to suppose these variables affect all living things, including our cats.

The only way we can assist them in healing and cleansing their own bodies is to look for clues to appropriate natural remedies or methods of healing. The more aware we become of feline traits and actions, the better equipped we'll be to help our animal companions. Often, studying the sun signs—each of which governs a different part of the body—helps me select effective homeopathic remedies. (However, the widely respected holistic veterinarian Christina Chambreau, D.V.M., cautions us to remember that this method diverges from the classical curative approach to homeopathy.)[1]

When I plan a litter of kittens, I give careful consideration not only to what season they'll be born in, but to what sign of the zodiac will guide them. Beyond genetics, it's amazing to see how similar are the personalities among kittens in a litter, even taking into consideration differences in sex and pecking order.

The following chapter covers the personality traits associated with the signs of the zodiac in conjunction with various homeopathic treatments, among them Schuessler's tissue remedies or cell salts, Dr. Bach's flower remedies, and aromatherapy.

Though the serious astrological practitioner would develop a natal horoscope based on the exact time and place of the cat's birth (one of my clients actually times the birth of her kittens with a stopwatch and has a full chart on each kitten), this isn't absolutely necessary for our purposes. The in-depth approach can be extremely informative, and I myself have consulted periodically with experts in the field.[2]

But the care, feeding, and spiritual well-being of our cats can benefit enormously if we simply learn about their astrological archetype—a means to begin looking past their velvet fur and the sparkle in their eyes. On your own, you could cast a relationship chart determining your compatibility with your cat. Or you may wish to dig deeper, either learning how to set up a chart or working with those who can.

What if you don't know your cat's birthday or exact age?

Well, you could choose a sun sign to celebrate the day you adopted her or the sign closest to her in personality and likeness. If we look deeply enough, we can understand who each of our cats is from a spiritual point of view and then explore the many healing philosophies (such as the oriental system of yang and yin) and apply their principles to our animal friends.

AN ANCIENT HEALING SCIENCE

IT IS interesting to note that the Chaldean priests of ancient Babylonia were also physicians who incorporated the astrological knowledge of their time in their medical work. They helped women organize their lives to bring their children into the world under the best possible cosmic conditions. According to astrologer and author Richard Ebertin, the priests took water from different colored transparent vessels that corresponded to the time of birth, and sought medicinal plants that they thought resembled certain planets.[3]

In Greece during the sixth and seventh centuries B.C., the time of the Orphic mysteries, tonal vibrations, music, and consecrated oils were important components of ritual. Even that long ago it was understood that a beautiful and harmonious environment supported self-healing. The stars were said to be the handwriting of heaven.

Empedocles (about 493–433 B.C.), the Greek philosopher, poet, and statesman, taught that all life was derived from the "root of things."[4] The four elements—earth, air, fire, and water—created various mixtures out of which arose love and hate, and in turn these active forces were continually uniting and separating the elements.

To Hippocrates (about 460–377 B.C.), "the father of medicine," has been attributed a piece of writing relating the heavens and the human body. He required his students to study astrology, stating that "the man who does not understand astrology is to be called a fool rather than a physician." When a dreamer sees the stars dimmed or obscured by atmospheric influence, Hippocrates wrote, he or she can determine the severity of a disease, its cause, and the appropriate remedy. Many other ancients were concerned with zodiacal plants, which are said to develop their full potency if they are gathered, prepared, and used when the sun is positioned in the appropriate sign (see How to Make Your Own Flower Essences, in chapter 5).

During the reign of Alexander the Great, the theories of oriental and Grecian astromedicine were first integrated. Two centuries later the astronomer Hipparchus (about 190–120 B.C.) divided the zodiac into 360 degrees and expanded the concept of correlating body parts and organs to the zodiac and the planets. And about 196 B.C., through a cultural exchange between Greece and the Roman Republic, astrology became known in Rome.

However, it was in Rome that the practice began to deteriorate, when Augustus had all astrologers and wizards exiled. As is true today, there was a great gap between serious astrological study and superstition.

Known as the "king of astrology," the Alexandrian mathematician, astronomer, and geographer Ptolemy (Claudius Ptolemaeus, about A.D. 100–170) is considered to have been one of the last great scientists of antiquity. His work still forms the basis of many astrological textbooks.

When the Christians entered the scene, they taught that the stars do not rule fate but act as pointers to the future. It's interesting to note that the numbers three, four, seven, and twelve are significant numerologically in both astrology and Christianity (the trinity, the four elements, the four cardinal signs, the four evangelists, the seven days of creation, the twelve disciples, the twelve zodiacal signs, and so on).

Such early astrophysicians as G. W. Surya reiterated what the Swiss alchemist-physician Paracelsus (Phillippus Aureolus Theophrastus Bombast von Hohenheim, about 1493–1541) had taught: that astrology is one of the pillars of medicine. Surya quoted Cicero's dictum, "It is sufficient to experience what happens even if we do not know how it happens."

Even this brief history of astromedicine suggests that its principles are extremely deep-rooted. Our ancestors had the foresight to look beyond the medical philosophy of declaring war on disease which is the basis of modern allopathic practice. The mainstream medical system rarely seems to consider that we're responsible for our own condition and that of our animal companions. How can caregivers not see that all beings are the sum total of their diet, actions, genetics, and environmental conditions?

ASTROLOGY AND THE MODERN CAT

AS YOU'VE seen, people throughout the ages have applied these principles to every aspect of their physical and spiritual lives. In much the same way, you can explore the twelve sun signs to help you augment your relationship with your cat companions. Regardless of any suggestions given, your cat's symptoms must always be your guide. And remember, consult a holistic veterinary practitioner before embarking on any therapeutic course of

action. (See chapter 5, "Natural Remedies," for further information about the substances described below.)

Schuessler's Twelve Tissue Remedies (Cell Salts)[5]

IN THE following descriptions, the twelve tissue remedies, or cell
salts, developed by Dr. Schuessler are correlated to the twelve sun
signs, based on studies done by astrophysician Inez Eudora Perry,
who believed the human body was a microcosm of the cosmos.[6]
With their spiritual underpinnings, Perry's choices for these remedies seem more applicable to the cat than treatments suggested by
practitioners such as Dr. M. Duz and Dr. Fritz Schwab, who based
their recommendations solely upon human physical characteristics. Since there are twelve of these salts, each has been associated
with the appropriate astrological personality:

Aries	Kali phosphoricum (Kali phos.)	potassium phosphate
Taurus	Natrium sulfuricum (Nat. sulf.)	sodium sulfate
Gemini	Kali muriaticum (Kali mur.)	potassium chloride
Cancer	Calcarea fluorica (Calc. fluor.)	calcium (lime) fluoride
Leo	Magnesium phosphoricum (Mag. phos.)	magnesium phosphate
Virgo	Kali sulfuricum (Kali. sulf.)	potassium sulfate
Libra	Natrium phosphoricum (Nat. phos.)	sodium phosphate
Scorpio	Calcarea sulfurica (Calc. sulf.)	calcium (lime) sulfate
Sagittarius	Silicea (Sil.)	silica
Capricorn	Calcarea phosphoricum (Calc. phos.)	calcium (lime) phosphate
Aquarius	Natrium muriaticum (Nat. mur.)	sodium chloride
Pisces	Ferrum phosphoricum (Ferr. phos.)	iron phosphate

Bach Flower Remedies

ALSO INCLUDED in the discussions below are suggestions for the use of Dr. Bach's flower remedies. Based upon the work of author Peter Damian, who states that Dr. Bach treated the personality, character, and mood of his human patients,[7] I've selected twelve of the thirty-eight flower remedies to correspond with the sun signs and Bach's twelve states of mind:

Dr. Bach's Twelve States of Mind

1. Fear
2. Terror
3. Mental Torture or Worry
4. Indecision
5. Indifference or Boredom
6. Doubt or Discouragement
7. Overconcern
8. Weakness
9. Self-distrust
10. Impatience
11. Overenthusiasm
12. Pride or Aloofness

In my opinion, the twelve signs of the zodiac relate directly to the twelve Bach flower remedies, as each sign involves some weakness that we can help our cats overcome as they grow and evolve. However, other remedies apply as well.

Bach's seven classifications (Seven-Step Method) may also be applicable to the sun signs. Using this method, you can prepare combinations that cover a broad spectrum of emotional states. All thirty-eight essences are employed in this system:

1. Fear: Aspen, Cherry Plum, Mimulus, Red Chestnut, and Rock Rose

2. Uncertainty: Cerato, Gentian, Gorse, Hornbeam, Scleranthus, and Wild Oat

3. Insufficient interest in present circumstances: Chestnut Bud, Clematis, Honeysuckle, Mustard, Olive, White Chestnut, and Wild Rose

4. Loneliness: Heather, Impatiens, and Water Violet

5. Oversensitivity: Agrimony, Centaury, Holly, and Walnut

6. Despondency and despair: Crabapple, Elm, Larch, Oak, Pine, Star of Bethlehem, Sweet Chestnut, and Willow

7. Overconcern for the welfare of others: Beech, Chicory, Rock Water, Vervain, and Vine

Homeopathic Remedies

THE HOMEOPATHICS I've selected for each sun sign are only a sampling of remedies that might apply. I based my choices upon Ebertin's research pertaining to the sections of the body ruled by the governing sun sign, but have made some of my own suggestions as well.

Metals

I'VE ALSO included the eight metallic solutions corresponding to each of the heavenly bodies (the sun, the moon, and the seven planets known to the ancients:

Gold (Aurum)	Sun
Silver (Argentum)	Moon
Quicksilver (Mercurius)	Mercury
Copper (Cuprum)	Venus
Iron (Ferrum)	Mars

Tin (Stannum)	Jupiter
Lead (Plumbum)	Saturn
Zinc (Zincum)	Uranus

Paracelsus, who was also the father of the pharmaceutical industry, became interested in metals by watching his father, a mining engineer, bring ores up from the underground. He was struck by the idea of using minerals and metals as remedies.

Although we seldom hear of metallic solutions being used in modern medicine, such cures were employed in ancient times. However, today we do have colloidal silver and colloidal gold available to us (see My Special Supplements in chapter 4, "Nutrition"), as well as homeopathic dilutions of metals.

Aromatherapy and Sound Healing

ACCORDING to author Scott Cunningham,[8] there are plants and essential oils associated with each sign of the zodiac—more than one aroma for each sign because most planets and elements rule more than one sign. You can use aromas to strengthen or decrease the influence of your cat's sun sign. For example, offering a Leo cat a whiff of ginger oil would only serve to increase his in-born propensity for aggression—unless you specifically visualize otherwise.

Healing sounds are also pleasant additions to any household where felines and humans enjoy a celestial bond.

YANG AND YIN: HEAVEN AND EARTH

IN CHARTS based on the astrological system described above, the horizontal plane that joins the ascendant (rising sign) and the descendent (descending sign) separates the visible from the invisible part of the heavens. The upper half is regarded as positive, and the lower half as negative. If we were to drop a line from the meridian, it would divide east and west, with the eastern half designated as positive and the western as negative.

The Chinese, relying on a 5,000-year-old tradition, regard heaven as yang (the generation of all that exists in the world), and earth as yin (the recipient of heaven and the bearer of heaven's progeny). Yang and yin are represented by the symbol of a circular disk divided by a wavy line. One side is dark (yin), the other light (yang), but rather than being antagonistic, they flow into one another and unite in oneness. This interrelationship is also pictured as a six-pointed star formed by the overlay of two triangles—yang with its apex pointed upward, yin its apex pointed downward—the superimposition uniting positive and negative, male and female.

We can further classify yang as the ambient-oriented type (ambient referring to external surroundings) and yin as the internal- or interior-oriented type. C. G. Jung referred to them as "extrovert" and "introvert." The ambient cat may be completely consumed with his territory, and the interior cat withdrawn and introspective, sensitive and reserved. Ambients are centrifugal (outward) in force, interiors centripetal (inward). Yang is vertical, yin horizontal. Yang corresponds to the sun and day, yin to the moon and night. During the day, the cat is up on all fours (vertical). At night, he is down (horizontal). At night, in the yin position, both humans and animals absorb more cosmic energy, which we give out again during the day, in the yang position.

Male and female/day and night (yang and yin) signs alternate in the zodiac. The male and female sign (positive and negative charges) form a continuous circle all around the circle of the zodiac.

Aries	Male	Libra	Male
Taurus	Female	Scorpio	Female
Gemini	Male	Sagittarius	Male
Cancer	Female	Capricorn	Female
Leo	Male	Aquarius	Male
Virgo	Female	Pisces	Female

Yang is associated with bright, warm colors; yin with dark, cool colors. The range of the spectrum falls between them, uniting the two in a kind of yang-yin rainbow:

Yang—red, orange, yellow, green, blue, indigo, violet—**Yin**

The color of your cat may be significant. To create a balance you may, for example, tie a brightly colored cloth or a kerchief on your yin-colored cat (red or yellow on the blue [gray], or black). Buddhist monks wear saffron robes supposedly because it stimulates their minds.

Here's a summary chart of the properties of yang and yin:[9]

Yang	Yin
Male	Female
Summer	Winter
Ordered	Disordered
Day (Turns Into...)	Night
Dry	Wet
Positive	Negative
Hard	Soft
Heavy	Light
Condensing	Dispersing
Fertilizing	Fertilized
Concentrated Applied Energy	Diffused Misapplied Energy

When the balance of yang and yin is disturbed, imbalance in the body may result. Balance may be restored through the use of natural treatments (for instance, a yin disease may be cured with a yang remedy). However, we must not fall into the trap of thinking that yang and yin are clear-cut concepts or tendencies. Rather, they flow into one another, alternate, and change from moment to moment. Both diet and healing play a big part in this.

We can maintain or restore balance by supplying the appropriate yang and yin foods. When planning your cat's menu, you may obtain guidance from her birth chart or, at least, her sun sign. A Jupiter type needs to be restored by yang foods.

Heating, salting, and seasoning with bitter herbs make foods more yang. Cooling by adding liquids, flavoring with aromatic spices, grating and crushing makes foods more yin. When cereals are soaked in water or when they are sweetened, they become more yin. As for the foods themselves, some are more yang, others more yin.[10] Just think in opposites:

Yang Vegetables	Yin Vegetables
Lettuce	Asparagus
Carrots	Cauliflower
Dandelion Greens	Kale
Garlic	Peas
Turnip	Cabbage (Red and White)

Yang Meat	Yin Meat
Beef	Pork (never to be fed to cats)
Chicken	
Fertilized Egg	
Lamb	
Venison	
Veal	

Yang Fats/Oils	Yin Fats/Oils
Rapeseed (Canola)	Suet (Beef Fat)
Sesame	Butter/Margarine
Soy	Lard
Sunflower	Olive Oil
Wheat Germ	Palm Oil

Yang dairy products
Soft Cheeses
Camembert
Goat's Milk

Yin Dairy Products
Buttermilk
Cream (Fresh)
Kefir
Milk
Yogurt

Yin (Miscellaneous)
Honey

ASTROMEDICINE AND THE SUN SIGNS

PLEASE STUDY the information provided for all twelve signs, as each sign governs a different part of the body. Again, consult your holistic practitioner before beginning any treatment.

Aries (The Ram)

March 21–April 19 (also March 21–April 21[11])
Cardinal element: fire
Ruling planet: Mars
Earth colors: cerise, magenta
Astral colors: white, rose pink
Gems: amethyst, diamond
Mineral element: iron
Bach flower: Impatiens
Cell salt: Kali phosphoricum

Aries, the first sign of the zodiac, represents birth. The ram is the newly born Lamb of God. Aries effects the cerebral nervous system and whatever is dependent on it. The spinal chord, sensory nerves, pituitary, face, and lower jaw are also influenced. The planet Mars stimulates the cells, influencing diseases relating to inflammations, fevers, and organ lesions; there may be a predisposition to liver problems. An elementary quality of dry heat is associated with this cardinal fire sign.

In his mind the Aries cat, even when from a large litter, is an only child. Strong and assertive, he makes his needs known when he's hungry. When he wants something, he'll get it. When he's awake, everyone's awake. If he doesn't answer when you call, it's not that he doesn't know his name—the Mars-ruled cat is simply self-absorbed, and he'll get to you when it's convenient for him. All the world is seen from his point of view.

Aries's kitten charms and naiveté linger into old age. He's cunning and extremely hard to resist. Though he can be vulnerable, he nearly always gets his own way with people and other animals. He's also fearless, and somehow always able to land on his feet. The old motto "If at first you don't succeed" fits him to a T. If he ever gets lost, he'll find his way home through the worst conditions. He'll persevere to the end, even if he dies trying.

As a fire sign (he shares this element with Leo and Sagittarius), he's got a sunny disposition that will cheer you in your darkest hours. Though not usually a lazy, by-the-fireplace cat, Aries cat does seek warmth, and lies in your lap or by your side when you sleep.

The unneutered Aries male is the eternal night stalker and gets into brutal fights, as exemplified by the Graeco-Roman god of war, Mars (Ares). In fact, Aries can be so aggressive that the chances of his becoming seriously injured or dying in a cat fight are very high. So please keep Aries (and all other) cats indoors and spay or neuter them (unless they're part of a breeding program). Many of the aggression problems encountered in Aries cats disappear after this simple altering procedure. But, no matter what, they'll never stop believing they're top cat.

The Aries cat is extremely curious and can be accident-prone. He'll love you intensely and share his possessions, but don't try to take something away from him unless it's dangerous, as he will resent you for it. Aries is the sign of authority, after all.

As always, be gentle, as Aries's ego bruises easily. When led with love and given plenty of exercise, this cat will be a champion at everything he does. Whether purebred or household pet, the Aries cat is very outgoing and quite the showman. He enjoys the spotlight.

To call him extremely intelligent is an understatement. If he could speak in human words, he'd have an answer for everything and would need always to be right. As it is, your life with the Aries cat will be a contest of strength and wit, with never a dull moment.

The Bach flower remedy *Impatiens* is appropriate for this willful and aggressive cat. Either Impatiens or Rescue Remedy (which includes Impatiens) can be utilized when the Aries energy and egocentric nature becomes overbearing.

The cell salt *Kali phosphoricum* (potassium phosphate) can be especially helpful when the Aries cat seems despondent, depressed and irritable, or impatient. Perhaps he is grieving the loss of some close animal or human friend, or homesick after a change in residence. Cold aggravates these symptoms, and he doesn't want to be alone, but he seems better after he rests, eats, and finds warmth.

The element *iron* (ferrum), related to the planet Mars, has always been a tonic for anemia. An old folk remedy prescribed sticking a clean nail in an apple overnight and then eating the apple for breakfast. Homeopathically, iron is used for sore muscles and rheumatic disorders. It may also benefit worm infestations in kittens, symptoms of which include regurgitation of food immediately upon taking it in, and abdominal flatulence.

Consider the following homeopathic remedies for Aries:[12]

Aconite (*Aconitum napellus*) when the head, cranial nerves, or ears ache, or if there is nasal catarrh. One of the guiding symptoms is sudden fever or inflammation with a propensity toward anxiety, fear, and anguish.

Arnica for a headache or bruising condition (following surgery). Use alternately with *Hypericum*.

Belladonna for a hot head or face and fever (I often use it after *Aconite*), or when the skin becomes red and hot to the touch. Guiding symptoms include a full, pounding pulse and dilated pupils.

Bryonia alba when there is a reduction of temperature through exposure to cold and a great thirst for water. Symptoms include chills accompanied by fever.

Chamomilla for teething discomfort.

Hypericum for symptoms associated with head and face.

Nux vomica when a symptom associated with the head, jaw, or face leads to stomach upset that produces bad breath.

Pulsatilla for conjunctivitis of the eyes when yellow discharge is a guiding symptom.

Sulphur for extreme fear and aversion to light.

The plants and essential oils associated with Aries are clove, coriander, cumin, frankincense, ginger, neroli, pennyroyal, pettigrain, pine, and woodruff. The ruling planet Mars is enhanced by basil, coriander, cumin, garlic,[13] ginger, hops, nasturtium, onion, and rue.

Taurus (The Bull)
April 20-May 21 (also April 21-May 21[14])
Cardinal element: earth

Ruling planet: Venus

Earth color: cerise

Astral colors: red, scarlet, orange, lemon yellow

Gems: moss agate, emerald

Mineral element: copper

Bach flower: Gentian

Cell salt: Natrium sulfuricum

Taurus governs the cerebellum, the liver, gallbladder, thyroid, throat, and neck, with a possible relationship to kidney problems. The sign of purification, Taurus is ruled by Venus, which controls intercellular fluid and influences infectious diseases. Being an earth sign means vulnerability in the back of the head and down the spine to the liver. An elementary quality of dry cold associated with this sign.

The Taurean cat will do whatever she wants whenever she wants to. Her shyness is endearing, though it may be frustrating when you'd like to show off her charming ways to friends and neighbors, but she won't perform. Even to animal trainers the stubborn Taurus proves quite a challenge. However, outside this pigheadedness, Taurus cats are a delight to have underfoot and love to be cuddled on your lap. Taurus cats tend to bond with one person, but can be magnanimous with their affection.

Taurean people are very outspoken. Without speech, the Taurus cat needs to express herself through physical means, so she needs plenty of exercise. A cat tree made of natural wood and hemp placed next to a sunny window will please her. If you had an aviary or an aquarium, she would delight in watching the birds fly or the tropical fish moving about in the water.

Vibrations and harmony are very important to Taureans' well-being. Harsh or bright lights and colors upset them, as do loud noises, so keep the stereo turned low. But they do love sound, such as the jungle, bird, or whale sounds found on nature tapes and CD's. Buy one of these, or better yet, make your own audiotape, reading "The Owl and the Pussycat" in your gentlest voice. Actually, all cats appreciate audiotapes of human companions' voices played when they're alone.

Taurus cats have great powers of concentration. They try very hard to understand what you need, but this has to suit them or the bull emerges victorious. If you're lucky enough to adopt Taurus as a kitten, you'll delight in watching her grow into a magnificent cat. Taurus females make wonderful mothers.

The Bach flower remedy recommended for the Taurus personality is *Gentian*. Because of their typical obstinacy, they're usually slow but sure, and resistant to change—the bulls of the cat world.

The cell salt *Natrium sulfuricum* (sodium sulfate) can be used homeopathically in relationship to excess water. It occurs rather abundantly in nature (in sea water and saline springs). The mental symptoms to watch for in cats are wildness and irritability followed by restless, sleepless nights. The Taurus cat will seem disheartened. Since Taurus relates to the cerebellum, the nervous system, and the liver, these cats may experience dizziness (the top of the cat's head may be sensitive also) accompanied by the presence of bile (the tongue may be coated, and the matter produced by vomiting yellow tinged), and diarrhea tinged with yellow. Combing or brushing the cat in this condition may be painful to her, though she'd purr to be groomed when healthy. Her throat might be dry and sore, and she may develop a hacking morning cough with salty mucus. If your Taurus cat usually seeks warmth and symptoms arise during damp weather, you're at least on the right track with this remedy; Schuessler recommends the 6X potency. Remember, though, if these symptoms appear, consult a homeopathic veterinarian before administering the remedy.

Copper (*cuprum*) relates to the planet Venus. *Cuprum metallicum* and *Cuprum aceticum* are particularly valuable in treating kidney disease. *Cuprum arsenicum* is valuable as a therapy for diseases of the urinary tract in doses of 3X and 12X.

Consider the following homeopathic remedies for Taurus:[15]

Aesculus hippocastanum (horse chestnut) when the symptoms include dry nose and throat with scanty secretions, dry cough, catarrh of nose and throat, throat inflammation, coughing made worse by cold air, coughing in the morning, and liver conditions affecting the general circulation. The tongue may be coated.

Alumina for nasal catarrh and sore throat due to the weakening of vocal chords owing to excessive calling when in estrus (heat cycle). There could be straining before urination, with a white sediment occurring occasionally. The spine may degenerate and the claws become brittle.

Arnica for sore throat when there seems to be pain (yawning seems difficult), for bruising injury when skin is unbroken. Use after surgery or during birth,[16] as it lessens the danger of difficult labor. *Arnica* can also be used externally for bruising and swelling in cream form, when the skin is *not* broken.

Arsenicum for laryngitis, cat flu, and any sore mouth condition, as well as for vomiting and diarrhea with foul smell. It is valuable in treating feline enteritis and skin conditions that produce dandruff-like flakes. Guiding symptom is the aggravation of conditions toward midnight.

Belladonna for dry, inflamed sore throat, thyroid conditions, or inner ear disorders. Its early use can help prevent brain damage from fever. The skin usually feels dry, with generalized redness and heat, and the cat does not want to be touched and is thirsty. The pupils of the eyes dilate, and the cat shows an aversion to light, with a fixed, staring look. Use of *Belladonna* often follows *Aconite.*

Calcarea carbonica (calcium carbonate) for catarrhal involvement of mucous membranes leading to the discharge of mucus. Throat glands are enlarged and appetite is frequently irregular.

Camphora for nasal discharge and larynx-related breathing problems. Skin can be icy cold to the touch. *Camphora* is also of value for low immune response that creates susceptibility to salmonellosis.

Chamomilla for teething.

Hamamelis (witch hazel) for overactive thyroid and pharyngitis.

Hypericum (Saint John's Wort) is for mucus in the throat, dry cough, scraping sound in the throat. It is also indicated for liver dysfunction with jaundice. However, its primary use, both internally and externally, is with lacerated wounds. It can be alternated with *Ledum* or alternately with *Arnica* after surgery, and is ideal after spaying or neutering.

Ignatia for grief and sadness, or for when kittens are taken from their protective Taurus mothers and sent to adoptive homes.

Iodum (iodine) for thyroid disorders. Symptoms may include a ravenous appetite and loss of condition.

Pulsatilla when you see bland yellow discharge from eyes and nose, uterine discharge (tendency toward pyometra and false pregnancy), feline influenza with eye symptoms, including yellowish discharge.

The plants and essential oils indicated for Taurus are: apple, cardamom, honeysuckle, lilac, magnolia, oakmoss, patchouli, plumeria, rose, thyme, tonka, and ylang-ylang. The planet Venus corresponds to: apple, chamomile, cardamom, catnip, daffodil, freesia, gardenia, geranium, hyacinth, iris, lilac, magnolia, mugwort, narcissus, palmarosa, plumeria, rose, spider lily, thyme, tuberose, tulip, vanilla, vetiver, white ginger, wood aloe, yarrow, and ylang-ylang.

Gemini (The Twins)

May 21–June 21

Cardinal element: air

Ruling planet: Mercury

Earth color: orange

Astral colors: red, white, blue

Gems: beryl, aquamarine, dark blue stones

Mineral element: quicksilver (mercury)

Bach flower: Cerato

Cell salt: Kali muriaticum

Gemini, which has a predisposition to neurosis, is governed by the planet Mercury. The nervous system, as well as the respiratory system, glands, fibers and tissues, shoulders, paws, and toes are all governed by this sign. An elementary quality of wet heat is associated with Gemini.

Gemini is male and female, extrovert and introvert, aggressive and passive—all rolled into one cat. This animal is a lesson in duality, giving you a full range of emotions and physical attributes. *He'll* give you a nip asking you to pay attention, then *she'll* turn around and lick the same spot. He/she, she/he, back and forth. You'll think, "Oh well, this is a typical feline behavior." But no, it's not; it's just Gemini.

You may be hoping to have your very own lap cat, but the truth is, this one belongs to the world. When you leave Gemini with the house sitter, you may fret that he'll die without you. But he's happily bonding with the sitter just in case you don't come back, and if you don't, he'll cozy up to the real estate broker too. It's not that he's fickle, but that, just as the scorpion's nature is to sting, Gemini's is to be all things to all creatures. Maybe you should just pretend you're as special to him as he makes you feel.

The Gemini cat is a multifaceted, creative cat—poetry in motion. No doubt he'll create something, even if it's havoc. He's ruled by Mercury, the winged-footed Greek god, so prepare to fly with him as if he were a catbird. He can slip through your fingers like quicksilver. Gemini is an air sign, and air must circulate freely, so let him have the run of the house. But with a harness and leash, you can stroll with him in the garden (keep off the grass, please—that's where fleas live).

Gemini won't want to be out for long though, since he's always in conflict. Just watch that tail swish to and fro. It seems to say, "I'm here, but I'd really like to be there, wouldn't I?" He'll rarely finish anything, including dinner. Instead, he'll be off making mischief somewhere. Such curiosity!

Gemini is quick. A bird or mouse doesn't have a chance. He'd like to eat it, but his twin likes to taunt, torture, and play with it first—hunger and patience at odds. Could we call him fidgety? No, everyone else is slow. Just let him be, as he changes so fast all his little quirks are here and gone in an instant. His mind is like a computer sifting through so much fancy so fast that not even the most avid nonverbal communication expert can get it all.

The Bach flower remedy to consider for Gemini is *Cerato*. In China, Gemini is known as the monkey sign because of its restless nature. However, Gemini cats like company and are rarely loners. They're intelligent, but sometimes do foolish things because of their inquisitive nature.

The cell salt *Kali muriaticum* (potassium chloride) is recommended for Gemini. Said to be in constant conflict between its yang and yin personalities, this cat might just convince one of his alter egos to starve. Since the respiratory system is governed by Gemini, it doesn't hurt to look first at such symptoms as loss of voice, white tongue, asthma, white mucus that seems difficult to bring up, a spasmodic cough, wheezing sounds, and rattling pneumonitis, a common upper respiratory ailment in cats. Usually introduced through the kitten's vaccinations, this group of viruses overloads the immune system and shuts it down. As a result, upper respiratory symptoms may become chronic—and only made worse through the abuse of antibiotics. Other guiding symptoms include white mucus (could also be yellow or greenish as disease progresses) discharged from the eyes, white dandruff, white catarrh from the nose, skin eruptions after vaccination, and a sluggish constitution. Schuessler uses 6X and 12X potencies of *Kali Mur.* This remedy can also be applied to the skin for burns, dry white eczema, and even warts.

Quicksilver (mercury) is the mineral element that corresponds to Gemini, which is ruled by the planet and god Mercury. This remedy, prepared under homeopathic guidelines, is administered for agitation with fear, restlessness, and irritability. It's also used for conjunctivitis and bronchial catarrh. The recommended doses are 3X and 12X. A guiding symptom is abundance of slimy saliva, as with spongy gums and stomatitis (an acute condition of the gums).

Consider the following homeopathic remedies for Gemini:[17]

Aconite (*Aconitum napellus,* monkshood) if there are cramping pains in the limbs and the joints become swollen, hot, and painful in motion. Also for pneumonia conditions with heat of body, thirst, dry cough, and nervous excitability.

Arsenicum for cough, shortness of breath, restlessness, wheezing, even bleeding from the lungs.

Bryonia alba for gastritis, dry cough with thirst, nasal discharge, possible bleeding, extensive inflammation in the pleural surfaces. When the guiding symptom is deterioration from movement, the cat prefers to lie on the affected side during pneumonia or pleurisy.

Eupatorium perfoliatum (boneset) when the cat feels bruised, weak in the limbs. The bladder may also be affected, causing cystitis.

The aromas Gemini responds to include: benzoin, bergamot mint, caraway, dill, lavender, lemon grass, lily of the valley, peppermint, and sweet pea. Mercury corresponds to benzoin, bergamot mint, caraway, celery, clary sage, costmary, dill, eucalyptus, fennel, lavender, lemon verbena, lily of the valley, marjoram, niaouli, parsley, peppermint, spearmint, and sweet pea.

Cancer (The Crab)
June 22–July 23
Cardinal element: water
Ruling planet: Moon
Earth color: orange-yellow
Astral colors: green, russet-brown

Gems: pearl, black onyx, emerald

Mineral element: silver

Bach flower: Clematis

Cell salt: Calcarea fluorica

Cancer is ruled by the Moon, which governs cell modularity and the blood. This sign also relates to the breasts, stomach, digestive organs, spleen, and elastic tissues. It is predisposed to diseases of the head and abdomen. Wet cold is the elementary quality associated with this water sign.

The Cancer cat is a gentle creature prone to staring wistfully at you—or at what you may think is nothing—for what seems like an eternity. She's very happy you keep her inside, as she's most content sitting by the hearth or in any warm, cozy spot. She looks like she's posing for a Christmas card wherever she alights.

A strong individual, the Cancer cat often prefers to go off by herself, whether she's the only cat or one of many. However, if your spirits are low, she'll more than likely stay by your side. She's easy to spoil.

The Cancer cat's tenacity is unparalleled. Usually the first to arrive at the food bowl and the last to leave it, she'll never let you forget that her sign rules the stomach. The Cancer cat tends to put on weight easily, so control portions and see that she exercises regularly. Cancer is also the most sentimental sign of the zodiac. This means she gets strongly attached to people, animals, and things, so don't reassign a food dish or a bed without her permission.

As a kitten, the Cancer cat will tend to bond with one person. She may run and hide when someone new enters, or stand her ground and hiss if approached. Quite vulnerable, she can be so dedicated to protecting herself that the slightest input can cause her to withdraw. But when left alone at night or separated from her companions, she's likely to cry and moan for the duration.

My Chloe tends to play "top cat" even though she's the shyest of all my animal companions. Hissing and growling when provoked by her feline friends (or anyone else for that matter), she's merely masking her fear with aggression. The Cancer cat tends to feel alienated since she can't share herself for fear of a potential defensive reaction.

Lightning, thunder, earthquakes, new people, and dogs can set her off, even when cats of other signs aren't bothered at all. She's also very adept at picking up human fear, so it's important for you to remain calm through a crisis. She tends to need constant reassurance.

You may be dismayed when people come to visit and make disparaging remarks about your Cancer cat's moody or unfriendly behavior. It seems only you know that there's a loving creature behind that growl. But if you don't give this cat all the love and security she needs, she may become reclusive. A nonthreatening approach is always best to coax this cat from her shell.

The mythological ruler of Cancer is Diana, the Roman goddess of the hunt and the Moon. Cancer's symbol is the crab, an animal whose habits shed a lot of light on cats born under this sign. When the crab is frightened, she runs into the sea or behind a rock, emerging only when she has resolved her feelings.

The Cancer cat can change moods quickly and dramatically. Just as the Moon, to us the fastest-moving body in the heavens, may hide behind the clouds and then emerge as a beautiful globe of light in the darkest sky, so does the Cancer cat go through her changes. When she's in touch with the emotional needs of those around her, she can be a great comfort. When she's not in touch, or out of control, she can be miserable.

My mother's cat, Teddy, was born on the fourth of July, like my daughter. He was an only kitten at birth, and she an only child. Their similarities are amazing, even though they were born twenty years apart and are of different species. They can each be crabby and irritable at times, and then the personification of sensitivity.

Cancer cats make wonderful mothers. If your female Cancer cat is to be spayed, and especially if she is the only cat in the family, adopt a kitten for her to nurture. She'll sulk and make a fuss at first, but the bonding that occurs will be profound. Remember, when left alone, Moon cats tend to get morose, so having their own friend is especially important. To them, being the only cat in a human family is a little like our living with a rhinoceros. We may be nice to them, feed them and play games with them, but we're not their kind. It's nice to have someone your own size to play with, someone who speaks fluent feline.

The Cancer cat never forgets anything and is extremely sensitive. Never laugh at her, and be careful not to make her feel foolish. Your Moonchild may get clingy and overbearing sometimes, but she's so endearing that you're likely to love and need her just as much as she needs you.

The Bach flower remedy for Cancer is *Clematis*. The Cancer cat often has a faraway look in her eyes. When she withdraws, try Clematis, along with something to nurture. A kitten would work wonders, but a rabbit might intrigue her as well. At the same time, they like their solitude and, as their guardians, we must respect their space. Cancer lives more in the dream world, and requires more sleep than most other signs. Cancer is the mother sign of the zodiac, and Clematis helps revive their vitality when they wear themselves out caring for others.

The cell salt for Cancer cats is *Calcarea fluorica* (calcium fluoride). One of the guiding symptoms for this remedy is deep depression. She may vomit undigested food, be prone to gastritis, be constipated and strain during bowel movements. She may seem weak in the morning and be very fatigued all day, taking more than normal daily naps. When she sleeps, she dreams vividly of impending danger. She is worse in damp weather. Schuessler recommends a 12X dosage when these symptoms are present.

Silver (argentum) is governed by the Moon, and is used homeopathically primarily in the form *Argentum nitricum* (*Arg. nit.*). The Moon corresponds to the stomach and digestive organs, this remedy is useful in treating gastroenteritis, usually accompanied by abdominal bloating and diarrhea after eating and drinking. Involvement of the stomach leads to vomiting. Because *Arg. nit.* acts on the central nervous system, consider administering it to cats showing fear and nervousness toward other animals.

Consider the following homeopathic remedies for Cancer:[18]

Abrotanum (southern wood, or lad's lover) for stomachache or a constriction in the chest. Primarily in cats, it's used for eruptive skin conditions with bluish discoloration and a tendency to alopecia (hair loss). The appetite may remain good, but they may be alternating constipation, with a distended abdomen. Wasting may become progressive, developing low and traveling upward; emaciation of the lower limbs is a strong guiding symptom. The symptoms are relieved by movement. A newborn kitten in need of this remedy may show oozing from its umbilical chord.

Alumina (aluminum oxide) for older cats, especially those showing debility. Look for chronic conjunctivitis with aversion to light, but since Cancer governs the stomach, there may be cravings for abnormal substances such as charcoal. Also good for any condition producing emaciation and vomiting, together with weakness of lower limbs; excessive dryness of mucous membranes; feverish states in which temperature remains elevated; cracked skin in an eczematous condition which appears rough and bleeds easily; and straining during bowel movements, with feces hard and knotty following a bout of constipation.

Arsenicum for indigestion, gas, and tremendous thirst but with minimal drinking. The abdomen could be swollen, so consider the possibility of liver and/or spleen problems. Inflammation of the lower bowel produces straining, with a dysenteric stool and a cadaverous odor. *Arsenicum* works quickly to allay vomiting and diarrhea.

Belladonna when the mouth is red, with swollen papillae, and swelling of the throat makes swallowing difficult. The cat is the picture of misery, with colicky pains, noisy gas, and possibly fever.

Bryonia alba (white bryony) because Cancer also relates to fluid balance. You may wish to explore this remedy for dry cough, or extensive inflammation in the lungs. The guiding symptom is the cat's worsening from movement (such as with pneumonia or pleurisy), and the cat prefers to lie on its affected side, bringing pressure to bear and thus restricting movement. Joint swellings may also benefit from this remedy.

Chamomilla for nausea or a bloated stomach after meals (simply making the chamomile tea and setting it out in a water dish is soothing).

Ignatia (Saint Ignatius' bean) for the Cancer mother when she is grieving after her kittens are taken away to their new homes.

Iodum (iodine) for pancreatitis, thyroid, or other glandular conditions, as well as a ravenous appetite with loss of condition. The lymph glands may feel hard, the skin seems dry and withered looking, and there may be increased urination, perhaps dark and strong smelling.

Nux vomica for digestive disorders, including flatulence, indigestion, and vomiting. The area over the liver may be sensitive to touch, and the stool is generally hard. In cases of poisoning from certain plants, *Nux vomica* has been prescribed with success when abdominal symptoms occur.

Pulsatilla for the cat with a sweet disposition, usually a feminine personality. There may be uterine discharge, bland or mucous material; or a creamy yellow discharge from the eyes, ears, and nose. Excellent remedy for pyometra and feline influenza, when typical eye conditions are involved.

Sulphur when there is rattling in the lungs. *Sulphur* also aids the action of other remedies.

The plants and essential oils associated with Cancer are: chamomile, cardamom, jasmine, lemon, lily, myrrh, palmarosa, plumeria, rose, sandalwood, and yarrow. Those ruled by the Moon are influenced by jasmine, lemon, lily, melon, night-blooming cereus, sandalwood, stephanotis, and water lily.

Leo (The Lion)
July 22–August 21 (also July 22–August 22[19])
Cardinal element: fire
Ruling planet: Sun

Earth colors: yellow, gold
Astral colors: red, green
Gems: ruby, peridot, sardonyx
Mineral element: gold
Bach flower: Vervain
Cell salt: Magnesium phosphoricum

Leo is the sign governing the heart, circulation, blood, eyes, and vitality. The lion is Leo's symbolic image and is ruled by the Sun. The Sun cat needs to be careful of inflammations. An elementary quality of dry heat is associated with this fire sign.

Leos love to lie in the sun—it's almost impossible to keep them out of it. But be careful, they can burn through those luxurious coats and experience excessive shedding. Seeking warmth to an extreme, they'll lie so close to the fireplace and heat vents, that you fear they'll roast.

It would be presumptuous of me, being a Leo myself, to refer to feline Leos as the "king of beasts," even though they (and I) think it's true! They're the only sign in the zodiac whose symbol is a beast of prey. To say feline Leos are proud and loyal is an understatement.

They thrive in a positive environment, and need a tremendous amount of love and admiration. They never seem to get enough lap time or petting, and their appetite for food is also insatiable. They love to be spoiled, but give a great deal of love in return. However, it's usually on their terms. If you don't encourage and patronize them a bit, they'll withdraw and brood for a while. This little lion must be given incredible amounts of affection.

Leo cats are very verbal and will have long conversations with you. One meow is seldom enough. They're rarely shy and have a magnificent deep, throaty purr. They greet people at the door and follow them from room to room.

Always the instigator, Leo marches around your home like the Pied Piper, with everyone following behind. If another cat usurps his position, the lion will most likely stalk off and sulk, awaiting the fond caresses of his "subjects"—you and other members of your household. This little cub plays many roles; he'll be your mother or your baby, depending on whether he's in a giving or a receiving mood. He's sunny by nature and will play with, pounce on, and tease all who enter his kingdom.

Leo usually takes center stage. If you're giving affection to another person or animal, he's sure to get in the middle. I suggest you make a special effort to not let him push another cat away from you, correcting him gently and telling him he'll have his turn. He hates to be scolded or demeaned publicly. Leo doesn't understand the meaning of "wrong" or "bad"—he thinks he's always right. However, he does have a great sense of fair play. I could be guilty of projecting a bit here, but indulge me—I'm a Leo!

If you think one Leo cat is a handful, try two. My Colette, a blue mink Tonkinese, was born on my birthday (July 26). My Celina, a Siamese Leo, was born August 22. These two have worked out a truce. Whatever Celina has (the crook of my arm, a toy, or treat), Colette has to have it, too. Celina will share with her, but if Colette gets too aggressive, Celina will give her a quick don't-forget-your-manners nip. They'll end up sparring and eventually licking each other, and all will be well. Leos are not mean cats; they just have a strong desire to be number one. Somehow Celina and Colette worked out a joint royal family rule.

Leo cats have a great sense of dignity. Just like Leo people, they're as theatrical as they are regal, though, so they often show off with acrobatics and high jumps. Leo cats need a lot of stimulation and love new toys, tiring of old ones quickly. Guard against accidents with Leos, as they often don't think before they leap—they just like to be watched and admired. If your Leo does not fit this profile, he may have had less-than-perfect care during the critical first six weeks of his life.

His independent nature will sometimes make you feel you can never get him to do what you want. Be patient and remember to lavish him with praise and affection. You've got a star on your hands, so be prepared to be his fan.

The Bach flower remedy suited to Leos is *Vervain*. Cats born under this sign may suffer from exhausting overenthusiasm. Strong-willed Leos possessed of great courage (the heart of the lion) exemplify Vervain. They tend to be overly concerned for others (such as their kittens and close pals). When this trait becomes overbearing, Vervain is an excellent choice.

Magnesium phosphoricum (magnesium phosphate) is the cell salt choice for Leo when symptoms call for its use. This is a remedy for cramps, convulsions, and other such contractive disturbances. When involuntary twitching of the legs, general tendency to nervous chorea (such as Saint Vitus' dance), or spasmodic movements occur, this cell salt is one to look into. The eyelids may be twitchy, becoming heavy or droopy with tearing, and stomach cramps may cause the animal to paw at his abdomen. The heart may become easily excited, palpitating when spasmodic. Schuessler recommends the 6X trituration; for cats, dissolve one or two tablets or pellets in an ounce of distilled water at room temperature. The guides for this cell salt are symptoms relieved by pressure and rubbing, or those aggravated by cold air, cold food, and so on. The mental state of the Leo cat may seem constrictive, fearful, sorrowful, grieving, or worried. If a simillimum occurs (that is, the remedy corresponds to the totality of symptoms), try *Mag. Phos.*

The Sun is represented by the element *gold* (*aurum*), which is a normal constituent of the body primarily found in the brain, through which it enters the central nervous system and enhances vitality. As the ruler of Leo, the Sun has to do with the heart. *Aurum* is beneficial in treating palpitations and constriction around the heart indicated when the cat draws in deep breaths. *Aurum iodatum* and *Aurum sulfuratum* are also prescribed in 3X to 12X dosages.

Consider the following homeopathic remedies for Leo:[20]

Aconite when there is cardiac anxiety, a full pulse, and increased heartbeat, and in the early stages of all feverish states, when symptoms come on suddenly. Animals that exhibit fear of crowds or strange places will also benefit from *Aconite.*

Aesculus hippocastanum (horse chestnut) when the heart action is full and heavy, or for liver conditions associated with venous congestion affecting the general circulation.

Arnica when the heart becomes enlarged while a generalized cardiac dropsy appears. As a heart remedy, it restores tone to the weakened muscle. *Arnica* reduces shock and should be a routine prescription after surgical procedures and birthing, as it lessens the danger of difficult labor. It can be used externally as well in cream form, when the skin is not broken.

Arsenicum for diarrhea and vomiting, with symptoms worse after midnight, and for skin conditions with dry, scaly, itchy patches, loss of hair, and dandruff-like flakes. Also for restlessness, with the cat frequently changing positions and thirsty for small sips of water.

Camphora (camphor) in the event of shock when the pulse becomes weak and heart failure is threatened. Also for salmonella.

Hamamelis (witch hazel) any condition showing venous congestion and passive hemorrhage from veins.

Aromas associated with Leo are: bay, basil, cinnamon, frankincense, ginger, juniper, lime, nasturtium, neroli, orange, pettigrain, and rosemary. Bay, bergamot, calendula, carnation, cedar, cinnamon, copal, frankincense, juniper, lime, neroli, orange, pettigrain, rosemary, and saffron are attributed to the Sun.

Virgo (The Virgin)

August 22–September 22 (also August 23–September 22[21])
Cardinal element: earth
Ruling planet: Mercury
Earth color: chartreuse
Astral colors: gold, black
Gems: pink jasper, sapphire
Mineral element: mercury
Bach flower: Centaury
Cell salt: Kali sulfuricum

The Virgo cat is ruled by Mercury, which maintains the nerves. Virgo cats are prone to infections. Virgo governs the bowels, intestines (and everything dependent on them), and solar plexus. This earth sign has an elementary quality of dry cold.

Though quick and alert, Virgos tend to be the most tranquil of all cats, their personality making them the most able to handle unfavorable conditions. If you live in constant stress and chaos, the Virgo cat is probably well suited to your lifestyle. But don't forget that even she has her limits, so try not to overload her. She can distress you and then exhibit her own contradictory feline moods, such as wanting to be on your lap but not wishing to be held against her will. Win her trust by avoiding the use of force. She is naturally friendly and has a warm disposition, but can be irritable if you make fun of her. Perceptive and steadfast, she responds best to a gentle approach.

It's been said that contact with cats actively reduces stress in humans. When the human strokes the cat and the cat rubs against the human, bodies almost instantaneously release stress, providing a kind of feline psychotherapy for us humans. But it's more than just the touching of the animal. When you earn a cat's love, the bond is so deep that even people with deep emotional scars, who find it hard to trust, often find their way back to trust through their relationship with a cat. The companionship of a cat may actually reduce blood pressure and calm the overworked heart.

Like the Leo cat, Virgo will usually follow you all over the house as you do chores, content just to see you and be near you.

She may be shy with visitors or at crowded cat shows, but with family and regular visitors this cat certainly won't be at a loss for meows, especially if there is Siamese blood in her lineage. She tries to communicate with you with sound just as you do with words, but she'll also send you pictures with her beautiful eyes so listen with your heart as well as your ears. She may have a wonderful story to tell you. She'll chatter away, but then button up the minute a stranger appears. Mercurial is the word, as she is ruled by Mercury.

She is so well-mannered and easy to be with, you may tend to favor her. She'll announce herself to feline friends with a polite lick, meaning "May I join you?" If rebuffed, she'll retreat, so always be gentle and sensitive with this beautiful creature. She understands "no" very well and usually doesn't need to be scolded, but if she does, a water squirt bottle does the trick. Don't forget, always send a positive mental picture (see Nonverbal Communication in chapter 2, "Interacting with Your Cat").

The Virgo cat loves routine and dislikes having the furniture moved, let alone her litter box or water bowl, so leave things where they are. However, being a Virgo, she'll adapt to change when necessary. Extremely clean and fastidious, the Virgo cat will waltz around her food bowl pawing the ground, in a kind of ritual dance to clean up the crumbs. Every trace must be hidden from predators, who might discover she had dinner on this spot.

She'd probably love a little kitten as a friend, but don't buy a breed of cat larger than she is unless you introduce the new arrival as a small kitten. Virgo likes to mother things smaller than herself, and doesn't want her position to be usurped.

Inquisitive at all times, the Virgo cat must look in every drawer and cupboard, and she hates closed doors. She loves toys and exercise, and delights in something new. The paper bags are almost as much fun as the contents. Always give her the run of the house to explore.

Virgo cats love to learn, and often surprise us by mastering new tasks—such as walking on a leash or coming when called—on the first try. However, if you don't help develop Virgo's potential fully, she can become a sad little introvert.

They need physical affection and encouragement, and love to sleep with humans. Often, they can't wait until you sit down so they can join you on your lap. If another animal or person in the house infringes on her one-on-one time with human companions, Virgo is likely to bolt and sulk under a chair. She gets lonely easily, so remember to give her quality time in great quantities. Virgos also have a fear of falling, so don't throw or drop this cat, not even in fun. Set her down front legs first.

Since she's a good traveler, consider taking her with you when you go on vacation. She'll really appreciate that.

Your Virgo cat may be prone to upper respiratory problems, especially if she hasn't been cleared of the chronic diseases produced by typical feline vaccinations. Some research has actually shown that cats actually acquire the same physical maladies their human companions have or fear the most, so stay as positive as you can.

Centaury is the Bach flower choice for Virgos that are shy, timid, or anxious to please. Just as the Virgo human is meticulous, the Virgo cat is almost always grooming herself, or her feline or human companions. You may not even know when Virgos are out of sorts, as they rather calmly accept their plight. When your Virgo cat has difficulty standing up for herself and gets browbeaten by her pals, try Centaury.

The cell salt for the Virgo constitution is *Kali sulfuricum* (potassium sulfate). As with sulphur, a guiding symptom is irritability. Virgos are not irritable by nature, but rather, only when they don't feel well. When they are out of sorts, they really don't want to be fussed with. And that's the beauty of homeopathy: Sometimes one dose is all it takes; the remedies are easy to administer and don't taste bad. You might notice that Virgo cats in need of *Kali sulf.* feel better in open air. *Kali sulf.* has been used in the treatment of bronchial pneumonia. Certain types of ringworm may benefit from this treatment when the skin shows a shedding or peeling action, is scaly looking, or shreds—a kind of casting off known in homeopathy as *desquamation*. Because Virgo rules the intestines, you may find symptoms such as slimy yellowish diarrhea, as well as excessive thirst, vomiting, mucus and serous discharges that are profuse and yellow (slimy or watery). Loss of smell is typical when these symptoms are present. Remember, if she loses her sense of smell, she'll probably refuse to eat. You may also notice a hacking cough, indicating dryness and constriction. The latter stages of inflammation are served by this remedy. Schuessler recommends 6X and 12X dosages. Compare with *Pulsatilla* in your *materia medica* and choose whichever remedy is more appropriate. Symptoms for both are aggravated in a warm room, discharges are yellow to yellowish green, and there may be pressure and a feeling of fullness (bloating) in the stomach.

The more books you can collect on homeopathy (for both cats and people), the better equipped you'll be to self-diagnose and diagnose for your cats. I always confer with my homeopathic practitioner prior to taking or giving a remedy, but what I read and observe can help that practitioner find the best remedy. Virgo can be an especially sensitive cat, and choosing the wrong remedy—or even the right remedy in the wrong potency—can produce an aggravation. This said, consider the following homeopathic remedies for Virgo:[22]

Quicksilver (*Mercurius hydrargyrum*) in homeopathic dilution is the mineral to consider when Virgo's nerves are fraying. Just as the planet Mercury corresponds to the element, the element responds to the central nervous system.

Abrotanum because Virgo rules the intestines. You may notice anxiety and depression from digestive disorders, alternating constipation and diarrhea. Symptoms worsen at night.

Agaricus for treatment of postdistemper chorea (irregular spasmodic movements of the limbs or facial muscles) as well as eczema with nervous involvement.

Aloe to combat allopathic drug use in congestive states of liver disease. It will help the portal circulation and restore a normal bowel action.

Alumina when constipation occurs, or any condition producing emaciation and vomiting, together with weakness of the lower limbs.

Arsenicum, with its all-embracing quality, is useful in the treatment of many well-defined sets of symptoms or conditions. In gastroenteric conditions *Arsenicum* generally will allay vomiting and diarrhea quickly.

Belladonna when the guiding symptom is a full, bounding pulse during any feverish condition, or when thirst is prominent along with abdominal pain and gas.

Bryonia alba when a yellowish discharge covers the tongue, there is tenderness over the liver area, and in chronic conditions the stool becomes hard and dry. *Bryonia alba* is useful when the cat seems worse for movement, as with pneumonia or pleurisy. The animal prefers to lie on its affected side, bringing pressure to bear and thus restricting movement.

Calcarea carbonica (calcium carbonate) if your young Virgo is fat and lazy, with slow dentition. This remedy, made from the middle layer of the oyster shell, is an excellent way for establishing calcium in a system where difficulty exists.

Eupatorium purpureum for inflammation of the ovaries, together with a tendency to miscarry; pain and tenderness over the kidneys; and cystitis with blood-stained urine. This remedy seems to have an affinity with the urogenital system of both male and female.

Nux vomica for many digestive disturbances and conges-
tions, or when there is gas and indigestion, when vomiting takes
place, there is tenderness over the stomach, and the liver region is
sensitive to touch. Stool is generally hard, but diarrhea and constipation may alternate. *Nux vomica* has proved of value in the
treatment of umbilical hernia in young cats.

Pulsatilla when the mucous membranes are involved. A predominantly female remedy, especially for mild, gentle, yielding
dispositions. *Pulsatilla* types, like Virgo, are changeable. They usually feel better in open air, worse in warm or damp closed areas.
A thick, bland, creamy yellow discharge; lacrimation of the eyes;
and stoppage of the right nostril often occur.

Sulphur is an excellent clearing remedy that also aids the
actions of other remedies. The sulphur type can display irritability. The action of this remedy is centrifugal (outward from within). If Virgo's abdominal (or other) conditions don't respond to
other remedies, sulphur may give your cat the push she needs to
complete the healing process.

The scents associated with Virgo are: caraway, clary sage,
costmary, cypress, dill, fennel, lemon balm, honeysuckle, oakmoss,
and patchouli. Mercury's influential aromas are: benzoin, bergamot mint, caraway, celery, clary sage, costmary, dill, eucalyptus,
fennel, lavender, lemon verbena, lily of the valley, marjoram,
niaouli, parsley, peppermint, spearmint, and sweet pea.

Libra (The Scales)
September 23-October 22
Cardinal element: air
Ruling planet: Venus
Earth color: green

Astral colors: black, crimson, light blue

Gem: opal

Mineral element: copper

Bach flower: Scleranthus

Cell salt: Natrium phosphoricum

Libra, ruled by Venus, governs the bladder and kidneys. A cardinal air sign, it has an elementary quality of wet heat.

The eternal judge, the Libra cat is part angel, part devil. Usually the peacemaker, he has to be right in the thick of it or you'll find him surveying his territory from every conceivable angle. That way he can represent all sides of the equation. Only then can he make a decision—but Libra defines decisions as something you change your mind about constantly. He loves harmony but remains a paradox himself.

The lesson of this sign, if you will, is never to give Libra a choice. He hates to make decisions. With his tail always in motion, he's the eternal cat in conflict: "Should I come or should I go?" It's so difficult to choose, and it's so difficult to get him into the groove of a routine, but this is exactly what he needs. Just feed him the same well-balanced fresh foods at the same time in the same place every day because change will upset his sense of well-being.

Libra tends to be a bit slow. You call and call him for breakfast, but he's more interested in watching something out the window—a blade of grass or a Saint Bernard. It's not that he's stubborn, it's just that he'll come when he wants to. If he doesn't come for meals, let him miss a few. This won't hurt, as long as he has fresh purified water. Perhaps at this moment some serious meditation is more beneficial to his psyche than eating.

And don't rush Libra when he's in the litter box. He'll scratch every inch, before and after—and when you're cleaning, wondering where "it" went. He'll meditate in there, too.

He sleeps all day and plays all night. Always use a firm, gentle tone, and if you can sing, sing to him. Libras tend to be auditory and they like music. If you whistle a little tune, he'll come running. Try "Pop Goes the Weasel" or "You Are My Sunshine." If you have to leave him at home alone, call him often and let him listen to your soothing voice on your answering machine.

Loving and sweet, Libra tends to be a verbal cat, who'll purr sweetly, rub up against you, and roll over at your feet. He'll drive you crazy, but you'll end up living to please him and loving every minute. It's nearly impossible to say "no" to a Libra. And he's difficult to train, as he loses interest quickly.

He'd love to please you, but he'd rather please himself. If you have more than one cat, your Libra will eat out of everyone else's bowl and snooze in everyone else's bed. He'll shed on your favorite velvet chair even though you've said "No chair!" a thousand times. All he hears and sees in his mind's eye is "chair, velvet chair." Don't even try to yell at him; it hurts his ears. If you do, he'll forget what he's been doing anyway.

In the Bach flower repertory, *Scleranthus* is perfectly suited for Libras as they are hesitant, uncertain, and seesaw between moods. The Venus-ruled cat may benefit from Scleranthus when indecision is part of the picture. Scleranthus combined with Rescue Remedy or Centaury can restore balance to their lives during stressful times.

Natrium phosphoricum (sodium phosphate) is the cell salt for Libra, treating the blood, muscles, nerve and brain cells, and intestinal tissues. Nat. Phos. is the remedy for conditions arising from an excess of lactic acid. The liver is the prime and master laboratory of the animal body, and since this remedy emulsifies fatty acids, it's indicated for liver upsets, such as when the cat has eaten fatty cooked meat or poultry (see chapter 4, "Nutrition," for more about the harmful effects of such a diet). Often simply changing the diet to fresh raw foods restores feline health, but if the symptomatic picture fits this cell salt, it's worth considering. Only the fresh food diet ensures resistance to fungus and parasites in the intestinal tract, so if your cat has been on some other diet, you may want to take a stool sample to the veterinarian to check for worms. Anxiety and fear, a kind of dullness with irritability, may be present, and the Libra cat may become upset easily. Other guiding symptoms may be a creamy, golden yellow discharge that glues the eyelids together in the morning; yellow nasal discharge; and yellow coating on the tongue, palate, back of the throat, and tonsils, along with inflammation. The cat may strain in the litter box. Libra governs the bladder and kidneys, so diabetes is something to watch for in its hepatic form.

Copper (*cuprum*) is the metallic element suited to those ruled by Venus. It occurs naturally in blood serum as a catalyst for a series of enzymes, is a component of cellular protoplasm, and controls the activity of the blood-building cells. It is valuable in the treatment of kidney disease accompanied by spasms. The 3X and 12X potencies are usually recommended.

Consider the following homeopathic remedies for Libra:[23]

Aconite if the urine is hot and assumes a reddish color.

Agaricus muscarius when conditions affect the central nervous system. The renal system may be involved when polyurine (large amounts of urine) accompanies a mucous urethral discharge in the male cat's urinary tract.

Aloe to combat use of allopathic drugs as well as the effects of free feeding and the feeding of dry food, which often leads to feline urological syndrome. When the urine is scanty and high colored and urging is frequent, particularly at night, think of *Aloe*. It is also indicated for congestive states of the liver, helps portal circulation, and restores normal bowel action.

Arsenicum album, along with all of its other beneficial uses, for Bright's disease, a kind of chronic nephritis (inflammation of the kidneys). Urinary dribbling may also be noted.

Camphora for the cat that's unable to void a full bladder; for shock, when the pulse becomes weak and heart failure is threatened; or for salmonellosis.

Nux vomica if the urine is scanty and frequently contains blood.

Pulsatilla—besides all of its applications for creamy yellow discharge from eyes, nose, and so on—if increased urination is an additional symptom. Young (often female) animals of gentle but changeable dispositions are well suited to *Pulsatilla*.

Essential plants and oils pertaining to Libra are: chamomile, daffodil, dill, eucalyptus, fennel, geranium, peppermint, pine, spearmint, palmarosa, and vanilla. Aromas attributable to Venus are: apple, chamomile, cardamom, catnip, daffodil, freesia, gardenia, geranium, hyacinth, iris, lilac, magnolia, mugwort, narcissus, palmarosa, plumeria, rose, spider lily, thyme, tuberose, tulip, vanilla, vetiver, white ginger, wood aloe, yarrow, and ylang-ylang.

Scorpio (The Scorpion)
October 23–November 21
Cardinal element: water
Ruling planets: Pluto, Mars

Earth color: blue

Astral colors: golden brown, black

Gems: topaz, malachite

Mineral element: iron

Bach flower: Chicory

Cell salt: Calcarea sulfurica

Ruled by Pluto, Scorpio governs the reproductive organs. Symbolized by the scorpion (and sometimes by the white eagle or the gray lizard), this fixed water sign has an elementary quality of wet cold.

Scorpio is ruled by Pluto, lord of the underworld. The myth that describes Scorpion is that of the phoenix rising from the ashes. She seems to know she can achieve whatever she wants, visualizing the goal before she begins.

The most invincible of signs, she loves a good contest. Such an incredible little specimen, this cat—strong body, strong will. She'll take on the big guys, even the family dog! She'll scrap with her mates and usually win. Scorpio loves a good fight but, mostly, she likes to win—and she possesses the necessary strategy. If she loses the battle, just wait; she'll be hiding around the corner ready to pounce, and won't quit until she succeeds.

If your Scorpio cat is a Cornish Rex or an oriental, you'll swear you're living with a gymnast. To maintain her sinewy muscles, feed her fresh foods and keep her active. She needs to release tension with lots of play, but it's not unusual for her to sit by the sidelines watching others make fools of themselves, whether they're cats or humans.

Watch the Scorpio kitten trying to ascend the drapes (if your fabric holds up)—this is a real challenge, but eventually she'll make it. And then she'll demonstrate tremendous courage, jumping to the floor like a flying squirrel. Don't even let her get started. Buy a big squirt bottle, fill it with water, and holster it to your side.

Just remember, in your house, you're top cat! If you forget, you're likely to feel like a lady- or gentleman-in-waiting. She needs firm but loving discipline. So say it with conviction, right now, out loud, "I am the boss," otherwise your Scorpio cat will get what she wants when she wants it! But remember, the Scorpion can sting, so handle her with care and give her lots of love and affection along with your discipline.

Don't let this aloof little being fool you. She needs your love in lavish amounts. And how can you resist when she stares deep into your soul as only Scorpio can? Her penetrating eyes express an almost unfathomable depth, and she'll never reveal everything to you. That's part of her mystery and her charm. Her eyes will follow you wherever you go, just like the Mona Lisa—she'll even hypnotize you if she can. If you think she's enchanted, you may just be right!

Though you'll never completely understand her, she'll seem wise to things humans can only guess at—forces operating on different levels of consciousness. If you're blue, she's likely to be there for you, licking away your tears before anyone else has an inkling that something's wrong. She'll love to share this little secret with you, and you'll be laughing out loud sooner than you think. But don't take it seriously if sometimes she ignores you. She'll be ready to be social again before long.

She's loyal, but she can be tough, too. When crossed, she'll swipe out and warn you with her claws, but only just enough to let you know she isn't pleased. Don't push when you are warned by her. She may be fun and outgoing, but she never forgets and can hold a grudge against anyone who accidentally, or otherwise, inflicts pain. She'll get you back by scaring you with a jump or pounce when you least expect it. Afterward, she'll lick your hand, so there's no way you can stay angry with her.

The Scorpio cat loves company, but is okay as an only cat also. She bonds with one person easily. If you work at home, she'll be content to be with you. If not, she'd like a friend to torment—just a little. Get her a challenging companion, maybe an Aries or a Sagittarius. However, Scorpio cats are fond of the opposite sex, so be sure to spay or neuter them at six months, unless you're planning to breed them.

Scorpio is a sensuous cat and loves to be groomed. If she's short-haired, polish her gleaming coat with a chamois; she'll love it. She needs lots of stroking, and she'll rub and nudge you back to thank you.

She's likely to be a pack rat. Your favorite powder puff, hair ribbon, or sport socks may disappear and later be found behind the dresser. If you retrieve them, leave a little mouse toy in their place. On the other hand, the Scorpio cat may rediscover a treasured item you thought was gone forever.

The Bach flower remedy *Chicory* is ideally suited for cats whose energy is drawn inward. Chicory types can be jealous, controlling, and possessive, keeping those in love with them in a state of constant attachment. Even though we all cherish the unconditional love our cats offer us, Scorpios seem to have a few strings attached. Humans who are Chicory types harbor a strong need to be thought as significant, so they enjoy company that supports this need. If you find yourself worshiping your feline Scorpio or start to feel as if you're in bondage, consider Chicory and a little Walnut (the remedy for advancing stages and breaking the tie that binds) for yourself. A loving relationship with your Scorpio cat is based on mutuality: "I am in your debt; you are in my heart. I am in your heart; you are in my debt."

Calcarea sulfurica (calcium sulfate) is the cell salt selected for Scorpio. Consider it for septic conditions (the presence of toxins) in general, the chief guiding symptom being pus that has found an outlet (as in an anal gland abscess). Other symptoms include mucous diarrhea with occasional pus, yellow discharge and purulent crusts; a slimy discharge with the stool; changeable mood, fear. The cat's anus may itch, and she may drag her bottom across your carpet. Schuessler recommends 6X and 12X, low potencies for purulent eye troubles with a yellow discharge. The cat is better in open air.

Iron (ferrum) is the metallic element related to Pluto. Prepared homeopathically, this remedy is used to raise hemoglobin and red cell counts. It stimulates the bone marrow and accelerates the circulation of blood.

Consider the following homeopathic remedies for Scorpio:[24]

Alumina is for conditions producing both emaciation and weakness of limbs. A craving for an abnormal substance (such as charcoal) may be seen, as well as straining at stool, with hard, knotty feces.

Arnica is often used both before and after surgery. It can be used prophylactically prior to spaying or neutering and in any condition where bruising and injury occur, even when the skin remains unbroken.[25] It reduces shock. Consider using *Arnica* after teeth cleaning or extraction. (I've found that the teeth and gums of my raw-meat-eating cats stay much cleaner and healthier. However, routine dental care is always advised; try to find a practitioner who doesn't use anesthesia.) This remedy is also appropriate if hunger is constant but food is rejected; for gastric bleeding; and for dysenteric stools accompanied by colicky pain and much straining. The cat may have difficulty expelling urine owing to a weakness in the bladder wall.

Arsenicum album for foul-smelling diarrhea. In the male genital system, orchitis may occur along with swelling of the scrotal skin. In such cases, neutering may be advisable, and a veterinary surgeon should be consulted. When *Arsenicum* is indicated, the cat exhibits thirst for small quantities of water, and other symptoms exacerbate toward midnight.

Belladonna for retention of urine, with straining to pass. Urine could be dark and turbid owing to presence of blood. Use *Belladonna* for feverish conditions, when the cat's pupils are markedly dilated and she assumes a staring look. Glands may show swelling and tenderness. The skin is usually red and hot, and the cat resents being touched.

Chamomilla for a teething kitten. Also of value to the female when there is tenderness and swelling of the mammary glands.

Hamamelis for venous congestion and passive hemorrhage from veins, and possibly blood in the urine. The eyes may appear bloodshot due to congestion of blood vessels.

Hypericum for lacerated wounds. When Scorpio gets into a brawl with another cat, it can be serious. Wounds that may lead to tetanus indicate the use of this remedy, along with Ledum for punctures (Hypericum for lacerations or incisions). These remedies can also be used externally. I often make a lotion of Hypericum and Calendula,[26] and I keep Ledum ointment on hand as well as standardized grapefruit extract ointment.[27]

Ignatia for postpartum Scorpio female cats if they become

depressed when separated from companions or from their kittens. This remedy also has an affinity with rectal conditions such as prolapse.

Iodum for gland conditions in general. The keynotes are a loss of condition and a ravenous appetite, though loss of appetite may also be an indication.

Iris versicolor to control sluggish action of the liver. Can be used to control some types of vomiting.

Pulsatilla for the female cat with a tendency to pyometra, with yellow vaginal discharge; ovarian underactivity leading to infertility; feline influenza, with typical bland yellow discharges from one or both eyes or nostrils, usually the right.

Aromas influential to Scorpio are: cardamom, galangal, hyacinth, hops, pennyroyal, pine, thyme, tuberose, and woodruff. Pluto is affected by basil, broom, coriander, cumin, deerstongue, galangal, garlic, ginger, hops, nasturtium, onion, pennyroyal, pine, rue, and woodruff.

Sagittarius (The Archer)

November 23–December 21
Cardinal element: fire
Ruling planet: Jupiter
Earth color: blue
Astral colors: gold, red, green
Gems: turquoise, diamond
Mineral element: tin
Bach flower: Agrimony
Cell salt: Silicea

Sagittarius is ruled by Jupiter, the planet of expansion, which also affects cell regeneration. This sign relates to the musculature, the cardiac system, and the blood vessels. A mutable fire sign and the friendliest sign in the zodiac, Sagittarius has an elementary quality of dry heat.

Happy, playful, and clownlike from birth, the Sagittarian cat lives to be loved, petted, and appreciated. The eyes of this little archer are trusting, and he'll be your loving, faithful friend always, especially if you keep him busy learning new things and meeting new people. He's independent, but he'll never deny you your divine right to give him pleasure. This optimistic little cat will steal your heart and keep you smiling.

He doesn't possess a mean bone in his body, and will never reject you, your friends, and other pets. He'll cry if you leave him alone, so don't do it. He needs a companion cat from birth, and it's best to adopt a sibling from the same litter, as two Sagittarians are better than one.

He'll cuddle in your arms, go for a ride in the car (he loves to travel), and may enjoy cat shows. He'll be happy if you leave an article of your clothing on the floor or in his bed for him to sleep with when you're at work. Better yet, take him with you if you can. If you can't, he'll probably drag that clothing of yours all around the house. Basically, he loves to be wherever you are. But his need for attention is balanced by his desire for freedom, so never let him outside, or he may never come back.

The Sagittarian cat may just think he's a dog. If you have one, he'll be happy to be friends with it, if you start him young. Dogs and cats can make wonderful companions, despite what many people think. But if you have a doggie door, be careful your Sagittarian cat doesn't sneak out and call every feline in the neighborhood to come over and play.

He's forever curious. If this cat could talk, he'd never stop asking you questions. If he knew what hypocrisy meant, he wouldn't stand for it. If he sees you do it, he'll want to do it too. He may be clumsy, knocking over vases and pulling down tablecloths in his path. Get him a tall scratching post or kitty tree, as he loves to shred things. If he were a person, he'd tear into ideas as enthusiastically as he tears into your couch.

Sagittarius can also be obstinate, and he likes to challenge your authority, especially if he's a big cat. As he grows, he may become a bit overbearing. He just doesn't realize how heavy he is when he lands on your stomach and wants to cuddle like a kitten. Don't throw him down, just give him the bear hug he seems to crave.

At cat shows, people and commotion don't frighten Sagittarius one bit. If you're interested in showing him, get him used to being handled from an early age. The judges will love him whether he's a household pet or a purebred.

The Bach flower remedy for Sagittarius is *Agrimony*. The Agrimony type is good spirited and carefree, but these attributes may disguise inner worries, nervousness, and anxiety. Peace loving and good companions, they don't like to be alone, though they're highly independent. Because they love freedom and adventure, they may worry that you'll forget about them and lock them in a room or closet, or that you won't ever come home and feed them. They are dichotomous like the archer, which illustrates triumph over his animal nature. He knows he's an animal, but you treat him as if he were a person. Agrimony can work wonders for oversensitivity too.

The cell salt attributed to Sagittarius is *Silicea* (silica). It is recommended when the cat seems irritated, definitely a symptom that something is wrong, either mentally or physically.

Could this clumsy cat have fallen and injured himself? Silicea may be used for everything from acne to bronchitis. The cat may experience a loss of power in the legs and/or a contraction of the tendons. Caries (decay, ulceration, or inflammation of the bone) of spinal processes may indicate the use of this remedy. Symptoms are always worse at night and during a full Moon. Schuessler recommends the 6X and 12X potencies.

Tin (*stannum*) is Jupiter's element. Like Jupiter, tin has a close connection with the respiratory system as well as the digestive organs, including the liver. Tin is used for hoarseness of the throat, with accompanying rawness, obstruction of the air passages, and yellow-green phlegm. The recommended dosage is 3X.

Consider the following homeopathic remedies for Sagittarius:[28]

Arnica because of the potential to injure himself. *Arnica* is a good remedy to keep on hand for both internal and external use before and after surgery, including tooth extraction.[29]

Bryonia alba for a feeling of weakness in the limbs. This remedy is extremely useful in the treatment of many conditions when the main guiding symptom grows worse from movement, such as pneumonia or pleurisy, where the animal prefers to lie on its affected side, bringing pressure to bear and thus restricting movement.

Chamomilla for mild pain in the extremities and for teething in the young kitten.

The essential plants and oils associated with Sagittarius are: bergamot, calendula, clove, hyssop, lemon balm, mace, nutmeg, oakmoss, rosemary, and saffron. Jupiter is enhanced by clove, honeysuckle, hyssop, lemon balm, meadowsweet, nutmeg, oakmoss, sage, star anise, and tonka.

Capricorn (The Goat)

December 22-January 20

Cardinal element: earth

Ruling planet: Saturn

Earth color: blue-violet

Astral colors: garnet, silver, gray, brown, black

Gems: garnet, white onyx, moonstone

Mineral element: lead

Bach flower: Mimulus

Cell salt: Calcarea phosphoricum

Ruled by Saturn and represented by the goat (and sometimes the fish or the unicorn), Capricorn rules the digestive tract and the bones. This sign has an elementary quality of dry cold.

Capricorn is an elegant cat, with one of the most intriguing personalities of all the signs. Because of her depth and complexity, she may appear aloof or remote, but this only masks an inherent shyness and introspection.

Renoir, my white oriental shorthair, was born January 16. When I first adopted him, he was so timid he hid under the bed, where no one could reach him. I was determined to make him my friend, but I didn't rush it. I practiced nonverbal communication with him by picturing him coming to me. He never purred or rubbed up against me, and I thought I'd never break through the barrier he had built around himself.

With astrology as my guide, I realized that Saturn indicates security, caution, and reliability. Capricorn, represented by the mountain goat, takes one step at a time, checking for sure ground or a firm foundation before making a move.

I decided some remedial work was in order, and so took Renoir, accompanied by his pal Celina, to College Fur Cats, a training class in the Los Angeles area that teaches cats operant behavior—just like that taught to movie and television cats. Little by little, he started to come out of his shell. One day, when I was making my bed, he meowed—a first!—and then he nudged me and purred, so I ran my nails gently down his back. Those simple gestures broke the ice. After that he actually seemed to enjoy the camaraderie of the class, which was great fun.

Slowly, I earned his love and trust, and now I can even take him to cat shows—he actually became a CFA Grand Premier. The moral of the story is that Capricorns may be slow to give you their love, but once they do, the bond is everlasting.

Capricorn is a feminine sign and forever youthful, but there's something stoic about her even when she's playing. Such intense eyes—when she looks at you, her eyes tell the whole story. Just be receptive to it.

She's strong-willed and tenacious, with a mind of her own. She doesn't like to be embarrassed and hates to lose. Though she's the most conservative sign in the zodiac, energy is one thing she doesn't conserve. Like the mountain goat, she likes to climb to the highest vantage point, and assume dominion over everything and everyone. When it comes to play, she's nonstop and downright silly.

The Capricorn cat will try hard to be a person for you, but remember, she's still a cat. A tidy animal, she'll rarely get dirty or break anything. If she does, she'll be very sorry, as she wants to be liked and admired.

Watch her weight, as she loves to eat. Also, watch for hairballs, as Capricorns are meticulous groomers, not only of themselves but of everything else, including you. She loves to let you groom her, bathe her, and brush her teeth, but if she thinks your guard is down, she'll bolt in a flash. She may sneak out-of-doors, so be sure she always wears a collar and tag. With patience you can teach her to walk on a leash. She may skulk, cower, slink, or lie down, but ultimately, she'll enjoy the trip.

She dreams about birds and anything that will keep her agile body and quick mind moving. She seems to sleep less than most cats, but boredom will knock her right out.

The Capricorn cat matures quickly, but still wants to be the baby and may be jealous of a new kitten, so think twice before bringing home a pal. She'd rather have you all to herself for a playmate. But when her supremacy isn't threatened, Capricorn loves other cats, perhaps more than people. And when she challenges a "top cat," she'll end up on top through sheer persistence, and the former ruler won't even realize his position has been usurped.

If you do bring home a new friend, just be patient. Capricorn will come around eventually, but she'll hiss at the intruder every chance she gets—and may even ignore you for a while. She's quite serious about her aggression and can do damage to the new cat, so be careful. Try changing the subject by giving her catnip or a new toy.

The Capricorn in need of *Mimulus*, the Bach flower remedy selected for this sign, suffers from fears of unknown origin, and insecurities caused by past experience. Her home, human guardians, and animal friends are all-important to her sense of security. She may be withdrawn, yet dislike being alone. Unless you look closely, you may think she's not the warmest cat you've ever known, but her sense of play will usually warm your heart. When fear gets the better of her, incorporate Mimulus into her regime, along with Rescue Remedy for extreme situations.

The cell salt for Capricorn is *Calcarea phosphoricum* (calcium phosphate). When Dr. George W. Carey allocated *Calc. phos.* to Capricorn, he may have done so because the Latin word calcium means (in addition to lime) "end" or "goal." This corresponds beautifully to the sign of Capricorn, as its season closes out the Roman calendar year and brings in the new. Capricorn rules the limbs and the digestive tract. Discuss this remedy with your practitioner if your cat seems especially anxious or has been grieving a loss or perhaps from a vexation. A change in weather may exacerbate rheumatism in the joints, accompanied by pain and swelling; there may be pain in the extremities during movement. Symptoms are worse from cold, wet, or motion; the cat feels better lying down. There may even be brittleness of bones. Corneal opacities and ulceration of the eyes, with a tendency to cataracts, may be present. A young kitten may display colicky diarrhea after feeding. In the adult, diabetes insipidus may benefit from this remedy. Think of *Calc. phos.* for an animal whose development was delayed because of improper diet. This remedy has an affinity with tissues concerned with the growth and repair of cells. The lower potencies of 3X and 6X are usually prescribed.

The metal for Saturn is *lead (plumbum)*. This remedy has proven useful for intermittent limping and for arteriosclerosis (a painful disorder in which fibrous tissue thickens the arteries so smaller ones may become blocked). This condition can lead to other conditions, such as epilepsy and kidney disorders. Since lead is not broken down metabolically (yet another reason not to feed food from cans, which contain lead), this element is eliminated from the body with great difficulty. Only dilutions from 6X and up should ever be considered.

Consider the following homeopathic remedies for Capricorn:[30]

Bryonia alba when there's a weakness in the limbs or pain with any movement. Joints are painful and swollen.

Calcarea carbonica (*calcium carb.*) for joint pain and poorly developed bones due to calcium deficiency. This is a good constitutional remedy for the treatment of skeletal disorders, perhaps exacerbated by too-close breeding of purebred cats. It's essential to include adequate bonemeal for calcium in the diets of pregnant and nursing queens. They, as well as nursing kittens, can require twice what other cats utilize on a daily basis.

Pulsatilla for feline influenza with typical eye symptoms. Again, pain in the limbs accompany other symptoms.

Aromas influencing Capricorn are: cypress, honeysuckle, lilac, mimosa, myrrh, patchouli, tonka, tulip, and vetiver. Cypress, mimosa, myrrh, and patchouli are attributed to the ruling planet, Saturn.

Aquarius (The Water Carrier)

January 21-February 19

Cardinal element: air

Ruling planets: Uranus, Saturn

Earth color: violet

Astral colors: blue, pink, nile green

Gems: amethyst, sapphire, opal, turquoise

Mineral element: zinc

Bach flower: Water Violet

Cell salt: Natrium muriaticum

Ruled by Uranus (a planet added to the astrological literature after its discovery in the eighteenth century), Aquarius is a fixed air sign, with an elementary quality of wet heat. This sign governs the legs, ankles, circulatory system, and blood.

My Romeo, a platinum point Tonkinese and an Aquarian, thinks he's a little king (and so do I). You can hold him like a baby, put him over your shoulder, walk him on a leash. He loves everybody, and in so doing turns staunch cat haters—even those allergic to cats[31]—into cat lovers, and cat lovers into avid Tonk lovers. How much of this is Aquarius and how much Tonkinese? The breed is known for affection, but the combination of breed and sign is even more powerful!

Aquarius is strong, trusting, fearless, and courageous, but also sensuous and sensitive. The Aquarian cat is incredibly psychic—he seems to know, without knowing how he knows. There is nothing average about Aquarius. He's the most precocious cat in the house, and becomes top cat before you know it. He knows when he's being good and when he's being bad—and has extremes in both directions. He loves freedom and is very independent.

Male or female, Aquarian cats will talk to you incessantly. They love people and tolerate other pets nicely, but they know you love them best and share that secret with you. They'll ignore you sometimes when you call, but come running when they're ready (just a few moments later than you'd like). They're unpredictable and contradictory—one moment calm and docile, and suddenly wound up like a tornado.

Great eaters as well as very good athletes, they love to climb as high as they can and dive-bomb from the top of the shutters, drapes, or cat trees. They'll jump into the air and expect you to catch them. They'll ride on your shoulders like a scarf. They do somersaults and roll over on their backs (sometimes falling asleep in that position, a hilarious sight).

With this perpetual clown, you'll never know what to expect. He can become best friends with a dog, a pot-bellied pig, even a horse or a goat! He's so outgoing and fearless that these other creatures just accept him as one of their own. Aquarius has a capacity to love beyond that of any other sign in the zodiac.

The Bach flower remedy selected for Aquarius is *Water Violet* because, despite his wonderful charms, this cat can be proud and aloof. He also can feel lonely if there's no one around to give him constant admiration. If he suddenly withdraws a bit, consider Water Violet, which will, when used with Rescue Remedy, help him handle whatever he's going through. He may also be quite headstrong and a bit indifferent. Water Violet may assist with any of these negative states of mind.

The cell salt selected for Aquarius is *Natrium muriaticum* (sodium chloride). Symptoms may include acrid lacrimation of the eyelids, which may be swollen. Cataracts or generalized opacities of the cornea may occur. There may be a thin watery discharge from the nasal passages, with difficulty breathing and an attendant cough. The cat may vomit a whitish gray material. An indifferent appetite and constipation may be present, as well as a generalized weakness of limbs. The skin may be itchy, and bald spots may occur on various body parts. *Nat. Mur.* is useful in the treatment of eczema in debilitated cats. Salt retention leads to thirst, which may indicate kidney problems, probably from years of the consumption of dry food.

Associated with Uranus, *zinc* (zincum) is a relatively new metal, first extracted from its ore in the mid-eighteenth century, about the same time that the planet was discovered by Herschel. The amount of zinc in organs seems to be higher when cell growth is vigorous. Uranus relates to the cerebellum, and many have regarded zinc as a brain remedy. Its main action is on the central nervous system, when tiredness and weakness alternate with restlessness and excitement. There is a tendency for the animal to lean to the left side. Lameness and weakness in the legs, with trembling and twitching, may be noticeable. Vomiting can occur, as well as enlargement of the liver, with signs of gas and colic. Eyes may twitch, and the conjunctiva become red and inflamed. This is a useful homeopathic remedy in veterinary practice for suppressed feverish conditions with long-standing septic (toxic) states.

Consider the following homeopathic remedies for Aquarius:[32]

Abrotanum for circulatory disorders and for emaciation of the legs.

Aconite as it relates to the veins.

Arnica for injuries, especially to the legs.

Ceanothus for conditions involving the spleen, such as Feline Leukemia virus. A course of 30C for fourteen days may help if pathological involvement of this organ is suspected.

Kali iodatum or *Kali hydriodicum* for various symptoms indicating eye and respiratory conditions, such as pneumonia. Stiffness of the joints, with pain that makes the cat cry out suddenly, is also a symptom. The skin may produce nodules, with swelling. I have used *Kali* for incessant itching when nothing else seems to help.

Ledum when the extremities become swollen and the feet feel hot. There can be tenderness and stiffness in the shoulder area.

Rhus toxicondedron for stiffness in joints alleviated by moving.

Aromas associated with Aquarius are: costmary, hops, lavender, lemon verbena, parsley, patchouli, pine, star anise, and sweet pea. Uranus is influenced by cypress, mimosa, myrrh, and patchouli.

Pisces (The Fish)

February 20–March 20
Cardinal element: water
Ruling planets: Neptune, Jupiter
Earth colors: cerise, magenta
Astral colors: white, pink, emerald green, black
Gems: chrysolite, pink shell, moonstone
Mineral element: tin
Bach flower: Rock Rose
Cell salt: Ferrum phosphoricum

Pisces, the twelfth and last sign of the zodiac, is ruled by Neptune and Jupiter, and represents change and the consciousness of the soul. This sign governs the arterial blood, the red corpuscles, and the feet. Cats born under this sign may be susceptible to diseases of the chest. Pisces is a mutable water sign, with an elementary quality of wet cold.

Sweet, gentle, endearing, and magical—part elf, part leprechaun—she grabs at your heartstrings, and before you know it, you're the proud adoptive parent of a Pisces cat.

Pisces are truly fanciful creatures. You expect to see them leaping from lily pad to lily pad in pursuit of the elusive butterfly. And, oh, those dreamy eyes—made of stardust, to be sure. They see, hear, and smell many things, such as spirits, that we don't know are there.

Pisceans are the keepers of thousands of years of secrets. Tune into them, and you'll be amazed at what they'll tell you. When you see their sleeping little bodies twitch, they're dreaming of chasing brightly colored birds, rainbows, and butterflies, for color is extremely important to them. They need it to express the higher attributes of their spirit. Try it yourself sometime, and maybe you'll meet your Pisces on the astral plane playing in the cool blue-green grass among the buttercups.

The Pisces cat needs to remain still for periods of time, and through this occasional stillness, she can bring the correct response directly to the surface of the psychic sea. Otherwise, she's pulled in opposing directions, constantly in conflict. Her sign is symbolized by two fishes—one swimming toward the source of the water, the other toward the sea.

Her tendency to be dreamy makes it easy for her to leave her body. Your Pisces cat may learn this technique early in life in order to avoid reprimands. She simply tunes out, traveling to realms of safety on the wings of fantasy. Give her lots of attention and encourage her to be outgoing, for if you don't, she'll be shy forever. But respect her privacy when she's in a mysterious mood, and let her be.

Pisces loves to love, but she gets stressed easily. Fortunately, you'll rarely need to reprimand her. She seems perfect—though you might be letting her get away with a lot. She'll charm you into getting her own way, so you may as well surrender. But she'll never abuse you for this or let you spoil her too much— she's too loving for that. Because she makes up her own rules, you must gently let her know what yours are. Use positive rein-forcement, and avoid the negative. Tell her she's good, and that's what she'll be.

Pisces cats have their own schedules. They'll sleep when they want to, eat when they want to, play when they want to—so you may just have to adjust your schedule to theirs.

It's important to protect her from bullies, animal or human, as she doesn't understand and can't tolerate aggression or violence. The music of Chopin or Mozart (both Pisceans) will soothe her.

Rock Rose is the Bach flower remedy of choice for Pisces. One of the five ingredients in Rescue Remedy, Rock Rose is usually prescribed for acute or accumulated fear. The Pisces/Rock Rose can be a target for abuse and is easily panicked. A hotbed of neurosis renders them prone to diseases of the psyche. For these reasons, also consider Rescue Remedy for the Pisces cat.

Ferrum phosphoricum (iron phosphate) is the cell salt attributed to Pisces. This remedy is especially useful in the early stages of inflammatory conditions that develop less quickly than those calling for Aconite, and a soft, full pulse is symptomatic, as opposed to the Aconite type. Throat involvement may be a consideration. Ferrum phosphoricum may prove useful in the treatment of heat stroke, ailments of the feet, and muscular stiffness, when joints become swollen.

Neptune also responds to the element *tin* (stannum). This metal has a close connection with the respiratory system, and so is employed for hoarseness and raw conditions of the throat, a weak chest, obstruction of air passages, and when yellow/green phlegm is expectorated with each cough. Tin is also associated with digestive organs such as the liver. The mental state of the Pisces cat may seem sad or anxious, and she may hide from people. Her symptoms worsen with anger, a loss of fluids, and even the slightest touch on affected parts. She feels better after her breakfast. She seeks warmth, and is improved by rest at night.

Consider the following homeopathic remedies for Pisces:[33]

Aconite because of Pisceans' propensity toward fear.

Bryonia alba when chills and fever accompany a thirst for large quantities of water. Nasal discharge may show bleeding, a yellowish deposit may cover the tongue, and vomiting may occur. The liver may be affected, leading to hepatitis, with jaundice and swelling or tenderness over the liver.

Calcarea carbonicum (*Calc. carb.*) can be used for muscular spasms, since Pisces controls the feet. Its application to the extremities in general is beneficial. Calcium, in homeopathic potency, is the only sure way to establish this element in the system.

The essential plants and oils influencing Pisces are: apple, cardamom, gardenia, hyacinth, jasmine, lily, mugwort, myrrh, palmarosa, sandalwood, vanilla, and ylang-ylang. Neptune's essential aromas are: clove, honeysuckle, hyssop, lemon balm, meadowsweet, nutmeg, oakmoss, sage, star anise, and tonka.

In Summary

THIS SECTION has touched on the application of only a few homeopathic remedies, Bach flowers, cell salts, and plant essences[34]—each of which may or may not have specific relationships to various aspects of the twelve sun signs. I encourage you always to look to your cat's specific symptoms, referring to your homeopathic repertory book (I use J. T. Kent's) and then working with your *materia medica* to find which remedy is the best to try (I use Boericke).

This is the homeopathic approach, so rather than trying to conquer disease, you may match as many symptoms as you can to the descriptions given for the homeopathic types in order to discover the constitutional and acute remedies that fit the overall picture of your cat's condition. Again, be sure to consult your homeopathic veterinarian or practitioner prior to administering any remedy.

Chapter Nine

Saying Goodbye
to the Ones We Love

COPING WITH THE LOSS
OF AN ANIMAL COMPANION

FOR ME, the loss of a cat is as agonizing an experience as anything I can imagine. My animal companions are every bit as important to me as my human family. I meet so many people at cat shows or through referrals who have lost an animal companion or who presently have an old or infirm cat for whom they would like a young friend, but I know in my heart they want that kitten to be there to help them grieve when the inevitable happens.

If you've read my introduction, you know I've grieved the loss of many animal friends. My mother tells me the first death I ever witnessed was that of a sparrow in my backyard. She says I stood right over that little bit of fluff and feathers and, when asked what I was doing, responded that I was waiting to be sure its soul would fly up to heaven.

As a cat breeder now, I still cry when I lose a kitten, at birth or days later. There never seems to be enough time for these precious little spirits. It can be hard to find people who understand such a deep attachment, but I've been blessed with friends and clients who love their animal companions and so can truly empathize with me.

The mourning process, the time needed to grieve, is a personal thing, but we must go through it, as denial is even more painful. I feel flower remedies are helpful at times like these. The Grief Recovery Hotline (800-445-4808) may be of help to some. For others, adopting a kitten, puppy, or adult cat or dog from the pound or Humane Society may be the answer, for surely our love doesn't die when our loved ones do. With so many animals dying needlessly at shelters every day, these adoptions are beneficial to both the adopter and adoptee. You may find the image of your deceased companion, or you may adopt a very different little being. Either way, trust yourself, follow your heart.

Be sure to allow yourself to progress through the stages outlined by Elisabeth Kubler-Ross in her excellent book.[1] They are, not necessarily in this order: **1.** denial and isolation, **2.** bargaining, **3.** anger and depression, and **4.** acceptance. Barbara Meyers, a certified grief therapist at the Holistic Animal Consulting Center in New York City, adds reinvestment to this list. After all, what good is love if you don't give it away? Other stages commonly experienced are guilt and the feeling of not being able to go on.

The decisions that plague us at the end are heavy burdens to bear, for instance, is it too late to seek alternative healing therapies when the animal has been through so much? Should we choose euthanasia, or permit our animals to endure until the end? Most homeopathically treated animals can die at home and not need to be euthanized.

COMMUNICATE WITH YOUR SICK
OR AGING CAT

ULTIMATELY, you and your animal friend need to make these choices together. Now is the time for spiritual work: meditation, prayer, and nonverbal communication. You'll receive guidance when your heart and mind are open. Do what you think is best, then let it go. Animals have their own paths and their own spiritual journeys, says Dr. Chambreau. So when the end is near, the best thing you can do for them is to release them. Tell them, out loud, that it's okay for them to pass on. This will help them follow their own path.

The psychic Laurel Steinhice tells us that animals reincarnate in tandem with their human companions and with each other. The closer the interspecies bonding, the more likely and more frequent such reincarnation is to occur. Steinhice believes the species are interchangeable. The Egyptians must have known this too, as their cats were often mummified and entombed with their human guardians. Steinhice also recommends telling your animal companions you understand that they wish to leave this body and that you will welcome them in their new one, so their spirit may continue its bond with you.[2]

Someone once told me I might view death as a departure on a great ship. Just as the ship sails away from us, and we wave goodbye from the shore, so it is that someone waits on the other side and is waving hello. Our animals make this journey with such grace if we only allow them this dignity, which is their birthright. So before you allow your beloved animals to be drugged, poked, and prodded, or surgically explored, communicate with them and try to ascertain what they want.

My dearest friend Imelda's nine-year-old cat, Mica, was diagnosed with acute liver failure. She was hospitalized and, because she refused food, was put on an IV. She was anesthetized for ultrasound and a liver biopsy only to be told that she had fatty acid liver disease. Our local veterinarian allowed us to administer homeopathics to Mica, but she appeared to be slipping away from us.

This went on for eight days, and the only treatment offered, both by our consulting holistic veterinarian and our local allopathic veterinarian, was to surgically insert a feeding tube through her cheek down to her stomach. Mica would be fed a thin food through this tube, which would be shielded by her wearing a large protective collar as well as being sequestered from the other cats in the household. There was no guarantee that this treatment would work, or even of how long she'd have to endure it.

Imelda asked Mica if she wanted to live this way, and the answer was definitely "No!" She and her husband decided to euthanize with dignity, sparing the cat from the humiliation of force-feeding. Sobbing, Imelda went off to have Mica put to sleep. But, as I was doing some errands, I suddenly felt Mica saying, "I just want to go home, not to heaven." And it seems that, when they got to the animal hospital, someone offered Mica some baby food, and this cat, which had all but shut down, wanted to eat it, so they took her home.

One more homeopathic was administered, and she ate some very bland food. Now she's well again, eating, playing, and enjoying life with her feline and human companions. Miracles do happen. The moral of this story is, listen to your heart and let yourself communicate heart to heart with your pet.

As with living, we can learn so much from our animal friends about death and dying. They have no fear of it but seem to view it as a natural progression. I'm sure they're sad to leave us, just as we're sad to lose them, but finally, we must, after we grieve, say farewell to the dead and concentrate on giving our love to the living.

Dr. Chambreau says we've been changed permanently by living with our animals, and in that way they live forever in how we interact with the world. Machaelle Small Wright suggests that animals, like humans, are not of this earth, but rather souls that have chosen to use this planet as their setting for an evolutionary experience. Animals have chosen not to operate in the same complicated way as humans, but rather to participate through nature. This, of course, does not make them lesser beings than us—it simply makes them different.[3]

As long as we remain in our steward relationship to them, they must trust us to do what's best for them. And that, of course, is all we can do.

Chapter Ten

In Summary

I HOPE the information I've gathered here will benefit your cat. Perhaps it will even motivate you to explore, both for you and for your companion animal, the fascinating world of holistic health care. I trust you can feel the passion and excitement I have for this ever-expanding field, which I believe is every bit as important as mainstream medicine.

Though along the way I've probably offended some well-meaning institutions and their schools of thought, my intent has merely been to present the many alternative treatments and therapies that exist today. I am in no way attempting to prescribe, give medical care, or replace anyone's practitioner. I just wish to arm you with all the information you need to make well-informed choices.

Indeed, many conventional veterinarians and pet food manufacturers mean well. They've spent years studying their specialties, and they deserve to profit from our use of their goods and services—as long as we and our companion animals benefit from their care.

Isn't it time we took back the responsibility for our health and that of our cats? I would never be so narrow-minded as to deny completely the usefulness of allopathic medicine, but I make sure that I exhaust every natural method available before I risk the use of drugs or surgery. And when I must resort to utilizing these methods of treatment, I'm glad I know how to help the body repair whatever toll they take.

Many of the things discussed in these pages may seem a little "far out" to you, and nothing works for everyone. Explore the Resources section that follows, and call or write for more information about whatever seems appropriate or interesting. In conjunction with your veterinarian, make your own determination when working with alternative consultants and practitioners, and always ask for references.

Finally, share this book, as well as your insights and concerns, with your health care providers; such a partnership will benefit you, them, and your cat. You may be surprised at how open to new ideas your providers are. But if they're not, the decision about whether to use holistic care still belongs to you.

I welcome you to the world of *Cat Care, Naturally*, and want you to know that I'm committed to continuing my journey and sharing my findings with those who have an open mind and heart, and are willing to listen. Just remember, the truth is not of much use to us if it comes too late.

Notes

Chapter One

1. Desmond Morris, *Cat Watching*, p. 13.
2. My favorite is *The Legacy of the Cat* by Gloria Stephens.
3. Roger De Haan, D.V.M., *What Is Holistic Veterinary Care? Natural Care of Pets: Alternative Therapies in Companion Animal Health,* 1982, p. 23.
4. Compiled by Drs. Richard Pitcairn, Jeffrey Levy, Christina Chambreau, Charles Loops, and Don Hamilton; and provided by Dr. Chambreau.
5. Cats that eat dry food drink more water because of its low moisture content; see Water section in chapter 4, "Nutrition."

Chapter Two

1. Machaelle Small Wright, *Behaving As If the God in All Life Mattered*, p. 165.
2. According to Yolanda LaCombe in "On the Floor with Cats: Cindy Wood's Feline Communication Advice," *Tiger Tribe*, March-April 1993, p. 19.
3. Adapted from Drs. Foster and Smith's "A Catalogue about Pets and People Too." This is a mail order catalog for canine, feline, and equine products selected by pet professionals (800-826-7206).

Chapter Three

1. Unless otherwise noted, all further quotations of Dr. Chambreau come from her conversations/correspondence with the author.
2. John Fudens, D.V.M., "Vaccinations," *Natural Pet*, p. 9-11.
3. W. Jean Dodds, D.V.M., *DVM*, Dec. 1990.
4. Richard Pitcairn, *D.V.M.*, Address to the American Holistic Veterinary Medical Association (AHVMA), September 1993; text available from AHVMA on audiotape or in written proceedings of conference. This condition has also been identified in people, and was written about extensively by J. Compton Burnett, M.D., in *Vaccinosis and Its Cure by Thuja, with Remarks on Homeoprophylaxis* and in his other books.

5. Richard Pitcairn, D.V.M., "A Foolish Practice," *Tiger Tribe*, Jan.-Feb. 1994, pp. 24-26.

6. C. Edgar Sheaffer, D.V.M., "Hooked on Homeopathy," *Tiger Tribe*, Nov.-Dec. 1993. pp. 8, 15–17.

7. Jeff Levy, D.V.M., "Feline Miasms," *Tiger Tribe*, May-June 1993, pp. 20-21.

8. National Health Federation, *Health Freedom News*, Feb. 1989.

9. Sue Marston, *The Vaccination Connection*, p. 5.

10. Ibid., p. 30.

11. Ibid., p. 30.

12. Ibid., p. 9.

13. Ibid., p. 9

14. Ibid., p. 6

15. Ibid., p. 28.

16. Ibid., p. 28.

17. Ibid., p. 28.

18. Ron Shultz, D.V.M., Conversation/correspondence with the author, Dec. 1994. Dr. Fudens ("Vaccinations," *Natural Pet,* Mar.-Apr. 1994, pp. 9-11) explains that vaccines are composed of either killed or modified live viruses. Killed viruses have been inactivated by chemicals or heat, but the protein membrane covering the virus has been left intact so the immune system will react against that protein, thinking it's a live virus, and produce antibodies. Modified live viruses have been changed by growing them on animal tissue through many life cycles, weakening the viruses by introducing them in tissue they don't normally infect. When a modified live virus is injected into the body, the immune system recognizes it as living, and produces antibodies long before the virus can restore its normal strength. John Saxon, M.A. Vet. (in Sue Marston's, *The Vaccination Connection*) says that, to our bodies or those of our animals, the difference between live and killed virus vaccines is "rather like asking a man about to be hanged whether he would prefer to be dropped six or eight feet."

19. Personal communication with Dr. Chambreau.

20. John Fudens, D.V. M., "Vaccinations," *Natural Pet,* Mar.-Apr. 1994, pp. 6–9

21. Elizabeth Terrell, "Post-Vaccinational Tumor Development in Cats," *Cat Fanciers Almanac—CFA Health Committee News*, Dec. 1993, p. 90.

22. Tom R. Phillips D.V.M., Ph.D., and Ronald D. Schultz, D.V.M., Ph.D., "Canine & Feline Vaccines," in *Kirk's Current Veterinary Therapy*, vol. 9 (1992 ed.), pp. 202-6.

23. Pat McKay, "Vaccinations," *Nutricare News*, Aug. 1988, p. xi.

24. *Isopathy* is the practice of administering potentized substances (which seem to be directly associated with the disease) from the patient's surrounding environment or from the patient himself.

25. Proving is the homeopathic procedure for ascertaining the effects of substances by administering them to healthy subjects in order to observe and record symptoms.

26. In a second speech at the 1993 AHVMA convention, Dr. Pitcairn addressed

research on and clinical experience using nosodes, mentioning the writing of Hahnemann (cholera), Boenninghausen (thuja in smallpox), Shepherd (homeopathy in epidemic diseases), Jervis (treatment of canine distemper), Day (stillbirths in pigs; bovine mastitis). Other studies on nosodes (or microdoses) conducted with human and animal subjects include those by Bastide, Daurat, Carriere, Karouby, Doucet-Jaboeuf, and Saxton. Don't confuse the prophylactic use of nosodes with their use in treating different diseases, as they are often used as remedies in treating disease.

27. Christopher Day M.R.C.V.S., "Isopathic Prevention of Kennel Cough, Is Vaccination Justified?" *International Journal for Homeopathy*, vol. 2, no. 1, Apr. 1987, pp. 45–50.

28. Per his address at the 1993 AHVMA meeting.

29. The source of the information in this section is, "Danger: Toxic Chemicals in the Home," *Natural Pet*, July-Aug. 1993, pp. 18-19.

30. Also see Marina McInnis, "Are Clumping Litters a Deadly Convenience?" *Tiger Tribe*, Jan.-Feb. 1993, pp. 18-21.

31. Diane Stein, *Natural Healing for Dogs and Cats*, p. 180.

32. Joanne Stefanatos, *Holistic Pet Care*.

33. Ann Miller, "Does Your Dog Food Bark? A Study of the Pet Food Fallacy," *Natural Pet*, March-April, 1995, pp. 58–59.

34. Richard Pitcairn, D.V.M., and Susan Hubble Pitcairn, *The Complete Guide To Natural Health For Dogs & Cats*, p. 13.

35. Pat McKay, *Reigning Cats and Dogs*, p. 3.

36. Diane Stein, *Natural Healing for Dogs and Cats*, p. 50.

37. Francis M. Pottenger, Jr., M.D., *Pottenger's Cats*, pp. 39–42. This book is available through the Price-Pottenger Nutrition Foundation (see Resources), as are edited versions of Dr. Pottenger's many research reports, books, pamphlets, and tapes. The foundation is a nonprofit educational organization that conducts worldwide research and disseminates information about natural nutrition.

38. *The Cornell Book of Cats: A Comprehensive Medical Reference for Every Cat or Kitten,* "Effects of Food Processing on Amino Acids," p. 73.

39. Alfred Plechner, D.V.M., and Martin Zucker, "Pet Allergies: Remedies for an Epidemic," *D.V.M.*, Mar. 1985, p. 11.

40. Ibid., p. 13.

41. *The Cornell Book of Cats: A Comprehensive Medical Reference for Every Cat or Kitten,* p. 73.

42. Ibid.

43. R. L. Wysong, D.V.M., *Fresh and Raw* (available from the Wysong Company— see Resources).

44. Ibid.

45. Tribal News "Don't Zap the Cat," *Tiger Tribe* (Nov.-Dec. 1993), p. 9.

46. Ibid.

47. Ibid.

48. Ibid.

Chapter Four

1. Pat McKay, *Reigning Cats and Dogs*, p. 1.
2. Among the holistic veterinarians, authors, institutions, and publications recommending a fresh raw food diet are Drs. Jeffrey Levy, Christina Chambreau, John Fudens, Russell Swift, Nancy Scanlan, N. G. Wolff (author of *Your Healthy Cat*), and Richard Pitcairn (*Complete Guide to Natural Health for Dogs and Cats*); Pat McKay (*Reigning Cats and Dogs*); Anitra Frazier (*The New Natural Cat*); Pat Lazarus (*Keep Your Pet Healthy the Natural Way*); Juliette de Bairacli Levy (*The Complete Herbal Handbook for Dogs and Cats*); Diane Stein (*Natural Healing for Dogs and Cats*); Nelly Grosjean (*Veterinary Aromatherapy*); *Tiger Tribe* magazine; the Wysong Pet Food Company; and the Los Angeles Zoo. See Resources section for contact information.
3. Anitra Frazier, *The New Natural Cat*, p. 54.
4. Elizabeth Marshall Thomas, *Tribe of the Tiger*. Marshall gives an in-depth look at the similarities, dietary and otherwise, among the thirty-two species in the cat family.
5. The zoo uses Nebraska Brand Feline Diet, which consists of raw horse meat and horse meat by-products, along with the soy grits, vitamins, and minerals. Rich Freitag, Vice President of Animal Spectrum, Inc., the makers of Nebraska Brand, tells me most of their clients use the horse meat-based mixture, but Animal Spectrum also supplies a few zoos with a beef-based product called Spectrum Feline. These items are acquired frozen, as are the mice.
6. Cooked bones can splinter and cause serious problems.
7. Conversation with the author.
8. John Fudens, D.V.M., *The Affinity Holistic Veterinary Clinics Layman's Handbook to Holistic Care*, chapter on diet and nutrition.
9. See Pat McKay's *Reigning Cats and Dogs*, as well as further discussion in the present book, for a complete breakdown on meats, vegetables, and grains.
10. For a more complete list, see Pat McKay, *Reigning Cats and Dogs*, pp. 27–49.
11. Anitra Frazier, *The New Natural Cat*, p. 52.
12. Ibid.
13. If you don't have access to a health food store or can't afford the prices, you'll be relieved to hear that Dr. Chambreau feels most animals do okay even on grocery-store-quality raw foods. For cheaper organic produce, you might try your local farmer's market; organic vendors display a standard logo.
14. Along with many other helpful hints, Anitra Frazier offers a wonderful chicken broth recipe in her book *The New Natural Cat*, pp. 243–44.
15. Never microwave food, as microwaving alters the molecular structure (see chapter 3).
16. Anitra Frazier, *The New Natural Cat*, p. 256.
17. *The Cornell Book of Cats: A Comprehensive Medical Reference for Every Cat and Kitten*, p. 90.
18. Pat McKay, "Raw, Raw, Raw," *Tiger Tribe*, Sept.-Oct. 1993, pp. 23-24.

19. Unless your cat has a medical condition that warrants special care. Check with your holistic veterinarian if in doubt.
20. As provided by Dr. Chambreau.
21. Pat McKay, *Reigning Cats and Dogs*, pp. 17–18.
22. See Supplements section for a partial list of organisms this invaluable additive controls, as well as a discussion of other uses to which it may be put.
23. Richard Pitcairn, D.V.M., and Susan Hubble Pitcairn, *Complete Guide to Natural Health for Dogs and Cats*, p. 15.
24. Beth M. Levy, *Dr. John Willard's Catalyst Altered Water: A Health Learning Handbook.*
25. Pat McKay, *Reigning Cats and Dogs,* p. 77.
26. Adapted from Pat McKay, *Reigning Cats and Dogs*, pp. 76–102; and "Your Complete Vitamin Guide for the 'Natural' Pet," *Natural Pet,* Mar.-Apr. 1994, pp. 16-18.
27. Russell Swift, D.V.M. distributes an excellent liquid supplement called AniMinerals, an all-natural source of essential and trace minerals. Suspension of the minerals in desalinated water makes the minerals easy to digest. Melinda Leeson recommends this product highly.
28. Montmorillonite clay is also known as Redmond clay. The following trace minerals are found in it: antimony, arsenic, barium, beryllium, bismuth, boron, bromine, cadmium, calcium, cerium, cesium, choline, chromium, cobalt, copper, dyprosium, erbium, europium, fluroine, gadolinium, gallium, germanium, gold, hainium, holmium, indium, iodine, iridium, iron, lanthanum, lithium, lutecium, magnesium, manganese, molybdenum, neodymium, nickel, niobium, osmium, palladium, phosphorus, platinum, potassium, praseodymium, pihenium, rhodium, rubidium, ruthenium, samarium, scandium, selenium, silicon, silver, sodium, strontium, sulfur, tantalum, tellurium, terbium, thallium, thorium, thulium, tin, titanium, tungsten, uranium, vanadium, ytterbium, yttrium, zinc, zirconium.
29. Conversation with the author.
30. If you can't find All Blend, combine $^1/_4$ cup each safflower, soy, peanut, and wheat germ oil. You may also include flaxseed oil, if you like. Store in the refrigerator in a brown glass bottle.
31. Conversation with the author.
32. Sunrider's excellent line of herbal foods were created for people, and I've taken them for years myself. See Resources for how to obtain Simply Herbs.
33. I recommend holistic therapy such as homeopathy or herbs over the use of allopathic drugs because antibiotics and steroids only suppress symptoms and just push disease back into the system (see chapter 3, "The Dangers of Conventional Care," as well as the chapters on alternative healing). Obviously, you should follow the advice of your cat's health practitioner, as there are times when you may be forced, as I have been, to use conventional drug therapies.
34. Pat McKay, *Reigning Cats and Dogs*, pp. 110–113.

35. Alfred J. Plechner, D.V.M., and Martin Zukor, *Pet Allergies: Remedies for an Epidemic*, p. 20.
36. Pat McKay, "Brewer's Yeast: Abused and Overused," *Sis Sewell's Healthy Pets—Naturally*, Feb. 1994.
37. Anitra Frazier, "Notes for a Natural Cat," *Tiger Tribe*, Jan.-Feb. 1994, p. 7.
38. Michael Lemmon, D.V.M., "Your Pet's Health," *Animal Guardian*, vol. 7, no. 3 (1994), pp. 11-12.
39. Conversation with the author.
40. R. Daniel Foster, "The Mushroom," *Los Angeles Magazine*, Nov. 1994, pp. 118-123. Gunther Frank, who has collected a wealth of information about kombucha, publishes a magazine on the subject and has written a book entitled *Kombucha: Healthy Beverage and Natural Remedy from the Far East*.
41. I'm impressed with Cell Tech's entire line, including their digestive enzymes. The Animal Connection Network has reported very good results with these products (see Resources). As I write this book, I'm enjoying another Cell Tech product, Omega Sun, which helps keep me focused.
42. See "Super Blue-Green Algae—Not Just for Fish," *Tiger Tribe* Nov.-Dec. 1994, pp. 14-16.
43. Richard A. Passwater, Ph.D., *The New Super Antioxidant Plus: The Amazing Story of Pycnogenol, Free-Radical Antagonist and Vitamin C Potentiator* (see Resources). I give a copy of this little book to each of my clients.
44. There are other types of colloidal silver, but they are manufactured through a chemical process and may contain animal proteins.
45. Including acne, AIDS, allergies, arthritis, bladder inflammation, blood parasites, blood poisoning, boils, bubonic plague, burns, cancer, candida, cholera, colitis, conjunctivitis, cystitis, diabetes, dysentery, eczema, gastritis, gonorrhea, hay fever, herpes, impetigo, indigestion, keratitis, leprosy, leukemia, lupus, lyme disease, malaria, meningitis, parasitic infections (both viral and fungal), pleurisy, pneumonia, prostate problems, rheumatism, rhinitis, ringworm, septic conditions (of the eyes, ears, mouth, and throat), skin cancer, staph and strep infections, syphilis, thyroid, tonsillitis, toxemia, tuberculosis, virus warts, and yeast infections.
46. Manufactured by the same company that makes Silverloid™ colloidal silver.
47. Remember, O_2 (oxygen) is a completely different substance from H_2O_7 (hydrogen peroxide); for a discussion of the use of H_2O_2, see How to Prevent Contamination and Spoilage, page 90.
48. Pat McKay, "Have You and Your Cat Had Your Oxygen Today?" *Tiger Tribe*, Sept.-Oct. 1993, pp. 21-22.
49. With various other brands of O_2, such as Homozon, the package directions give suggested dosages for humans. Make sure to adjust the dosage appropriately for your cat if you use these products.
50. Conversation with the author.
51. Research on DMG and the immune response was conducted at the Medical University of South Carolina under the directorship of Charles D. Graber,

Ph.D. Dr. Graber's group demonstrated that DMG may enhance both humeral (antibody production) and cellular (cellular lymphocyte production) immunity, making an individual less prone to infections and able to respond more quickly to invasion by various viral and bacterial organisms. Their research also showed a normalized or substantially raised immune response in the blood of patients with diabetes and sickle cell anemia. Many health practitioners are reporting that DMG is an effective antiinfectious agent for their patients. See Charles D. Graber, Ph.D., *Journal of Infectious Diseases 143* (1981), pp. 101–105.

52. J. W. Meduski, M.D., Ph.D. at the University of Southern California School of Medicine.

53. Including bacteria (salmonella, e-coli, streptococcus, bacillus, vibrio cholera, staphylococcus, clostridium, coryne bacteria, diplococcus, lactobacillus, mycobaterium, shigella dysenteria, chlamydia, brucella, cloaca, haemophilus, klebsiella, legionella, moraxella, neisseria, pseudomonas, sarcina, proteus, alcalingenes, campylobacter, pasteurella, serratia, aerobacter, helicobacter); fungi (candida albicans, trichophyton, epidermophyton, aspergillus, niger, chaetomium, deratinomyces, monilia albicans, trichoderma, saccharomyces, fusarium, pencillium, neurospora); and virus/amebiasis (giardia lamblia, influenza a, african swine fever, entamoeb histolytica, swine vesicular, herpes simplex, foot and mouth disease).

Chapter Five

1. John Fudens, D.V.M., *The Affinity Holistic Veterinary Clinic's Layman's Handbook to Holistic Care*, p. 21.
2. The Resources section at the back of this book contains names of organizations that can help you find holistic veterinarians. You can also contact me for a list.
3. Penelope Ody, *The Complete Medicinal Herb: A Practical Guide to the Healing Properties of Herbs with More Than 250 Remedies for Common Ailments*; Penny C. Royal, *Herbally Yours*; and Louise Tenney, M.H., *Today's Herbal Health* (see Resources section).
4. John Fudens, D.V.M., *Layman's Handbook*, "Herbal Medicine and Pet Health."
5. Note that powdered herbs are also sold in capsule form. You may remove the contents of the capsules to use in herbal recipes.
6. Concentrated herbs are also available. They are processed in the same way as extracts but are subjected to dehydration in order to remove the moisture, resulting in a solvent-free product. Concentrated herbs are four to six times as potent as extracts.
7. There are three companies whose products I use often, both for myself and my cats, and distribute to my clients: Sunrider Whole Food Herbs, Nature's Sunshine, and Systemic Formulas, Inc. See Resources for further information.
8. See My Special Supplements section in chapter 4, "Nutrition," about the dangers of preservatives used with aloe vera.
9. Check with your own health practitioner before fasting.
10. Deepak Chopra, M.D., *Quantum Healing*, p. 17.

11. Other examples of functional disturbances include: a lot of scratching, but no bumps, redness, or scabs showing; a slight red line along the tooth-gum margin; appetite changes, finickiness at mealtime; behavioral changes (too sweet, too aggressive); vomiting (or gagging) hairballs; any other symptoms out of the normal range for healthy cats.

12. The Bach flower remedies associated with the sun signs (see also Flower Essences in chapter 5, "Natural Remedies") work very well alongside homeopathic treatment.

13. Homeopathic Education Services (which reports that homeopathy is sometimes called the "royal medicine" because the British royal family has used these remedies since the 1830s) produces a catalogue through which you may order remedies and tapes by phone or mail; in addition, they have a store in Berkeley, California. Standard Homeopathics and Washington Homeopathic Products are also quite reliable, according to Dr. Chambreau.

14. Conversation with the author.

15. There are now many excellent holistic and homeopathic veterinarians across the country. A number of them may be of help by phone even though they're not local (see Resources or contact me for a list).

16. See Books, Publications, and Tapes in Resources for further sources of information on the preparation of homeopathic remedies.

17. Remedies made from diseased tissue are known as *nosodes*, and are discussed in more detail in the section on vaccination (see chapter 3, "Dangers to Your Cat").

18. Recommended readings and sources for purchasing cell salts are included in the Resources section. See also chapter 8, for the relationship of the cell salts to the sun signs.

19. H. G. Wolff, D.V.M., *Your Healthy Cat: Homeopathic Medicines for Common Feline Ailments*, p. 7.

20. Dr. Chambreau demonstrates this process in her video (see Resources).

21. Conversation with the author.

22. Adapted from a chart by Raul Ibarra, M.D. in "Chronobiology: A Possible Explanation for Homeopathic Aggravation," the *Townsend Letter for Doctors*, February/March, 1990, p. 99.

23. Kirlian photography allows us to see this energy field, which surrounds all living things. A Kirlian photograph of a leaf, part of which has been cut off, shows light still glowing around the portion of the leaf that's no longer there (see the Auras and Chakras of a Cat in chapter 7).

24. Many flower remedies contain alcohol as a preservative. Always dilute them in purified or spring water, as recommended on the label.

25. Numerous human case studies are detailed in Phillip M. Chancellor, *Bach Flower Remedies*. If you're interested in studying Dr. Bach's approach in depth or in prescribing his remedies for yourself or your cats, I recommend his book *The Bach Flower Remedies* as well as *Practical Uses and Applications of the Bach Flower Remedies* by Jessica Beal, Ph.D., N.D. (see Resources).

26. The founders of FES, Richard Katz and Patricia Kaminsky, have written

Flower Essence Repertory, a comprehensive selection guide for the natural health practitioner. This book describes the FES remedies as well as English flower essences produced by Bach's company as well as by Healing Herbs (see Resources).

27. Sheehan publishes a booklet entitled "A Guide to Green Hope Farm" (see Resources).

28. I consult with Yolanda LaCombe (see Resources), who prefers to work with healing herbs and North American flower essences, but I use the Bach remedies as well.

29. The remedies are preserved in alcohol, so you must dilute them in spring water before administering, especially orally, as most cats will have a strong negative reaction to the taste.

30. This type of dosage bottles may be sold wherever you purchase your flower remedies, or you may order bottles directly from Ellon USA or FES (see Resources).

31. Researched from *Practical Uses and Applications of the Bach Flower Remedies* by Jessica Beal, Ph.D., N.D.; *The Flower Remedies Handbook* by Donna Cunningham, and *Flower Essence Repertory* by Flower Essence Services.

32. Conversation with Christina Chambreau, D.V.M.

33. Healing Herbs's emergency formula is called 5 Flowers. I feel it's even more effective than Rescue Remedy; however, I use them both.

34. I also make up special formulas for my clients and kitten buyers by appointment and through telephone consultation.

35. Diane Stein, *Natural Healing for Dogs and Cats*, p. 146-47.

36. Diane Stein suggests placing the bottles under a copper pyramid for two hours. Again, do this one flower essence at a time. However, in my opinion, this step is optional.

37. Contact Perelandra for a catalogue and information about their books and remedies (see Resources).

38. The Burton Goldberg Group, *Alternative Medicine: The Definitive Guide*, pp. 52-61. The authors of this work also cite information from John Steele, Ph.D., and Robert Tisserand, both leaders in the field of aromatherapy. I use John Steele's oils myself, available through Capital Drugs (see Resources).

39. Scott Cunningham, *Magical Aromatherapy*, pp. 25-39.

40. One source for live aromatic plants, herbs, seeds, and other products is Capriland's Herb Farm in Connecticut (see Resources).

41. Eye of the Cat in California is a good source of good dried herbs.

42. You may also purchase essential oils from Aroma Vera, Inc., in California (see Resources).

43. Nelly Grosjean, *Veterinary Aromatherapy*, p. 30. This is an excellent work to keep on hand for reference and recipes.

44. Hydrosol is a type of homeopathic aromatherapy; see Nelly Grosjean, *Veterinary Aromatherapy*, pp.17-18.

45. A poultice made of some powder, such as clay, mixed with water to form a thick paste. It's applied with gauze and secured with a bandage. See also Herbs section in this chapter.
46. Grosjean supplies diffusers and natural mixtures for them through La Chevêche (see Resources).
47. *The Cornell Book of Cats: A Comprehensive Medical Reference for Every Cat or Kitten,* by the faculty and staff of the Cornell Feline Health Center, Cornell University, edited by Mordecai Siegal. Catnip produces the opposite effect in humans; it calms and soothes the nerves.
48. Scott Cunningham, *Magical Aromatherapy,* p. 45.
49. Diane Stein, *Natural Healing for Dogs and Cats,* p. 77

Chapter Six

1. Cited in Barbara Rosen, "Chiropractic For Cats," *Cats Magazine,* Feb. 1993, pp. 45-46.
2. Ibid.
3. Nancy Scanlan, D.V.M., "Needles for Cats, or How I Saw the Light and Became Holistic with the Help of Acupuncture," *Tiger Tribe,* Mar.-Apr. 1993, pp. 15-17; Jeanne Demyan, D.V.M., "The Case of Murasaki," in ibid., p. 18.
4. The validity of the meridian system was verified by the French researcher Pierre de Vernejoul, who injected radioactive isotopes into the acupoints of humans and tracked them with a gamma-imaging camera. These injections traveled 30cm. along the known acupuncture meridians within four to six minutes. Vernejoul then injected the isotopes into blood vessels at random places in the body; these injections did not travel in the same manner. Thus, Vernejoul saw that the meridians comprise a system of distinct pathways within the body (researched from the Burton Goldberg Group, *Alternative Medicine: The Definitive Guide,* 1993, p. 37). Moreover, Kirlian photographs of the energy field emanating from the body show changes after acupuncture treatment.
5. Richard H. Pitcairn, D.V.M., and Susan Hubble Pitcairn, *Complete Guide to Natural Health for Dogs and Cats, pp. 148–150.* See Yang and Yin, in chapter 8.
6. Ibid.
7. Diane Stein, *Natural Healing for Dogs and Cats,* p. 125; Stein's source for this information was Edith A. Uridel, "Alternative Therapies," *Dog Fancy,* Mar. 1992, p. 46.
8. The cats I myself have observed receiving acupuncture treatments tolerate the traditional procedure rather well.
9. I would also suggest Dr. Bach's Rescue Remedy (See Flower Essences in chapter 5, "Natural Remedies"). George Macleod, D.V.M., states that the predisposing factors that may produce a picture calling for Aconitum (see Homeopathy, in chapter 5) include shock, operation, and exposure to cold, dry winds or dry heat; see *Cats: Homeopathic Remedies.*
10. Daily activities are accomplished while the brain generates the beta pattern. An alpha state in felines is equivalent to that achieved by humans during meditation. Theta is achieved in deep trance, delta in sleep.

11. Developed by Moshe Feldenkreis, this method is based on the concept that each cell, through its life force or vital intelligence, is connected with the whole body— and with other life forms.

Chapter Seven

1. From *Alternative Medicine: The Definitive Guide*, p. 465. It's amazing how few practitioners are aware of the miracles that occur on a daily basis using alternative holistic care on both people and animals. You may wish to share this book with your veterinarian as a gift.
2. Joanne Stefanatos, D.V.M., "Holistic Pet Care" (videotape); see Resources.
3. In *Healing For the Age of Enlightenment*, pp. 116-119.
4. Dael, *The Crystal Book*, p. 13.
5. Diane Stein, *Natural Healing for Dogs and Cats*, p. 174.
6. Dr. Stefanatos shows an example of this energy halter, originally designed by Dr. Gloria Dodd, in her videotape "Holistic Pet Care" (see Resources for halter and videotape).
7. Human beings hear at approximately 20 kilohertz (kHz). Cats hear at 40-50 kHz.
8. Henry Sigerist, *Civilization and Disease*, 1962, p. 149.
9. John Craige, D.V.M., "Therapeutic Sound for Animals," *Pet and Horse Exchange*, vol. 10, no. 7 (July 1993).
10. Conversation with Dr. Craige.
11. Such as Richard Gerber, M.D., *Vibrational Medicine* (see Resources).
12. Wayne Perry, "Cosmic Choir" (audiotape); see Resources.
13. You may obtain the chart and tape by contacting Musikarma Productions (see Resources); the materials are meant to be used together.
14. Conversation with the author.
15. This is detailed in Perry's chart.
16. Study conducted by Frances Rauscher, University of California, Irvine; reported in "Tribal News," *Tiger Tribe*, Nov.-Dec. 1993, pp. 10-11.
17. This section was researched from John Fudens, D.V.M., *The Affinity Holistic Veterinary Clinic's Layman's Handbook*, "Magnetism"; and Joanne Stefanatos, D.V.M., "Holistic Pet Care" (videotape; see Resources).
18. This section was researched from John Fudens, D.V.M., *The Affinity Holistic Veterinary Clinic's Layman's Handbook*, "Radionics."
19. New Horizons also offers intensive seminars on identifying the vitamins, minerals, herbs, and homeopathic substances that will fit your specific body chemistry, and combatting the "electronic pollution" in your environment. Both the equipment and the training are expensive. At the time of this writing, the SE-5 sold for approximately $2,500, and a six-day training course cost $700. You may obtain more information by contacting New Horizons Trust (see Resources).

Chapter Eight

1. Throughout this chapter you'll see Dr. Chambreau's cautionary notes regarding the astrological use of homeopathy. Always consult a doctor of veterinary medicine before administering any remedy to your cat.

2. Though sun sign astrology can be entertaining and fun, it by no means provides the scientific depth or insight available through consultation with a trained astrologer. With the advent of computer technology, interdimensional astrological readings (which incorporate information from the several different systems of the zodiac) can now be offered at a reasonable cost. An astrological profile varies depending upon the system used, so combining perspectives allows us to understand more completely the personality, soul, and social aspects of an individual (human or animal). Interdimensional astrologer Eleanor Haspel-Porter, Ph.D., offers all levels of astrological consultations, some of which include the interdimensional use of color (see Resources).

3. Reinhold Ebertin, *Astrological Healing: The History and Practice of Astromedicine*, pp. 3–4. Ebertin's books contains a wealth of data documenting how, historically, astrology was incorporated into most healing sciences.

4. Ibid, pp. 37–38.

5. See William Boericke, M.D., and Willis A. Dewey, M.D., *The Twelve Tissue Remedies of Schuessler*, pp. 29–30.

6. Ibid., pp. 39–45. Perry observed that the work of Dr. George W. Carey, who wrote *The Relations of the Mineral Salts of the Body to the Signs of the Zodiac* (see *The Zodiac and the Salts of Salvation* in Resources), upon which Perry's work was based, unlocked the door to mental and physical well-being.

7. Peter Damian, *The Twelve Healers of the Zodiac*, pp. 2–3.

8. Scott Cunningham, *Magical Aromatherapy*, pp. 167–68.

9. Reinhold Ebertin, *Astrological Healing: The History and Practice of Astromedecine*, p. 138.

10. Jeffrey Levy, D.V.M., of Williamsburg, Massachusetts, has incorporated the yang/yin philosophy into his natural diet for cats. He refers to the protein portion of raw meat and organ meat as yang, the carbohydrate portion as neutral, and the vegetable portion as yin. He uses both yang and yin supplements.

11. The dates in parentheses are those given by Inez Eudora Perry in *The Zodiac and the Salts of Salvation*. Perry's astrological dating of this and certain other sun signs varies from the traditional system used by most prominent astrologers.

12. Dr. Chambreau reminds us that the best way to use homeopathy is to treat the animal with professional help, at the deepest (constitutional) level. This means giving one dose of a remedy and then often waiting weeks or months. Do not use these remedies without consulting your homeopathic veterinarian.

13. I only give my cats Kyolic garlic, as fresh garlic seems too bitter.

14. See note 10, above.

15. Dr. Chambreau asks us to remember that the goal is not to have to use these remedies. Ideally, your cat should be healthy enough to get a cough or cold

and get well on her own within two to seven days.

16. Caution: Do not use *Arnica* if anesthesia is to be used (such as with cesarean section).

17. As Dr. Chambreau reminds us, though, your homemade diet and the care of a homeopathic practitioner (both begun when the kitten is only a few weeks old), should keep your cat so healthy it probably won't need to be given any remedies.

18. You can help your homeopathic prescriber by noticing the characteristics of your cat's condition, even if the practitioner ends up choosing a different remedy. Always ask her or him about your selection before administering it.

19. See note 11, above.

20. See note 12, above.

21. See note 11, above.

22. As long as the cat is not already receiving deep constitutional treatment with another homeopathic remedy. Always remember to consult your homeopathic veterinarian before giving a remedy to your cats.

23. See note 15, above.

24. See note 17, above.

25. I don't recommend using *Arnica* on the day of surgery itself. Consider using *Aconite* the night before and the morning of surgery, and resume with *Arnica,* alternating with *Hypericum,* after surgery. However, Dr. Chambreau has stopped routinely recommending *Arnica* or *Aconite* for surgery, using them only if cats are sore. Often, they recover well without treatment.

26. One part tincture to ten parts distilled water.

27. One drop of the liquid to one ounce distilled water.

28. See note 18, above.

29. See note 25, above.

30. See note 22, above.

31. I've found a homeopathic remedy, Homeopathic Cat Hair, that I keep on hand to offer to people with allergies to cat dander. Contact Delisos for more information. (see Resources).

32. See note 12, above.

33. See note 15, above.

34. See chapter 5, "Natural Remedies," for more complete information about all these substances.

Chapter Nine

1. See Resources.

2. Cited in Diane Stein, *Natural Healing for Dogs and Cats,* p. 166.

3. Machaelle Small Wright, *Behaving As If the God in All Life Mattered.*

Resources

 PLEASE NOTE: at the time of this writing, the companies and practitioners supply one or more products and/or services that are acceptable within the guidelines of this book. This does not mean that I necessarily recommend all products and/or services made, sold, or provided by these companies and/or practitioners. Product and service quality can change, management, policies, and standards can change. I urge you to keep this in mind and to be alert. Read labels and product brochures carefully, even for products you have been using for a long time. Conduct your own interviews. There may be other fine suppliers and practitioners not listed here. My not listing certain suppliers and practitioners does not necessarily mean that I wouldn't recommend them if I knew about them.

Associations

American Cat Association (ACA)
Dept. CF, 8101 Katherine Avenue
Panorama City, CA 91402
(818) 781-5656
America's oldest cat registry

American Cat Fanciers' Association
(ACFA)
Dept. CF, P.O. Box 203,
Pt. Lookout, MO 65726
(417) 334-5430
One of the nation's largest registries of
pedigreed and household cats

American Holistic Veterinary
Medical Association
2214 Old Emmorton Road

Bel Air, MD 21014
(410) 569-0795
Referrals and information

The American Institute of
Homeopathy
1585 Glencoe Road
Denver, CO 80220
(303) 370-9164
This is the oldest homeopathic, and the
oldest medical association in the U.S.,
and publishes the *Journal of the American
Institute of Homeopathy.*

American Veterinarian
Chiropractic Association
P.O. Box 249
Port Byron, IL 61275
(309) 523-3995

A 100-hour course is taught on animal chiropractic to veterinarians and chiropractors.

The Animal Connection Network™
c/o Carol Bennett
P.O. Box 8084
Durango, CO 81301
(610) 259-4629
Conference call on the ninth day of each month at 5:00 pm Pacific Time and 8:00 pm EST. Using a touchtone phone, dial 1131 then after another tone, dial 415. Your cost (at the time of this writing) is the long distance charge for the call, which lasts approximately forty-five minutes. You can also subscribe to their newsletter for six months (April-September).

Bio-Integral Resource Center
P.O. Box 7414
Berkeley, California 94707
(510) 524-2567
Non-profit organization researching and promoting information on the least toxic methods of pest management.

Canadian Cat Association (CCA)
220 Advance Blvd. #101
Brampton, Ontario, Canada L6T4J5
(905) 459-1481
Canada's cat registry of pedigreed cats.

Cat Fanciers' Association (CFA)
1805 Atlantic Ave.
P.O. Box 1005
Manasquan, NJ 08736-1005
(908) 528-9797
World's largest registry of pedigreed cats. They publish the *Cat Fanciers' Almanac*, a montly magazine. Call for information on subscribing.

Cat Fanciers' Federation (CFF)
P.O. Box 661
Gratis, Ohio 45330
(573) 787-9009
A cat registry of purebred cats.

Delta Society
P.O. Box 1080
Renton, WA 95057
(206) 226-7357
National directory of grief counselors, books on grief, etc.

Flower Essence Society
P.O. Box 459
Nevada City, CA 95959
(800) 548-0075
Classes in flower essences and a newsletter.

The Foundation for Homeopathic Education and Research
5916 Chabot Crest
Oakland, CA 94618
(510) 420-8791
They sponsor homeopathic research, and educate health professionals and the general public about research on homeopathic medicine.

Grief Recovery Help Line
Grief Recovery Institute
(800) 445-4808
Monday-Friday 12 to 8 PM EST

Homeonet
18 De Boom Street
San Francisco, CA 94107
(415) 442-0220
For those with access to a computer and modem—human and veterinary homeopaths share cases.

Homeopathic Educational Services
2124 Kittridge Street
Berkeley, CA 94704
Order line: (800) 359-9051
Info. and catalogues: (510) 649-0294
Extensive list of books, tapes, information, and kits and helpful service.

Homeopathic Information
Resources, Ltd.
Oneida River Park Drive
Clay, NY 13041
(800) 289-4447
Books, tapes, remedy kits. Good veterinary homeopathy section.

Institute for Traditional Medicine
2017 S.E. Hawthorne
Portland, OR 97214
(800) 544-7504
Chinese herbs and books.

International Bio-Oxidative Med.
Foundation
P.O. Box 610767
Dallas/Fort Worth, TX 75261
(817) 481-9772
Promotes use of intravenous hydrogen peroxide infusion.

The International Cat Association
(TICA)
P.O. Box 2684
Harlingen, TX 78551
(210) 428-8046
First cat registry to register household pets and award them distinctive titles as well as purebreds.

International Foundation for
Homeopathy
2366 Eastlake Avenue E., Ste. 329
Seattle, WA 98102

(206) 324-8230
Directory of homeopaths who are graduates of IFH courses. Their journal, *Resonance,* contains occasional articles by veterinary homeopaths including Dr. Pitcairn and Dr. Levy. They also publish a yearly collection of "cured cases," which are very useful in studying homeopathy.

International Veterinary
Acupuncture Society
2140 Conestoga Road
Chester Springs, Pennsylvania 19425
(610) 827-7245/FAX (610) 827-1366
Referrals and information. Send SASE for veterinarians in your area.

National Center For Homeopathy
801 N. Fairfax Street #306
Alexandria, VA 22314
(703) 548-7790
Directory of homeopathic practitioners, pharmacies, resources, and study groups.

Network Chiropractic Veterinarians
Contact Dr. Mark P. Haverkos for referrals and information.
8 N. Huntersville Road
Batesville, Indiana
(812) 934-2410

New England School of Homeopathy
356 Middle Street
Amherst, MA 01002
(800) 637-4440
In-depth homeopathy courses and the wonderful *New England Journal of Homeopathy*.

The Pacific Institute of Aromatherapy
P.O. Box 6723
San Rafael, CA 94903
(415) 479-9121
Courses available to individuals and
companies interested in becoming certified in aromatherapy practice.

Price-Pottenger Nutrition Foundation
P.O. Box 2614
La Mesa, CA 91943-2614
(619) 547-7763)
"A non-profit tax-exempt education
organization dedicated to the promotion
of enhanced health through an awareness of ecology, lifestyle, and healthy
food production for good nutrition."
Catalog of books, pamphlets, and tapes.

Practitioners

Christina Chambreau, D.V.M.
908 Coldbottom Road
Sparks, MD 21152
(410) 771-4968
Member Academy of Veterinary
Homeopathy, courses given on veterinary homeopathy.

Lisa Bergon
c/o Westside Hospital for Cats
1844 14th Street
Santa Monica, CA 90404
(310) 452-9091
Licensed acupuncturist. Also available
for consultations on the use of herbs
and homeopathy in the treatment of
your cat.

Morgana Davies
2642 N. Calvert Street
Baltimore, MD 21218
(410) 235-7124

Certified Bach flower therapist and
Reiki practitioner. Lectures and workshops available.

John Fudens, D.V.M.
29296 US 19N # 104
Clearwater, FL 34621
(813) 787-6010
Affinity holistic clinic

Linda Goodman
2023 Chicago Avenue #B-25
Riverside, CA 92507
(909) 784-9070
Animal communicator and behavior
consultant.

Carol Gurney
3715 N. Cornel Road
Agoura, CA 91301
(818) 597-1154
Animal communicator and bodywork.

Donald K. Hamilton, D.V.M.
P.O. Box 67
Ocate, NM 87734
505/666-2091

Eleonor Haspel-Portner, Ph.D.
(310) 459-1886
Astrologer, psychologist, and Reiki
master.

Healthy Attitudes Holistic Health
Practice for You and Your Pets
Harrisburg, PA
(717) 541-8817
Jane Crowley, Reiki master, color therapist, and certified Bach Flower consultant available for treatments, classes, and
certifications using the PEMS approach
(physical, emotional, mental, and spiritual).

Lydia Hibby
18810 Bert Road
Riverside, California 92508
(909) 789-0330
Animal analyst available for consultations, lectures, and seminars. Newsletter: *Pet Network News.*

Samantha Khury
1251 10th Street
Manhattan Beach, CA 90266
(310) 374-6812
Therapist and educator available for
lectures, seminars, workshops, private
therapy.

Yolanda LaCombe/John Lowery
Glendale, CA
(818) 845-6570
Consultant working with healing herbs
and North American flower essences.

Michael W. Lemmon, D.V.M.
P.O. Box 2085
Renton, Washington
(206) 226-8418

Charles E. Loops, DVM
RT. 2, Box 568
Pittsboro, NC 27312
(919) 542-0442
Fax: (919) 542-0535

Loving Touch Animal Center
1975 Glenn Club Dr.
Stone Mountain, GA 30087
(404) 498-5956
Michelle Tilghman, D.V.M., manufacturer of Homeopathic Animal First
Aid Kit.

Pat McKay
372 Grace Drive
So. Pasadena, CA 911030
(818) 441-8415
Animal nutrition consultant. Author of
Reigning Cats and Dogs. Consultations,
natural health care products. She publishes *Nutricare News* for her clients.

Barbara Meyers
Holistic Animal Consulting Center
29 Lyman Avenue
Staten Island, NY 10305
(718) 720-5548
Grief therapist, certified Bach flower
remedies counselor.

Lisa Newman
3150 N. Lodge Rd.
Tucson, AZ 85715
(800) 497-5665
Holistic animal practitioner.

Richard Pitcairn, D.V.M., Ph.D.
1283 Lincoln Street
Eugene, Oregon 97401
(503) 342-7665

Sis Sewell
c/o Healthy Pets Naturally
(404) 475-4550
Holistic practitioner and publisher of
Healthy Pets, Naturally.

Mary Ann Simonds
Wisdom Stone Farms
17101 N.E. 40th Avenue
Vancouver, WA 98686
(360) 573-1958
Natural healing, consulting.

Laurel Steinhice
6712 Currywood Drive
Nashville, TN 37205
(615) 356-4280
Channeling and psychic work. Reiki
master.

Russell Swift, D.V.M.
3511 W. Commercial Boulevard,
Ste. 227
Fort Lauderdale, FL 33309-3322
(305) 739-4416

Linda Tellington-Jones
P.O. Box 3793
Santa Fe, NM 87501-0793
(800) 854-TEAM
T-Touch Therapy.

Marion Webb-Former
340 The Circle
Queen Elizabeth Street
London, SE1 2ND, England
Channeling and psychic work.

Celeste Yarnall
9875 Gloucester Drive
Beverly Hills, CA 90210
(310) 278-1385
Consulting on the natural diet and
alternative health therapies for cats and
dogs. Organic foods and supplements
available for delivery and/or shipping.
Distributor for: Advanced Enzyme
Technologies/Woolly 'n Wild's Pure
Comfort (aloe vera juice without sodium benzoate, Erigeron and Herbal
shampoos, conditioners and topical
sprays), Best Friends (supplements formulated by Pat McKay; Bio-C, Bonemeal with red marrow, MinerAll Plus,
and PuriZone), Cell Tech (Super
Blue-Green Algae), Emprise (DHEA,

Acemannon/Manapol), Kaire International (Pycnogenol), Life Plus (supplements), Nature's Sunshine (Chinese
herbs and herbal supplements),
Sedna/Withers Mill Company (Prog-
est, Essiac), Sunrider (Whole food supplements and herbal products), and
Threshold/Source Naturals (Colloidal
silver and supplements for people,
which I use for cats); Standardized
grapefruit extract, Kitty Lac, and Goat
A Lac milk replacer for kittens, and
much, much more.

At the time of this writing, I am
creating my own special feline supplements called Celestial Cats Feline Supplements formulated with Pat McKay.
The first will combine Bonemeal, MinerAll Plus, and Bio-C with additional
supplements, including Blue-Green
Algae. The second is a food enzyme
that I am working on with Dr. Russell
Swift. Please feel free to contact me
regarding their availability.

For a list of holistic veterinarians
and practitioners, send a stamped, self-
addressed envelope plus $3.00.

Suppliers:

Acuspark
P.O. Box 366
Swanee, GA 30174
(404) 822-0752
EMS unit (for practitioners), which
provides electro-muscle stimulation for
pain relief.

Agape Video Systems, Inc.
1325 Vegas Valley Drive
Las Vegas, CA 89109
Holistic Pet Care video by Dr. Joanne
Stefanatos.

Ainsworth Homeopathic Pharmacy
36 New Cavendish Street
London, WIM 7LH, England
011-44-7935-5330
Large choices of remedies, many that
are not available in the U.S., and animal
nosodes.

All The Best
8050 Lake City Way
Seattle, WA 98115
Mail order: (800) 962-8266
Store: (206) 524-0199
Natural pet foods, supplements, home-
opathics, and supplies.

Alpha Omega Labs
Box 291
Fort Benton, MT 59441
(800) 554-1961
Bio-Culture 2000, (L. Salivarius) and
other holistic products.

Alta Health Products
1979 E. Locust St.
Pasadena, CA 91107
(818) 796-1047
Outside CA: (800) 423-4155
Alta-Silica X.

Amrita Herbal Products
Rt. 1, Box 737
Floyd, VA 24091
(703) 745-3474
Herb tinctures and salves.

Analytical Research Labs
8650 N. 22nd Avenue
Phoenix, AZ 85021
(800) 528-4067
Heavy metal analysis and mineral
analysis.

Animal Health Options, Inc.
1724 Langhorne-Yardley Road
Yardley, PA 19067
(215) 493-0621
Manufacturers of Chinese herbal food
supplements.

Anitra's Natural Pet Products, Ltd.
c/o Halo Purely for Pets
3438 East Lake Road #14
Palm Harbor, FL 34685
(800) 426-4256/ (813) 854-2214
Offers Anitra Frazier's vita-mineral mix
and other fine natural products created
by Anitra Frazier.

Aromatherapy Seminars
1830 S. Robertson Boulevard
Los Angeles, CA 90035
(800) 677-2368 / (310) 838-6122
Certificate programs provided through
correspondence courses plus specialty
classes offered to those individuals
already certified. Videotapes and blend-
ing materials also available.

Aroma Vera, Inc.
5901 Rodeo Road
Los Angeles, CA 90016
(310) 280-0407
Essential oils

Aubrey's Organics
4419 N. Manhattan Avenue
Tampa, FL 33614
(813) 876-4879
Manufacturers of shampoos, conditioners, and grooming spray for pets.

Australian Bush Flower Essences
Box 531, Spit Junction NSW
Australia 2088

Avena Botanicals
20 Mill Street
Rockland, ME 04841
(207) 594-0694
Herbal supplements for animals, tinctures, and earmite formula (uses De Bairacli Levy formula).

Beckett's Apothecary
1004 Chester Pike
Sharon Hill, PA 19079
(800) 727-8188
Homeopathic remedies. Mail order.

Better Way Cat Litter
Sanex Corporation
P.O. Box 573073
Houston, TX 77259-3073
Makers of Calico, Grand Prize, and Better Way cat litters. Biodegradable, flushable clumping litter.

Bio-Botanica (New York)
75 Commerce Dr.
Hauppauge, NY 11788
(800) 645-5720
Herb extracts

Bio/Chem Research
865 Parallel Dr.
P.O. Box 238
Lakeport, CA 95453
(707) 263-1475
Makers of Citricidal brand of products for disinfection and control of intestinal parasites.

Biogenetics Food Corporation/Jesse Davis
3427 Exchange Avenue #8
Naples, FL 33942
(800) 477-7688
Manufacturers of nutritional and

antioxidant supplements, Bioguard for Pets, Bioguard Plus for Pets, Feline Balance, and Feline Vitality™.

Biovet International/Pacific Botanicals
1440 Kapiolani Blvd. #108-186
Honolulu, HI 96814
(800) 468-7578
Antioxidants from organically grown wheat sprouts.

Boericke & Tafel
2381 Circadian Way
Santa Rosa, CA 95407
(800) 876-9505
Homeopathic remedies. Automatic 2nd day mail for professionals.

Boiron-Borneman
#6 Campus Blvd.
Newtown Square, PA 19073
(800) 258-8823
Suppliers of homeopathic remedies.

Books From India, Ltd.
45 Museum Street
London, WC1A1LR, England
011-44-171405-3784

Capitol Drugs
4454 Van Nuys Boulevard
Sherman Oaks, CA 91403
(818) 905-8338
Homeopathic remedies, John Steele's oils, herbs, books, and more.

Capriland's Herb Farm
534 Silver Street
Coventry, CT 06238
(203) 742-7244
Live aromatic plants, herbs, seeds, and products. Send SASE for catalog ordering information.

Resources: Suppliers

Care Fresh
Absorption Corporation
1051 Hilton Avenue
Bellingham, WA 98225
(800) 242-2287
Fluffy, paper-based litter. Biodegradable, dust-free, flushable, and incinerable.

Cat-Chee Enterprises
1621 W. 25th Street #320
San Pedro, CA 90732
(310) 831-5901 / (800) 381-2121
Kitty Kamode custom-made wood cabinets to conceal your cat's litter box.

Cat Country Organic
Premium Litter for Cats Inc.
P.O. Box 778
Lewiston, MT 59457
(800) 752-8864
Biodegradable litter. Plant-based. Dust-free. Flushable.

Cat Fairies
Gail Colombo
3964 26th Street
San Francisco, CA 94131
(415) 550-7472
Sprouts, books, catnip, etc. Catalog available.

Cat Fence-In Kits
P.O. Box 795
Sparks, NY 89432
(702) 359-4575

Celletech Ltd.
518 Tasman
Madison, WI
(608) 221-9413 or (800) 888-4066
Ships single dose homeopathics, and more.

Citra-Fresh Pet Litter
Blossom Products Company
P.O. Box 4163
Scottsdale, AZ 85261
Fluffy, light-colored, dried citrus materials.

College Fur Cats
Sandi Wirth
(818) 597-8760
Behavior training classes. Fun for every cat companion.

Coyote Moon Herbs
Teresa Finkbeiner, M.H.
P.O. Box 312
Gainesville, FL 32602
(904) 377-0765
Herbs by mail order.

Critter Oil
The SuDi Company
P.O. Box 12767
St. Petersburg, FL 33733
(813) 327-2356
Natural flea-rid products, pet foods, supplements, and supplies.

Cybernetics Research Corp.
523 Caldwell Boulevard
Nampa, ID 83651
(208) 465-9092
World-wide health search. Their primary purpose is to provide access to all information concerning health and nutritional information. Referral services for health professionals and specialists.

Derma Pet
P.O. Box 59713
Potomac, MD 20859
(800) 755-4738

Manufacturers of Derma Pet Conditioner for Pets (a spray-on product) and Derma Pet Conditioning Shampoo for Pets.

Deva Flower Remedies
c/o Natural Labs Corp.
P.O. Box 230229
Encinitas, CA
(800) 233-0810

Gloria Dodd, D.V.M.
Everglo Ranch
P.O. Box 1242
Gualala, CA 95445
Audio cassettes. Dr. Dodd no longer offers consultations.

Dold Diagnostics
450 Porter Road, Ste. C
Dixon, CA 95620
(916) 678-1301
Services offered for home testing of blood and saliva for FelV (feline leukemia).

Dolisos America, Inc.
3014 Rigel Avenue
Las Vegas, NV 89102
(800) 365-4767
Homeopathic remedies. Free catalog.

Dr. Don's Formulas
P.O. Box 6153
Federal Way, WA 98063
(206) 838-3878
Manufacturers of homeopathic products: Stop Fleas, Stop Stress

Dr. Goodpet Laboratories
P.O. Box 4489
Inglewood, CA 90309
(800) 222-9932 / (213) 672-3269
Homeopathics and vitamins.

East Coast Herbs
1281 North Mt. Juliette Rd.
Mt. Juliette, TN 37122
(800) 283-5191
Herbs

Eco Safe Products
P.O. Box 1177
St. Augustine, FL 32085
(800) 274-7387
Herbal products and flea products.

Ellon USA, Inc
644 Merrick Road
Lynbrook, NY 11563
(800) 433-7523
Bach flower remedies

Energy Refractors
53166 State Rte. 681
Reedsville, OH 45772
(614) 378-6155
Hydrogen Peroxide

Enhanced Water Products, Inc.
8337 Penn Avenue South
Bloomington, MN 55431
(612) 881-7314
Crystal enhanced water

Felix Company
3623 Fremont Avenue N.
Seattle, WA 98103
Cat care products

FIELDFresh™ Cat Box Filler
The Andersons
P.O. Box 119
Maumee, OH 43537
(800) 537-3370
Organic, 100% Biodegradable, compostable, and flushable cat box filler.

Fleabusters, Inc.
6555 N.W. Ninth Avenue #411
Ft. Lauderdale, FL 33309
(800) 666-3532
This company will come to your home
and treat it with a nonpesticide flea
product.

Flower Essence Services
P.O. Box 1769
Nevada City, CA 95959
(800) 548-0075
Flower essences, aromatherapy, and
books available through mail order.

Frontier Cooperative Herbs
P.O. Box 69
Norway, CA 52318
Bach flower remedies. Source of gelatin
capsules, herbs, combination homeo-
pathics, and more.

Dr. Gary Glum
Silent Walker Publishing
P.O. Box 92856
Los Angeles, CA 90009
(310) 271-9931
Essiac Herb Formula

Green Hope Farm
P.O. Box 125, True Road
Meriden, NH 03770
(603) 469-3662
Flower essences by Molly Sheehan
including Bermuda essences, Adiron-
dack essences and vegetable/flower
essences from her divinely directed
garden.

Green Terrestrial Herb Farm
P.O. Box 266
Milton, NY 12547
Pam Montgomery
Wild, crafted, common and hard to
find tinctures. Catalog.

Gurudas
P.O. Box 868
San Rafael, CA 94915
Flower essences, gem elixirs, and
books.

Hahnemann Pharmacy
828 San Pablo Avenue
Albany, CA 94706
(510) 527-3003
Supplies the nosodes for animal disease
prevention (sold only to veterinarians).
Herbal formulas and remedies up to
30C.

Halo Products, Purely for Pets
3438 East Lake Road #14
Palm Harbor, FL 34685
(800) 426-4256 / (813) 854-2214
Manufacturers of Dream Coat, Derma
Dream, Natural Herbal Ear Wash, and
other natural pet care products.

Hanson Homeopathic
Herbal Medicine
4540 Southside Boulevard #5
Jacksonville, FL 32216-5458
(904) 641-6301
Largest stock of homeopathic remedies
and products in the South.

Harmony Farms
2824 Foothill Boulevard
La Crescenta, CA 91214
Bruce Oxford (818) 248-3068
Naturally grown meat and poultry.

Herb Farm
P.O. Box 116
Williams, OR 97544
(800) 348-4372
Liquid herbal extracts, herbal compounds, herbal glycerites (no alcohol),
books, and betonite (montmorillonite)
clay. Most of the herbs sold are organic
or wildcrafted (picked from nature).

Hi-Tor Dust-Free Cat Litter
Triumph Pet Industries
P.O. Box 100
Hillburn, NY 10931
Made from recycled newspaper that has
been processed and formed into pellets.
Biodegradable and dust-free.

Hobon Detoxifying Products
Naples, FL
(800) 521-7722

Holistic Pet Care Catalog for Dogs,
Cats, and Horses
Patty Swygert
1811 Franklin Avenue
McLean, VA 22101
(703) 536-2515
Fax: (703) 536-4070
The catalog includes natural foods, supplements, first aid, treats, homeopathic
remedies, herbs, aromatherapy products,
flower essences, books, and suggested
magazines, classes, and events.

Holistic Pet Center
15599 S.E. 82nd Drive
P.O. Box 1166
Clackamas, OR 97015
(800) 788-7387
Vet Line supplement for cats and dogs,
books, and Kitty Fishin' pole.

Helios Pharmacy
97 Camden Rd.
Turnbridge Wells
Kent TN1 2QR England
0892-536393/ 537254
Fax: 0892-546850
Homeopathic remedies including LM
potencies

J & B Catalog
(800) 526-0388
Wholesale pet supplies

J.D.'s Cat Habitats
P.O. Box 3237
Park City, UT 84060
(801) 649-0685
Cat trees made from natural (not live)
juniper trees.

Jerry Teplitz Enterprises, Inc.
219 53rd Street
Virginia Beach, VA 23451
(800) 777-3529
Books, tapes, and music on stress reduction.

Kyolic Garlic
Wakunaga of America Co., Ltd.
23501 Madero
Mission Viejo, CA 92691
(800) 421-2998 /
(800) 544-5800 (in CA)
Manufacturers of high-potency garlic
in capsule, tablet, and liquid form.

Laurel Farms
P.O. Box 7405
Studio City, CA 91614
(310) 289-4372
Kombucha tea

L & H Vitamins
37-10 Crescent Street
Long Island City, NY 11101
(800) 221-1152
Carries natural pet supplements, vitamins, herbs, homeopathics, and Bach
flower remedies at discounted prices.

Longevity Pure Medicine
9595 Wilshire Boulevard #502
Beverly Hills, CA 90212
(310) 273-7423
Suppliers of homeopathic remedies.

Lotus Light
P.O. Box 1008
Silverlake, WI 53170
(414) 889-8501
Dr. Good pet products, cat collars,
shampoo, and supplements.

Love Your Pets
15443 S. Latourette Road
Oregon City, OR 97045
(800) 258-8589 / (503) 631-7389
Manufacturer of Love Your Pet Calmer
and other supplements.

Magnetic Field Therapy
858 Third Avenue #126
Chula Vista, CA 91911
(619) 427-7231
Provide information on magnetic field
therapy.

Magnet Sales & Manufacturing, Inc.
11248 Playa Court
Culver City, CA 90230
(800) 421-6692
Magnetic specialties and more.

Mid-America Marketing
P.O. Box 124
Eaton, OH 45320
(800) 922-1744
Complete source for magnet therapy
products

Matrix Institute, Inc.
P.O. Box 336
Chesterfield, NH 03443
(603) 363-4916
Vibrational remedies, flower essences,
and gem essences. Publishes Gordon
Michael Scalion's newsletter.

Merz Apothecary
4716 N. Lincoln Avenue
Chicago, IL 60625
(800) 252-0275
Homeopathic pharmacy

Minimum Price Homeopathic Books
250 H. Street
P.O. Box 2187
Blaine, WA 98231
Orders: (800) 663-8272
Info.: (604) 597-4757

Morrill's New Directions
P.O. Box 30
Orient, ME 04471
(800) 368-5057
Natural pet care products. Free catalog
available.

Musikarma Productions/Wayne Perry
8391 Beverly Boulevard, Suite 333,
Los Angeles, CA 90048
(213) 655-7781
Healing charts and tapes for sound
therapy.

Natural Animal
P.O. Box 1177
St. Augustine, FL 32085
(800) 274-7387
Manufacturers of Natural Animal Coat
Enhancer, Ester C, and other natural
pet care products.

Natural Animal Nutrition
2109 Emmorton Park
Suite 113
Edgewood, MD 21040
(800) 548-2899
Nutritional supplements

The Natural Pet Care Company
8050 Lake City Way, N.E.
Seattle, WA 98115
(800) 962-8266
Free catalog available.

Nature's Herb Company
110 46th Street
Emeryville, CA 94608
(510) 601-0700.
Free catalog available.

Nature's Own Environmental Services
899 Brentwood
Venice, FL 34292
(813) 485-3115
Melinda Leeson consults on homeopathy, nutrition, and herbs for animals.

Necessary Trading Company
One Natures Way
New Castle, VA 24127
(703) 864-5103
All natural kelp, citrus oil, and sham-
poo.

Nelly Grosjean's Natural Products
La Chevêche
13690 Graveson-en-Provence, France
(33) 90 95 81 72 /
Fax: (33) 90 95 85 20
or in the U.S.: Vie Arôme distributed
by Aromatherapy Int'l
3 Seal Harbor Road, Suite 437
Winthrop, MA 02152
(617) 846-0285 /
Fax: (617)0 846-5474
Natural and organic quality aromatic
essential oils, hydrosols, aromatic diffusers, books, and Nelly Grosjean's aromatic specialties. Mail order facility.
Delivery within 48 hours in France, 5
days elsewhere.

N.E.S.S. (Nutritional Enzyme
Support Systems)
2903 N.W. Platte Road
Riverside, MO 64150
(800) 637-7893 for catalog
Manufacturers of Vet-Zimes (digestive
enzymes for pets). Sells to veterinarians.
Newsletter and product catalog including water filtration systems through
reverse osmosis. They also carry acuspark for pain relief.

New Horizons Trust
53166 St. Rt. 681
Reedsville, OH 45772
(800) 755-6360
Alternative health and all natural products. Free catalog available.

Newton Laboratories
P.O. Box 936
Lithonia, GA 30058
(800) 448-7256 / (404) 922-2644
Homeopathic combination line for
dogs, cats, and horses.

Noah's Park
13600 Wright Circle
Tampa, FL 33626
(800) 842-6624
Natural pet foods and products. Mail order.

Norfields
632-3/4 N. Doheny Drive
Los Angeles, CA 90069
(800) 344-8400
Manufacturers of magnetic health care products.

Northeast Homeopathic Products
563 Massachusetts Avenue, Route 111
Acton, MA 01720-2903
(800) 551-3611
Standard Homeopathic distributor pharmacy.

Nu Age Laboratories
4200 Laclede Avenue
St. Louis, MO 63108
(314) 533-9600
Suppliers of homeopathic remedies.

Nutri-Dyn Products, Inc.
(New Biologics)
2470 Wisconsin St.
Downers Grove, IL 60515
(708) 969-6700
Glandular supplements, herbals, home-opathics, amino acid supplements, and nutritionals.

Ocean Health Products
(800) 477-5108
Cartilade (shark cartilage)

Pampered Pets & People
Leisha & Mark Churchman
504 Indian Trail

Palm Springs, CA 92264-7623
(800) 243-2704 / (619) 778-7176
Fax: (619) 322-243.
Custom cat tree and habitats.

Peeskill Pet Products - PVT
2306 N.E. 7th Avenue
Ft. Lauderdale, FL 33305-2128
(800) 551-1495
PVT, a complete health care line for dogs and cats. Organic vitamin supple-ments, protein shampoo, and skin cream.

Pegasus Products, Inc.
P.O. Box 228
Boulder, CO 80306
(800) 527-6104
Flower and gemstone essences.

Perelandra Flower Essences
P.O. Box 3603
Warrenton, VA 22186
(703) 937-2153 / Fax (803) 937-3360
Flower essences, books by Machaelle Small Wright.

Pet Care Systems, Inc.
717 N. Clinton Street
Grand Ledge, MI 48837
(800) 794-3287
Wheat Scoop Litter- Recyclable clumping litter made from wheat and corn.

PetGuard, Inc.
165 Industrial Loop S.
Orange Park, FL 32073
(800) 874-3221/ (904) 264-8500
Provides one of the natural commercial pet foods.

Pet's Friends, Inc.
3511 W. Commercial Boulevard,
Suite 227
Ft. Lauderdale, FL 33309
(305) 739-4416
Dr. Russell Swift's enzyme formulas:
FlorazymeLP, FlorazymeEFA,
AniMinerals.

Pets Naturally
13459 Ventura Blvd.
Sherman Oaks, CA 91423
(818) 784-1233
Health food store that carries natural
products, homeopathics, and natural
supplements.

Pet Pyramind
Hollingsworth Technology
1341 N. Woodland Boulevard
Deland, FL 32720
(904) 736-4930
New age pet habitat

Santa Monica Homeopathic Pharmacy
629 Broadway
Santa Monica, CA 90401
(310) 395-1131
Homeopathic remedies, Chinese herbal
food supplements.

Sherpa's Pet Trading Company
357 E. 57th Street, St. 15A
New York, NY 10022
(800) 743-7723 / (212) 838-9837
Fax: (212) 308-1187
Travel carrier bags for pets accepted on
most major airlines.

Standard Homeopathic Company
P.O. Box 61067
Los Angeles, CA 90061
(800) 624-9659 / (310) 321-4284

Fax: (212) 308-1187
Remedies sold in amber bottles from
2 dram to 2 oz. size. You can request
any size pellet, from #10 to #35, or
tablets. Wide selection of lotions and
creams, too.

Standard Process Laboratories
(800) 558-8740
1200 W. Royal Lee Drive
Palmyra, WI 53156
Immuplex, thyrotropin, glandulars, etc.

St. John Pet Care Products
1656 W. 240th Street
Harbor City, CA 90710
(800) 969-7387
Manufacturers of Petrodex Dental Kit.

Systemic Formulas
P.O. Box 1516
Ogden, UT 84402
(800) 445-4647
Food supplements, grandulars with
herbs, and homeopathics. (For veterinarians only). Free catalog available.

Taylor's Pharmacy
230 North Park Avenue
Winter Park, FL 32789
(407) 644-1025
Homeopathic pharmacy.

Tonkatinkers Kreations
1403 Carolbeth Ave.
Macomb, IL 61455
(309) 837–3150
Posts and purches.

Vetri Science Labs
20 New England Drive
Essex Junction, VT 05453
(800) 882-9993

Manufacturers of NuCat supplement with digestive enzymes, and vetri-liquid DM6.

VideoRemedies
(800) 733-4874
Dr. Chambreau's video: homeopathic first aid for pets and two for treating humans (see publications).

Vita Fons II
P.O. Box 178
Metaline, WA 99152
(509) 446-4107 / (800) 468-VITA
Vibrational healing

Vita-Lite—Duro-Lite Lamps, Inc.,
Duro-Test Corp.
9 Law Drive
Fairfield, NJ 07004
(800) 526-7193 / (201) 808-0902
Full-spectrum natural lighting.

The Vitamin Shoppe
4700 Westside Avenue
North Bergen, NJ 07047
(800) 223-1216
Natural vitamins, herbs, homeopathics, and Bach flower remedies at discounted prices.

Vita Plus Industries
953 E. Sahara Ave. #218
Las Vegas, NV 89104
(702) 733-8805
Overnight, Supertabs and Coenzyme Q-10 supplements.

Washington Homeopathic Products
4914 Del Rey Avenue
Bethesda, MD 20814
(800) 336-1695
They make veterinary nosodes and carry remedies, ointments, some books.

The Whole Animal Catalog (A Subsidiary of the Uptown Veterinarian)
3131 Hennepin Avenue South
Minneapolis, MN 55408
(800) 377-6369
Supplements, herbal formulations, kelp, books, and the wonderful Tiger Cat Toy, a mobile with a mouse!

Williams Pet Products
P.O. Box 7203
Rocky Mount, NC 27804
(919) 442-3160
In Canada, contact Phero Tech
7572 Progress Way
Delta, B.C. V4G 1E9
(604) 940-9944
Manufacturers of Williams Flea Trap.

Wow-Bow Distributors
13 B Lucon Dr.
Deer Park, NY 11729
(516) 254-6064
Natural pet foods, supplements, and products. Free catalog.

Wysong Corporation
1880 N. Eastman
Midland, MI 48640
(517) 631-0009
Educational materials and tapes. Also the manufacturer of Litter Lite, a pelleted cat litter box filler that is dust-free, natural, and biodegradable. Natural pet foods and supplements.

Mc ZAND Herbal, Inc.
P.O. Box 5312
Santa Monica, CA 90409
(310) 822-0500
(800) 800-0405
Manufacturers of herbal formulas for pets and people. Brochure available.

Books, Publications, Tapes

Alternatives in Healing
by Simon Mill, and Steven J. Finando,
New York: Plume/NAL Books, 1988.

Alternative Health Care Resources
by Brett Jason Sinclair.
Englewood Cliffs, NJ: Parker Publishing Co., 1992. Although this directory contains only two listings for veterinary care (the AHVMA and the IVAS, both listed in this section), its 500-page list of resources contains organizations, journals and practitioners that could prove useful.

Alternatives for the Health Conscious Individual (newsletter). Mountain Home Publishing, P.O. Box 829, Ingram, TX 78025. (512) 367-4492.

Alternative Medicine: The Definitive Guide
The Alternative Medicine Yellow Pages: A Comprehensive Guide to the New World of Health
The Alternative Medicine Digest, the Voice of Alternative Medicine
Puyallup, WA: Burton Goldberg Group/Future Medicine Publishing, Inc., 1994.

The Animal Guardian
Distributed by the Doris Day
Animal League
227 Massachusetts Avenue N.E.
Suite 100, P.O. Box 96829
Washington, D.C. 20090-6829.

The Animal Press
Monthly publication published by Four Star Industries, 4180 Ruffin Road #110, San Diego, CA 92122
(619) 268-7082.

Aromatherapy: To Heal and Tend the Body
by Robert Tisserand. Santa Fe, New Mexico: Lotus Light Press, 1988.

Astrological Healing: The History and Practice of Astromedicine
by Reinhold Ebertin. York Beach, ME: Samuel Weiser, Inc., 1989.

The Bach Flower Remedies
by Edward Bach, M.D., and F.J. Wheeler, M.D. New Canaan, CT: Keats Publishing, Inc., 1979. Available through Ellon USA, Inc.

Bach Flower Therapy: Theory and Practice
by Mechthild Scheffer. Rochester, VT: Inner Traditions Int'l, Ltd., 1984.

Behaving As If the God in All Life Mattered
by Machaelle Small Wright.
Perelandra, Ltd., P.O. Box 3603,
Warrenton, VA 221860. A beautifully written book dealing with the story of the author's ability to see and hear the invisible forces of nature.

The Betrayal of Health: The Impact of Nutrition, Environment, and Lifestyle on Illness in American
by Joseph D. Beasley, M.D.
New York: Times Books, 1991. A highly readable condensation of a report made to the Kellogg Foundation.

The Biochemic Handbook
by J.B. Chapman and Edward L. Perry M.D. St. Louis: Formur International, 1976.

A Cancer Battle Plan
by Anne E. Frahm with David J. Frahm.
Colorado Springs: Pinon Press, 1992.

The Cat Fancier's Almanac
The monthly magazine of the Cat
Fanciers' Association. Contact the association for subscription information
(see associations).

The Cat Lover's Cookbook
by Franki B. Papai.
New York: St. Martin's Press, 1993.
More approaches to preparing food for
cats. Most recipes are for cooked food
but could easily be adapted to the Natural Diet program by using raw meat
and increasing the protein percentage.

Cat Nips! Feline Cuisine
by Rick & Martha Reynolds.
New York: Berkley Books, 1992.
Recipes for "snack-like" foods that can
be stored easily in the refrigerator.

Cats: Homeopathic Remedies
by George Macleod. New York: Beekman Publications, Inc., 1990. A highly
respected British veterinary homeopath.

*Cats Naturally: Natural Rearing for
Healthier Cats*
by Juliette De Bairacli Levy.
Winchester, MA: Faber and Faber, Inc.
1991. The mother of holistic veterinary care on the subject of cats. The
original source book for many holistic
veterinarians.

Cat Watching
by Desmond Morris. New York:
Crown Books, 1986.

Civilization and Disease
by Henry Sigerist. Chicago: University
of Chicago Press, 1962.

*Common-Sense Pest Control: Least Toxic
Solutions for Your Home, Garden, Pets, and
Community*
by William Olkowski, Sheila Daar, and
Helga Olkowski. Newtown, CT:
Taunton Press, Inc., 1991.

*The Complete Herbal Handbook for the
Dog and Cat*
by Juliette De Bairacli Levy. Winchester, MA: Faber and Faber, 6th edition,
1991. A companion to *Cats Naturally.*

*The Complete Medicinal Herbal: A Practi-
cal Guide to the Healing Properties of
Herbs with More Than 250 Remedies for
Common Ailments*
by Penelope Ody. New York: Dorling
Kindersley, 1993.

*The Cornell Book of Cats, A Comprehen-
sive Medical Reference for Every Cat and
Kitten* by the faculty and staff of Cor-
nell Feline Health Center, Cornell
University, edited by Mordecai Siegal.
New York: Villard Books, 1991.

The Crystal Book
by Dael Walker.
Sunol, CA: The Crystal Co., 1983.

*Cunningham's Encyclopedia of
Magical Herbs*
by Scott Cunningham. Saint Paul, MN:
Llewellyn Publications, 1985.

Death: The Final Stage of Growth
by Elisabeth Kubler-Ross. Englewood
Cliffs. NJ: Prentice-Hall, 1976.

On Death and Dying
by Elisabeth Kubler-Ross. New York:
Macmillan, 1969.

*Discovering Homeopathy: Medicine
for the 21st Century*
by Dana Ullman.
Berkeley: North Atlantic Books, 1991.

*The Diviner's Handbook: A Guide to the
Timeless Art of Dowsing* by Tom Graves.
Rochester, VT: Destiny Books, 1990.

*Dr. Pitcairn's Complete Guide to Natural
Health For Dogs & Cats* by Richard Pitcairn, M.D., Ph.D. and Susan Hubble
Pitcairn. Emmaus, PA: Rodale Press,
1982. Another great book to use often.

Echo, Inc. (Educational Concern for
Hydrogen Peroxide). A newsletter.
P.O. Box 126 Delano, MN 55328.

Encyclopedia of Magical Herbs
by Scott Cunningham. St. Paul, MN:
Llewellyn Publications, 1992.

*Enzyme Nutrition: The Food
Enzyme Concept*
by Dr. Edward Howell. New York:
Avery Publishing Group, Inc., 1985.

*Everybody's Guide to
Homeopathic Medicines*
by Stephen Cummings, M.D., and
Dana Ullman. Los Angeles: Jeremy P.
Tarcher, 1991.

The Family Guide to Homeopathy
by Alain Horvilleur, M.D. Norwood,
PA: Health and Homeopathy Publishing, Inc., 1986.

The Family News (quarterly newsletter
on Oxygen Therapies), 9845 N.E. Second Avenue, Miami Shores, FL 33138,
(800) 284-6263.

Feed the Kitty—Naturally
by Joan Harper. PETPRESS, Rt. 3,
Richland Center, WI 53581

Flower Essence Repertory
by Richard Katz and Patricia Kaminsky. Nevada City, CA: Flower Essence
Society, Division of Earth-Spirit, 1992.

*Flower Essences: Reordering Our Under-
standing and Approach to Illness and
Health* by Machaelle Small Wright.
Warrenton, VA: Perelandra Ltd., 1988.

*The Flower Remedies Handbook—Emo-
tional Healing & Growth with Bach and
Other Flower Essences* by Donna
Cunnningham. New York: Sterling
Publishing Co., Inc., 1992.

*Food Enzymes: The Missing Link to Radi-
ant Health* by Humbart Santillo.
Prescott, AZ: Hohm Press, 1987.

Food Is Your Best Medicine
by Dr. Henry G. Bieler and Maxine
Block. New York: Ballantine Books,
Inc., 1987.

*Free Radicals, Stress and Antioxidant
Enzymes —A Guide to Cellular Health*
(booklet) by Peter R. Rothschild, and
William J. Fahey. Honolulu: University
Labs Press, 1991

Fresh and Raw
by Dr. Wysong. Midland, MI: The
Wysong Company, 1990.

*Healing For the Age of Enlightenment: Bal-
anced Nutrition, Vita Flex, Color Therapy.*
by Stanley Burroughs. Newcastle, CA:
self published, 1976.

The Healing Herbs: The Ultimate Guide To The Curative Power Of Nature's Medicines by Michael Castleman. Emmaus, PA: Rodale Press, 1991. A "user-friendly herbal guide."

Healing Music: The Harmonic Path to Inner Wholeness by Andrew Watson and Nevill Drury. Dorset, England: Prism Press, 1989. A Nature & Health Book.

The Healing Touch: The Proven Massage Program for Cats and Dogs by Michael W. Fox. New York: Newmarket Press, 1981.

Healing Wise by Susan Wood. P.O. Box 64, Woodstock, New York 12498 (914) 246-8081. She consults on Tuesday eves. between 7:30-9:30, Apr.-Oct., or you can send her $1.00 for a catalog or newsletter.

Health and Healing by Andrew Weil, M.D. New York: Houghton Mifflin, 1988.

Healthy Homes, Healthy Kids: Protecting Your Children From Everyday Environmental Hazards by Joyce M. Schoemaker, Ph.D. & Charity Y. Vitale, Ph.D. Washington, D.C.: Island Press, 1991. What's good for your kids is even better for your cats.

Healthy Pets, Naturally: The Holistic Newsletter with Natural Remedies For Treatable Ailments. 3000 Old Alabama Road, Suite 119-329, Alpharetta, GA 30202 (404) 475-4550.

The Herb Book by John Lust. New York: Bantam Books, 1974.

Herbal Handbook for Farm and Stable by Juliette De Bairacli Levy. Emmaus, PA: Rodale Press, 1976.

Herbally Yours by Penny C. Royal. Hurricane, UT: Sound Nutrition, 1982.

"Holistic Pet Care: A Video with Dr. Joanne Stefanatos." Produced by Agape Video Systems, Inc. Las Vegas, NV. An amazing survey of the holistic therapies available for animals.

The Holographic Universe by Michael Talbot. New York: Harper-Perennial, 1991. About physics, but with lots of miracle stories. Dr. Pitcairn recommended this book to *Tiger Tribe Magazine,* and it has obvious relevance to understanding how homeopathy works.

"Homeopathic First Aid For Pets" (Video) featuring Christina Chambreau, D.V.M., explaining the use of six homeopathic remedies for animals. The videotape and the remedies she describes can be ordered through Video Remedies, Inc., P.O. Box 290866, Davie, FL 33329-0866, (800) 733-4874.

Homeopathic Medicine in the Home by Jonathan Brewlow. Ashwin Publications, P.O. Box 1686, Ojai, CA 93024, (805) 646-6622. This book was intended to be used as part of a correspondence course, but can stand alone.
  It uses as a companion volume,

Homeopathic Medicine at Home by Maes-imund B. Panos, M.D. and Jane Heim-lich (Los Angeles: Jeremy Tarcher, Inc., 1980), which includes a section on homeopathy and animals). Topics covered in the Brewlow book include *materia medica,* use of the repertory, and use of remedies in acute conditions. Short section on prescribing for animals. Useful resource listings.

The Homeopathic Treatment of Children by Paul Herscu. Berkeley, CA: North Atlantic Books, 1991. Modern, in-depth work on eight remedies. Gives insights that are applicable to animals.

How To Heal the Earth in Your Spare Time by Andy Lopez. The Invisible Gardener, 29169 Heathercliff Road #216-408, Malibu, CA 90265, (302) 457-6658.

How Natural Remedies Work by Jo Serrentino, 1991. Hartley & Marks, Inc. Box 147, Point Roberts, WA 98281. Interesting discussions of the "active" ingredients in natural remedies including vitamins, minerals, nutrients, homeopathic and naturo-pathic remedies.

How To Live The Millenium: The Bee Pollen Bible by Royden Brown. Prescott, AZ: Hohm Press, 1993. Encyclopedic examination of research done on bee products by the founder of CC Pollen. Available through CC Pollen (800-875-0096).

Immunizations: The Reality Behind The Myth by Walene James.

New York: Greenwood, 1988. Available through The American Natural Hygiene Society, P.O. Box 30630, Tampa, FL 33630, (813) 855-6607.

Keep Your Pet Healthy the Natural Way by Pat Lazarus. New Canaan, CT: Keats Publishing, 1986. Contains references to many holistic veterinarians.

Kinship With All Life by J. Allen Boone. San Francisco: Harper SF, 1976.

Kirk's Current Veterinary Therapy by Robert W. Kirk. Philadelphia: Saunders, W.B., Co., 1994.

Lectures On Homeopathic Philosophy by James Tyler Kent, M.D. Berkeley: North Atlantic Books, 1979. If you are going to care for your animal companions holistically, you have to change your thinking. This book, written in 1900, explains how homeopathy works and how best to use it.

The Legacy of the Cat by Gloria Stephens. San Francisco: Chronicle Books, 1990.

Magical Aromatherapy: The Power of Scent by Scott Cunningham. Saint Paul, MN: Llewellyn Publications, 1989.

The Magical Staff: The Vitalist Tradition in Western Medicine by Matthew Wood. Berkeley: North Atlantic Books, 1992. An understanding of how the use of "energy" medicines came about historically. Offers an interesting perspective on homeopathy from someone trained in both homeopathy and herbalism.

The Magic of Massage: A New and Holistic Approach 3rd, Revised Ed.
by Ouida West. Mamaroneck, NY: Hastings House Publishers, 1990.

Natural Healing For Dogs & Cats
by Diane Stein. Freedom, CA: The Crossing Press, 1993. Everything from physical anatomy to non-physical anatomy and reincarnation. Very useful book includes surveys of nutritional, herbal, and homeopathic approaches to healing animals.

Natural Health, Natural Medicine
by Andrew Weil, M.D.
New York: Houghton Mifflin, 1990.

Natural Pet Magazine
P.O. Box 351, Trilby, FL 33593
(904) 583-2770

Nature Healing Conings for Animals
by Machaelle Small Wright.
Warrenton, VA: Perelandra, Ltd., 1993.

The New Holistic Herbal
by David Hoffman.
Rockport, MA: Element Books, Inc., 1990. Contains a precise and detailed herbal as well as good sections on the preparation of herbs, the actions of herbs, the chemistry of herbs, and an overview of each body system and its relationship to herbs.

A New Model For Health and Disease
Berkeley, CA: North Atlantic Books, 1991. Gives greater understanding of the dangers of overusing antibiotics.

The New Natural Cat: A Complete Guide For Finicky Owners

by Anitra Frazier with Norma Eckroate. New York: Plume/NAL Books, revised edition, 1990. A well-researched book. I keep it handy for reference.

The New Super Antioxidant Plus: The Amazing Story Of Pycnogenol, Free-Radical Antagonist & Vitamin C Potentiator
by Richard A. Passwater, Ph.D. New Canaan, CT: Keats Publishing, Inc., 1992.

Nontoxic, Natural & Earthwise
by Debra Lynn Dadd. Los Angeles: Jeremy P. Tarcher, Inc., 1990. Over 600 mail order sources for non-toxic, recycled, cruelty-free, natural and other products. See also her book, *The Nontoxic Home and Office.* Los Angeles: Jeremy P. Tarcher, 1992.

Nutricare News
A newsletter published by Pat McKay for her clients. Call (818) 441-8415 for information.

The Organon of Medicine
by Samuel Hahnemann, M.D. Translated with preface by William Boericke, M.D., New Delhi, India: B. Jain Publishers, 1976. From the master's mouth. A must for the serious student.

Perfect Health: The Complete Mind-Body Guide
by Deepak Chopra, M.D. New York: Crown Publishing Group, 1991.

Pet Allergies: Remedies for an Epidemic
by Alfred J. Plechner, D.V.M. and Martin Zucker. Inglewood, CA: Very Healthy Enterprises, Inc., 1986.

Pottenger's Cats: A Study In Nutrition
by Francis M. Pottenger, Jr. M.D. San
Diego: Price-Pottenger Foundation,
1983.

*Practical Uses and Applications of the
Bach Flower Remedies*
by Jessica Beal. Las Vegas: Balancing
Essentials Press, 1989.

Prescription for Nutritional Healing
by James F. Balch, M.D., and Phyllis A.
Balch. New York: Avery Publishing
Group, 1990.

The Principles of Light and Color
by Dr. Edward D. Babbitt.
Santa Fe: Sun Publishing Co., 1992.

A Quick Guide to Food Additives
by Robert Goodman.
San Diego: Silvercat Publications, 1990.

*Quantum Healing: Exploring the Frontiers
of Body, Mind, Medicine*
by Deepak Chopra.
New York: Bantam Books, 1990.

Reigning Cats and Dogs
by Pat McKay. South Pasadena, CA:
Oscar Publications, 1992. An excellent
book describing the formula and
options for the Fresh Food Diet. Also
dessert recipes, herbs, and homeopathy.
Highly recommended.

*The Reiki Handbook: A Manual For Stu-
dents & Therapists Of The Usui Shiko
Ryoho System Of Healing*
by Larry Arnold and Sandy Nevius.
Harrisburg, PA: PSI Press, 1982.

Rodale's Illustrated Encyclopedia of Herbs
by Claire Kowalchik and William H.
Hylton, Editors. Emmaus, PA: Rodale
Press, 1987.

"Samantha Khury: I Talk
To Animals" (Video).
1251 10th Street, Manhattan Beach,
CA 90266, (310) 374-6812.

The Science of Homeopathy
by George Vithoulkas.
New York: Grove Atlantic, 1980.

Stories the Animals Tell Me
by Beatrice Lydecker. San Francisco:
Harper, San Francisco, 1979.

*The Tellington T-Touch: A Breakthrough
Technique to Train and Care for Your
Favorite Animal* by Linda Tellington-
Jones with Sybil Taylor. New York:
Viking Penguin, 1992. A system of body
work based on Feldenkreis for people.

Tiger Tribe Magazine
1407 East College Street, Iowa City,
Iowa 52245-9905, (319)/ 351-6698.
Holistic health and more for cats.

Today's Herbal Health
by Louise Tenney.
Woodland Books, P.O. Box 160,
Pleasant Grove, UT, (800) 777-BOOK.

Tribe of the Tiger
by Elizabeth Marshall Thomas.
New York: Simon & Schuster, 1993.

The Twelve Tissue Remedies of Schuessler
by William Boericke and Willis A.
Dewey. New Delhi: Jain Publishing,
1982

The Vaccination Connection
by Sue Marston. Woodland Hills, CA:
People for Reason in Science and
Medicine (PRISM), 1993.

Veterinary Aromatherapy
by Nelly Grosjean. Saffron Walden,
England: C. W. Daniel Co., Ltd., 1994.

*Vibrational Medicine: New Choices for
Healing Ourselves*
by Richard Gerber, M.D.
Santa Fe: Bear & Co., 1988.

*What is Holistic Veterinary Care? Natural
Care of Pets* by Roger De Haan, D.V.M.
This is a booklet available from Dr. De
Haan at (508) 521-1899

What Your Doctor Won't Tell You
by Jane Heimlich.
New York: Harper-Collins, 1990. A
tremendous overview of alternative
medical therapies. Contains a good listing of resources for further exploration.

Your Body Doesn't Lie
by John Diamond, M.D. New York:
Warner Books, 1980. Also published
under the title *BK: Behavioral Kinesiology*.

Your Cat Naturally
by Grace McHattie. New York: Carroll
& Graf, 1992. While there are some
major flaws in the discussion of diet in
this book, there are some useful herbal
and homeopathic tidbits. Nice pictures
and an easy-to-use first aid chapter.

*Your Healthy Cat: Homeopathic Medicines
For Common Feline Ailments*
by H.G. Wolff, DVM.
Berkeley: North Atlantic Books, 1991.

The Zodiac and the Salts of Salvation
by G.W. Carey and Inez E. Perry.
York Beach, ME: Samuel Weiser, Inc.
1989.

Repertories and Materia Medica

Allen, H.C., M.D., *Allen's Keynotes.:
Keynotes and Characteristics with Compar-
isions of Some of the Leading Remedies of
the Materia Medica.* New Delhi, India:
Jain Publishing Co., 1977. Nosode
materia medica.

Barthel, H., *Synthetic Repertory*, vol. 2.
Heidelberg, Germany: K.F. Haug Ver-
lag, 1973. A modern repertory, many
additions. Volume 2 is general and very
useful with animals.

Boericke, William, *Materia Medica with
Repertory.* St. Louis, MO: Formur International, 1982.

Clarke, J.H., *Clinical Repertory.*
New York: Beekman Publications,
Inc., 1979. Three-volume set, detailed
symptoms from provings.

Coulter, Catherine, *Portraits of Homeo-
pathic Medicine, vols. 1 and 2.* Berkeley,
CA: North Atlantic Books, 1986, 1988.
On human personality of remedies.

Hahnemann, S., trans. by R.E. Dud-
geon, *Materia Medica Pura,* 2 vols. New
Delhi, India, Jain Publishing Co.

Hering, Constantine., *Guiding Symptoms to Our Materia Medica.* A ten-vol-
ume set. New Delhi: Jain Publishing
Co., 1879–91. The best for animals.
From the provings, you'll often find
your specific animal symptoms.

Kent, James, *Repertory of the Homeopathic Materia Medica with Word Index.* New Delhi, India: Jain Publishing Co., 1993. The most popular index of symptoms, affordable and a must for prescribing.

Kunzli, J., M.D., *Kent's Repertorium Generale.* New Delhi, India: Jain Publishing Co., 1987. An expanded Kent, with many new additions. If you can, get this one instead of Kent.

Mac Repertory. Kent Homeopathic Associates, P.O. Box 39, Fairfax, CA, 1986. A repertory for Macintosh computer that helps homeopaths repertorize their cases. Free info packet available: (415) 457-0678.

Macleod, G., M.R.C.M.V.S., *A Veterinary Materia Medica and Repertory with a Materia Medica of the Nosodes.* Saffron Waldon, England: C.W. Daniel Co., 1983.

Morrisson, Roger, *Desktop Guide to Keynotes and Confirmatory Symptoms.* Albany, CA: Hahnemann Clinic, 1993. Modern, concise.

Murphy, Robin, *Homeopathic Medical Repertory: A Modern Alphabetic Repertory.* Pagosa Springs, CO: Hahnemann Academy of North America, 1993. An even more modern repertory, with many new additions. Some people like much more, some much less. Slightly cumbersome for animal work, but sometimes gives critical, additional remedies.

Phatak, S.R., *Concise Repertory of Homeopathic Medicines.* New Delhi, India: Jain Publishing Co.

Schuessler, W. H., M.D. *Materia Medica* An abridged therapy manual on the biochemic treatment of diseases.

Wolff, H.G., D.V.M., *Veterinary Materia Medica & Clinical Repertory,* Saffron Walden, England: C.W. Daniel Co., Ltd., 1983.

Vaccinations and Nosodes

Bastide, M. et al, "Immunoinodulator Activity of Very Low Doses of Thymulin in Mice," *International Journal of Immunotherapy,* III, 1987.

Boiron, J., J. Abecassis, and P. Belon, *Aspects of Research in Homeopathy,* vol. 1. Paris: Editions Boiron, 1983.

Burnett, J. Compton, M.D.. *Vaccinosis and its Cure by Thuja with Remarks on Homeoprophlaxis,* London, 1884.

Day, C.E. I, "Isopathic Prevention of Kennel Cough—Is Vaccination Justified?" *Journal of the Int. Assoc. for Vet. Homeopathy,* vol. 2, no. 1.

Day, C.E. I., "Isopathic Prevention of Kennel Cough—Is Vaccination Justified?" Clarification of kennel cough article in vol. 2, no. 1, *Journal of the Int. Assoc. for Vet. Homeopathy,* vol. 2, no. 2.

Day, C.E. I., "Clinical Trails in Bovine Mastitis Using Nosodes for Prevention," *Journal of the Int. Assoc. for Vet. Homeopathy,* vol. 1, 1986 and *British Homeopathic Journal,* 75, 1986.

Day, C.E. I., *The Homeopathic Treatment of Small Animals: Principles and Practice.* London: Wigmere Publishing, 1984.

Cat Care Naturally

Dodds, Jean W., "*Vaccine Safety and Efficacy*," *Kennel Healthline* vol. III, no. 2, Feb. 1991.

Dodds, Jean W., "Vaccine Safety and Efficacy Revisited. Autoimmune and Allergic Disease on the Rise," *Veterinary Forum,* May 1993.

Dodds, Jean W., "More on Vaccines," *AKC Gazette,* March 1994.

Dodds, Jean W., "Killed Versus Modified Live Virus Vaccines," *AKC Gazette,* Aug. 1991.

Frick, O.L. and D.L. Brooks, "Immunoglobulin E Antibodies to Pollen Augmented in Dogs by Virus Vaccines," *American Journal of Veterinary Research,* vol. 44, no. 3, March 1983.

Julian, A.O., *Materia Medica of New Homeopathic Remedies.* Beaconsfield, England: Beaconsfield Publications, Ltd., 1979.

Karougby, Y. et al, "Immunostimulating and Antitumoral Properties of Thuyone," *Immunology,* vol. 173, 1986.

McDonald, I.J., "Factors That Can Undermine the Success of Routine Vaccination Protocols," *Veterinary Medicine,* March 1992.

Oehen, S., H. Hengartner, R. Ziukernagel, "Vaccination for Disease," *Science,* vol. 251, January 1991.

Phillips, T.R. and R.D. Schultz, "Canine and Feline Vaccinations," in *Current Veterinary Therapy XI,* Robert W. Kirk ed., Philadelphia: W.B. Saunders, 1986.

Phillips, T.R. et al, "Effects of Vaccines on the Canine Immune System," *Can. Journal of Veterinary Research,* 53, 1989.

Pitcairn, R.H., "Homeopathic Alternatives to Vaccines," Proceeding of the American Holistic Vet. Med. Assn. 1993.

Ray, W.J., "Vaccine Safety and Efficacy Revisited," *Vet. Forum,* August 1993.

Rude, T et al, "Safety, Efficacy Heart of Vaccine Use; Experts Discuss Pros and Cons," *DVM Magazine,* Dec. 1988.

Singh, Gupta Girish, "Antiviral Efficacy of Homeopathic Drugs Against Animal Viruses," *British Homeopathic Journal,* vol. 74, vo. 3, July 1985).

Tizard, I., "Risks Associated with Use of Live Vaccines," *JAVMA,* vol. 196, no. 11, June 1990.

Wilford, Christine, "Vaccines Revisited," *AKC Gazette,* vol. III, no. 1, Jan. 1994.

Index